MRI of Gynaecological Diseases

Guofu Zhang
Editor

MRI of Gynaecological Diseases

Illustrations and Cases

SSTP

Springer

Editor
Guofu Zhang
Radiology
Obstetrics and Gynecology Hospital of Fudan University
Shanghai, China

ISBN 978-981-99-3643-4 ISBN 978-981-99-3644-1 (eBook)
https://doi.org/10.1007/978-981-99-3644-1

Jointly published with Shanghai Scientific and Technical Publishers
The print edition is not for sale in China (Mainland). Customers from China (Mainland) please order the print book from: Shanghai Scientific and Technical Publishers.

This Springer imprint is published by the registered company Springer Nature Singapore Pte Ltd.
The registered company address is: 152 Beach Road, #21-01/04 Gateway East, Singapore 189721, Singapore

Paper in this product is recyclable.

Preface

With the rapid development of economic construction and improvement of people's living standards and quality of life, women's health has been widely concerned by the whole society. Nevertheless, targeted professional reference books on imaging of gynecological diseases are still rare.

Obstetrics and Gynecology Hospital of Fudan University, as a tertiary specialized hospital of obstetrics and gynecology, is also an affiliated hospital of Fudan University. It provides clinical service to over 1,700,000 outpatients and 74,000 inpatients throughout China and from the rest of the world. Obstetrics and Gynecology Hospital of Fudan University is responsible for the clinical diagnosis and treatment of difficult patients in Shanghai, East China, and some domestic areas. Obstetrics and Gynecology Hospital of Fudan University was equipped with 1.5 T MRI system in 2009, which is the first MRI installation unit in Shanghai specialized hospital of obstetrics and gynecology. In 2021, the hospital was further equipped with a 3.0 T MRI system.

Abundant clinical case data and many years of experience in MRI diagnosis of gynecological and obstetrics diseases have prompted us to summarize and edit some common and difficult cases into a book, hoping to further increase the understanding of gynecological diseases spectrum and improve the level of imaging diagnosis with extensive readers.

The book is divided into 12 parts, 49 cases, covering the basic gynecological common, rare diseases. I would like to thank every editor for their joint efforts. It is your efforts that enable the final publication of this book.

It is also necessary to thank Shanghai Scientific and Technical Publishers and Springer for their efficient and orderly work in publishing this book.

Our experience and ability are limited, and there are inevitably shortcomings or even mistakes in the book. Readers are welcome to criticize and correct, which will be of great benefit to enrich the content and improve the level of this book when it is republished in the future. Thank you!

Shanghai, People's Republic of China — Guofu Zhang

Editorial Board

Contents

Part I

Imaging Technique

1 Magnetic Resonance Imaging of Female Pelvis

Minhua Shen and Qing Zhou

1.1 Female Pelvic MRI Examination Techniques

1.1.1 Routine Protocols

Examination of MRI for female pelvis requires relatively long time. However, because the uterus and ovaries are located in the pelvic cavity, respiratory movement and intestinal peristalsis have little influence on imaging quality, so satisfactory images can be obtained with the patients in a of calm breathing state. Although there is no need for filling the bladder to complete MRI examination of the uterus ahead, uterine serosa is thin, and the adjacent myometrium has similar signals to abdominal wall muscle. The bladder that stores a certain amount of urine can help to distinguish them, so as to better display the contour of uterus.

MRI can be imaging in any orientation and has excellent soft tissue contrast resolution, so it can accurately display the size, number, shape, location of lesions, and the adjacent relationship with surrounding structures. Female reproductive system tumors such as cervical cancer, uterine fibroids, and ovarian teratoma have good soft tissue contrast with surrounding structures, and multidirectional imaging makes the anatomical relationship between various organs and structures in the pelvic cavity clearly displayed. Sagittal imaging along the long axis of uterus can better display the contour of uterus than other orientations and can clearly display zonal anatomy of uterine body and cervix, which provides an intuitive anatomical basis for determining the protruding direction of uterine fibroids and the extent of cervical cancer invasion. The best orientation to show ovaries is coronal.

Abundant MR imaging sequences and various imaging techniques can well display the histological characteristics of lesions and make qualitative diagnosis. Since the signal contrast of each layer of uterus is not obvious on T1WI, T2WI is the main scanning sequence for female reproductive system. Multi-sequence imaging shows good contrast due to signal differences, not only between various organs, between organs and surrounding structures in the pelvic cavity, but also within the organs. The application of flow compensation technique can greatly reduce the interference of vascular pulsation artifacts. Fat-suppressed sequence is used to identify fat component in lesions and distinguish fat from hemorrhage.

Primary and secondary ovarian tumors are common diseases of female reproductive system, which seriously endanger women's health. MRI has no ionizing radiation damage and is an ideal examination method for women of childbearing age. MRI can make accurate diagnosis for ovarian tumors and show internal structure of the tumor, anatomical structure of surrounding normal tissue, and spread of tumor, which is helpful for qualitative diagnosis of tumors and differentiation of benign and malignant tumors and assisting in clinical staging of malignant tumors [1, 2].

1.1.2 Dynamic Contrast-Enhanced MRI (DCE-MRI)

Being a noninvasive method, DCE-MRI can achieve characterization of tissue vascular system, blood volume, and permeability through continuous and rapid acquisition of images before, during, and after administration contrast agent, thereby providing information on tumor angiogenesis and quantifying the pharmacokinetic characteristics of contrast agent. It mainly uses T1-weighted 3D (three-dimensional) gradient echo fat suppressed sequence to reflect the changes of T1 signal intensity. It can not only improve the image spatial resolution of displaying tumor but also has important clinical value in the diagnosis of peritoneal diseases and differentiation of benign and malignant adnexal diseases and is helpful for evaluation of endometrial carcinoma. There are also researchers using both multiphase and multiplanar small angle fast spin-echo (FSE) imaging sequence to analyze

M. Shen · Q. Zhou (✉)
Department of Radiology, Obstetrics and Gynecology Hospital, Fudan University, Shanghai, People's Republic of China

G. Zhang (ed.), *MRI of Gynaecological Diseases*, https://doi.org/10.1007/978-981-99-3644-1_1

contractions of the uterus, which can completely eliminate influence of respiratory movement and intestinal peristalsis, so as to improve detection rate of uterine small lesions. 3D contrast-enhanced imaging sequence is a very effective method for endometrial carcinoma staging with the sensitivity and specificity of as high as 95% for evaluating both myometrium and cervix invasion.

1.1.3 Diffusion Weighted Imaging (DWI)

DWI reflects thermal movement of water molecules, detecting cell-level molecular displacement, which is mainly affected by integrity of cell membranes in biological tissues, extracellular microstructure, active transport mechanisms, and microcirculation. DWI is one kind of noninvasive method that can detect diffusion movement of water molecules in living tissue [3]. Ovarian endometriosis cysts, simple ovarian cysts, ovarian serous and mucinous cysts, malignant cystic ovarian tumors, and benign cystic ovarian tumors similar to malignancy often lack characteristic MR imaging features. Apparent diffusion coefficient (ADC) values of different cystic lesions are helpful for both identification of lesions and analysis of cystic contents. DWI can also help to distinguish tumor recurrence and inflammatory changes, improves the detection rate of early recurrence of uterine malignant tumors, and also plays an important clinical role in detection of peritoneal carcinoma. Studies have shown that the combination of DCE-MRI and DWI can significantly improve the accuracy of the diagnosis of pelvic diseases [3–5]. For young patients who plan to preserve their fertility, it is necessary to evaluate the extent of cervical cancer before surgery. The application of DWI for preoperative evaluation can greatly improve the success rate of vaginal-cervical isthmus anastomosis. DWI is also of great significance for differentiation of normal lymph nodes and metastatic lymph nodes.

1.1.4 Contrast-Enhanced MR Angiography (CE-MRA)

Rapid intravenous injection (bolus injection) of paramagnetic substances reduces T1 relaxation time of blood from 1200 ms to less than 100 ms, which is significantly shorter than adipose tissue (250 ms), using ultra-fast and heavily weighted T1WI sequence to record this T1 relaxation difference, so that blood vessels and surrounding tissues have a strong contrast, resulting in a bright blood vessel image. When contrast agent circulates through target blood vessel area for the first time, and within a period of peak concentration, the image data of region of interest is quickly collected from three-dimensional direction, and through various post-processing techniques, a multi-angle projection or volume reconstruction is generated 3D CE-MRA. On the basis of conventional CE-MRA sequences, major manufactories have developed TR CE-MRA (time-resolved CE-MRA) sequences [6]. Scanning time of each circle period is reduced from 15 to 20 s to less than 5 s. Repeated multiple scanning can obtain images with high time resolution.

CE-MRA can be used to observe direction of blood flow and determine feeding arteries and draining veins. Compared with ultrasonography technology, CE-MRA has a larger field of view and higher spatial resolution and can display blood vessels in multiple phases and angles.

Compared with CTA technology, CE-MRA has higher soft tissue resolution and no ionizing radiation. Multi-phase scanning can be repeated and get higher resolution imaging of veins. Compared with pelvic venography and retrograde ovarian venography, CE-MRA does not need to change direction of normal blood flow and has higher specificity. CE-MRA can also be used to show origins of uterine arteries before interventional angiography [7, 8] and diagnose uterine arteriovenous malformation (UAVM) [9] and pelvic congestion syndrome (PCS) (Figs. 1.1 and 1.2) [10, 11].

1.1.5 3D-T2WI Sequence

3D-T2WI sequence of the pelvis, allowing multiplanar reformatting (MPR) of uterus, can be more precisely diagnose Müllerian duct anomalies compared to conventional MRI alone [12]. 3D reconstruction by MRI has excellent advantages since its soft tissue resolution and multiplanar imaging capabilities allow the construction of a close to exact model that can assist surgeons in explaining the complex nature of the lesion to patients and in suggesting the course of action or further examination needed [13]. MR urography (MRU) is added in cases of congenital anomalies of genital system (Fig. 1.3) [14].

1.1.6 MR Spectroscopy (MRS)

MRS can use tiny differences in atomic nuclear magnetic resonance frequency to noninvasively detect content changes of various compounds in the body and provide relevant metabolic information. Different from the distribution map formed by MRI based on the spatial position of signals, MRS is formed by displaying many signals in a space with different peak curves. Single-voxel MRS only provides chemical composition information of one region of interest at a time, but it uses complete fat and water suppression, and is not interfered by adjacent tissues and relatively the results are reliable. Multi-voxel MRS can compare the spectra of different tissue types among voxels, but it inevitably contains the

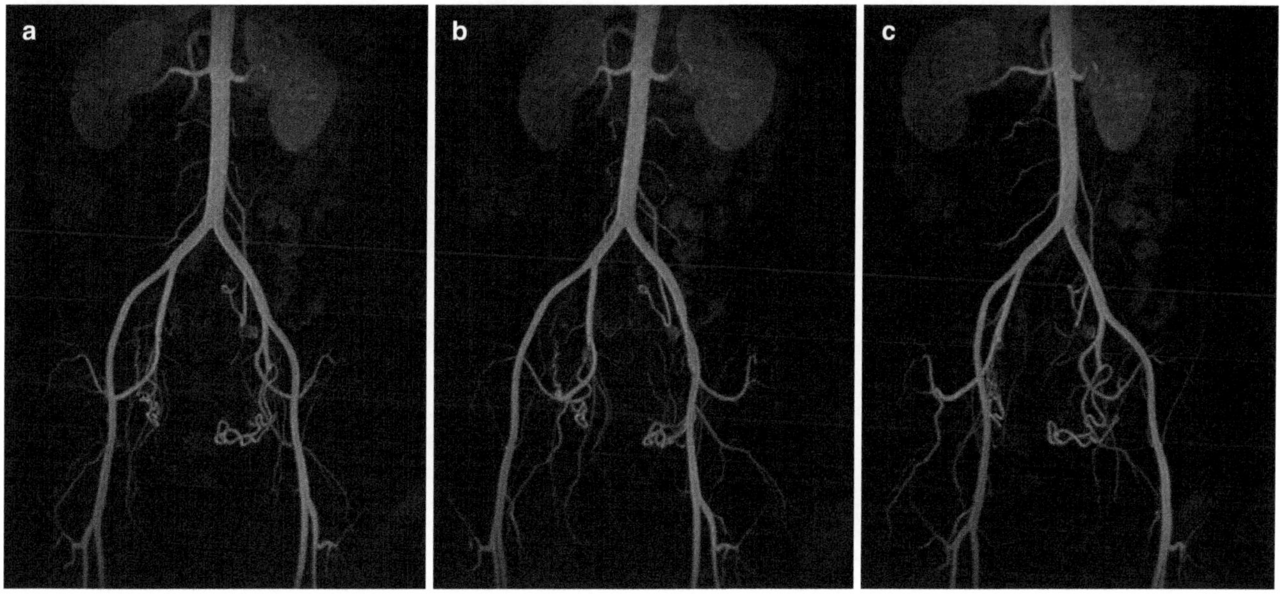

Fig. 1.1 Before interventional surgery, CE-MRA technique was used to observe the opening position and angle of uterine artery by rotating 3D images from different angles (**a**: frontal position; **b**, **c**: oblique position)

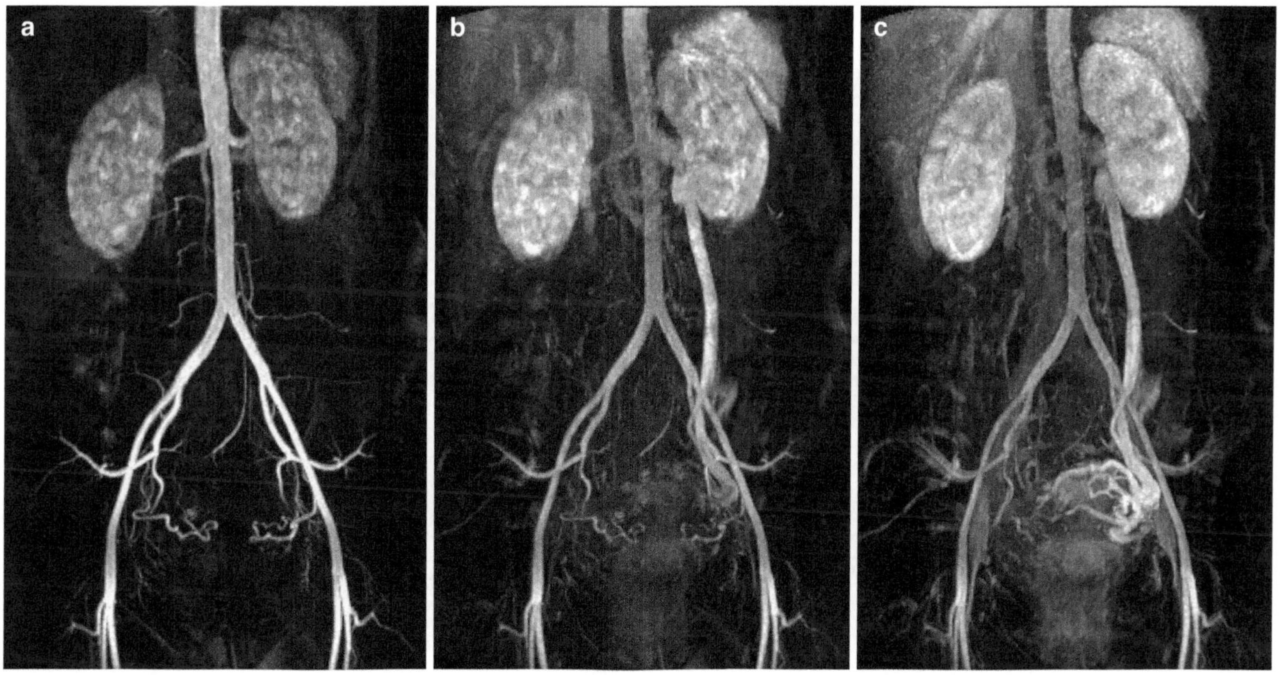

Fig. 1.2 CE-MRA in a 42-year-old woman with left ovarian vein reflux and dilated veins. Dilation of left ovarian vein was shown in arterial phase (**a**, **b**). Dilated ovarian vein communicating with pelvic vein was seen during early venous phase (**c**)

components of adjacent voxels. Most of malignant adnexal tumors have elevated concentrations of choline compounds and lactic acid. However, the probability of these metabolites being detected in omental metastases is less than 50%, because spectroscopy analysis in metastatic diseases is more sensitive to techniques (including magnetic field heterogeneity, intestinal peristalsis, small voxels in the region of interest, and spectra of the omentum contaminated by adjacent adipose tissue, etc.). The content of total choline and lipids in cervical tumors is also elevated, which may be helpful to identify aggressiveness of tumors or determine residual or recurrence of tumors [15]. MRS is mostly used as a research tool, and its clinical applications are gradually being developed (Fig. 1.4).

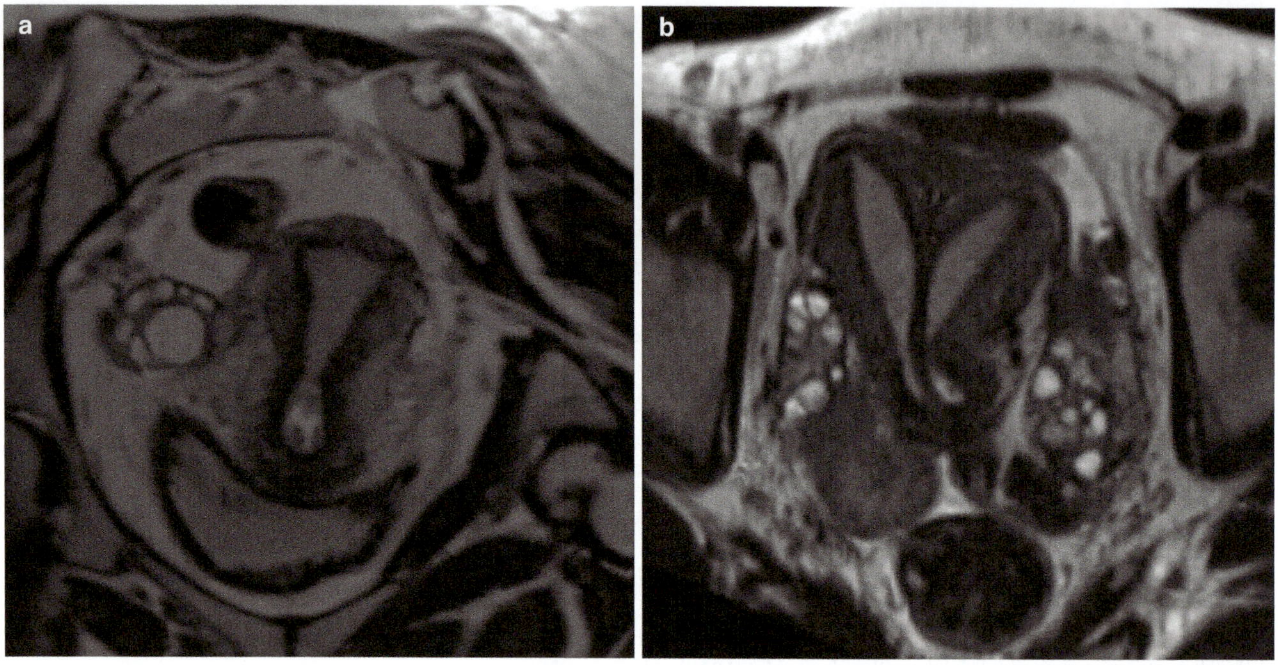

Fig. 1.3 MPR imaging of 3D-T2WI sequence was used to observe the contour of uterine cavity. A normal uterus (**a**) and a complete septate uterus (**b**) were shown

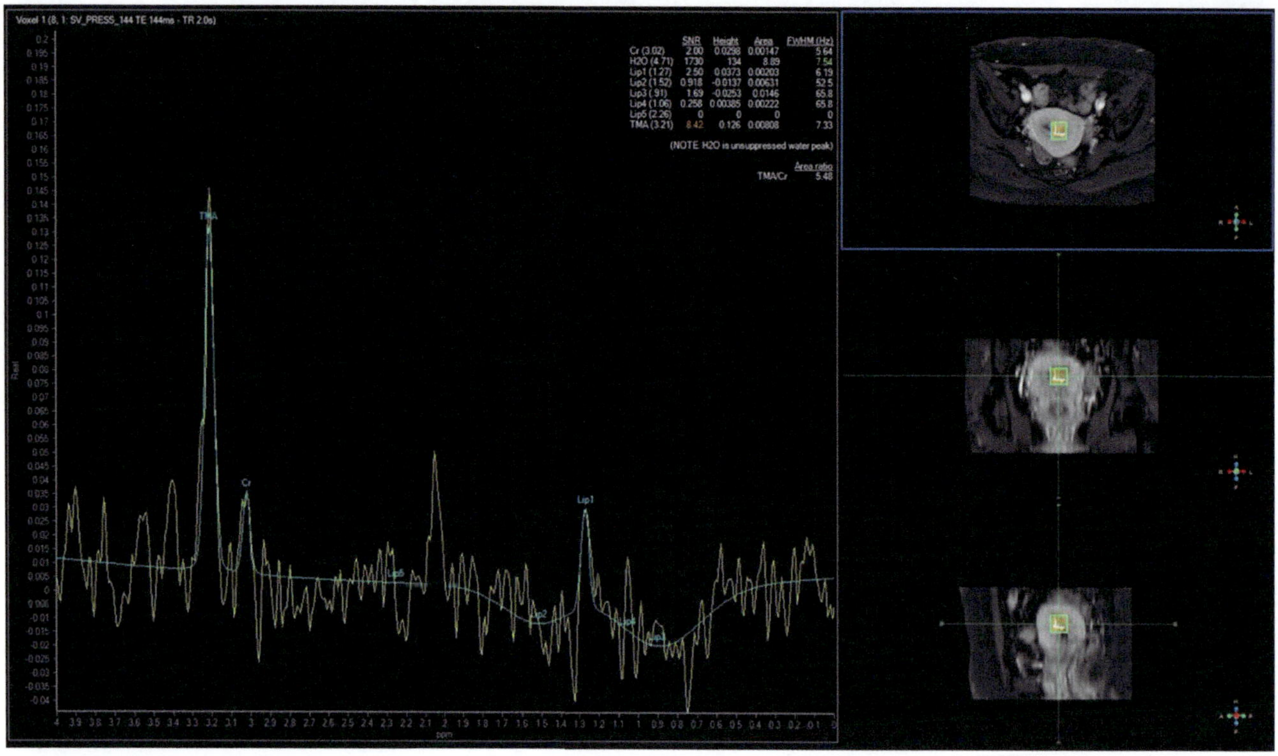

Fig. 1.4 MRS (3T MR scanner) was used to analyze the nature of the tumor in a 31-year-old woman with endometrial cancer

1.2 Female Pelvic MRI Examination Proposal

There are various sequences available for female pelvic MRI scanning. In general, fat-suppressed T2WI sequence is the most important sequence. Because of the great variations in orientation, shape, and location of uterus and ovaries, oblique sagittal and coronal scanning or perpendicular to the long axis of uterus are often required to more clearly show uterus, ovaries, fallopian tubes, and the related tumors. For patients with endometrial carcinoma, sagittal and axial are the main scanning orientations; while for patients with cervical cancer and ovarian diseases, axial and coronal are the main scanning orientations [5]. Scanning protocols with and without fat-suppressed technique could complement each other. For staging of ovarian tumors, the scanning range should be as large as possible, and it is often necessary to evaluate coexistent ascites, retroperitoneal lymph nodes, and distant metastatic lesions. In our institution, the routine sequences, special techniques, and imaging parameters of both 1.5T and 3T MR scanners are shown in Tables 1.1, 1.2, 1.3, 1.4, and 1.5.

Table 1.1 Routine female pelvic MRI scanning sequences in our institution

Scanning sequences	Coil	Center point of positioning	Upper and lower range	Effects
Three plane localizer	Body coil	5 cm above pubic symphysis	Diaphragm to lower renal pole	Orientation
Sagittal T2WI	TORSOPA	Fundus of uterus	Whole pelvic cavity	Lesions display, staging
Axial T1WI, T2WI	TORSOPA	Uterus	Whole pelvic cavity	Lesions display, staging
Coronal T2WI	TORSOPA	Fundus of uterus	Whole pelvic cavity	Lesions display, staging

Table 1.2 Scanning parameters of conventional MRI sequences in female pelvis

	Sequences	FOV	TR/TE (ms)	Bandwidth (Hz)	Slice thickness/slice spacing (mm)	Matrix	Flip angle
TIWI	TSE	350	550/10	178	4/1.2	320 × 240	150
T2WI	TSE	350	4000/83	260	4/1.2	320 × 320	144
FS-T1WI	VIBE	380	4.9/2.4	400	4/0.8	320 × 192	10
FS-T2WI	TSE	350	8000/83	260	4/1.2	256 × 256	150
DCE-MRI	VIBE	380	4.9/2.4	400	4/0.8	320 × 192	10

Note: *FS* fat suppressed

Table 1.3 Scanning parameters of DWI in our institution

	Strength (T)	Sequences	FOV	TR/TE (ms)	Bandwidth (Hz)	Slice thickness/slice spacing (mm)	Matrix	*b* value
DWI	1.5	EP2D	320	2800/81	1250	5/1.5	292 × 320	0–800
DWI	3	EPI	240	2919/66	52.8	5/1.5	292 × 320	0–800

Table 1.4 Scanning parameters of special MRI sequences of uterus and adnexa

	Sequences	FOV	TR/TE (ms)	Pixel (mm)	Slice thickness/slice spacing (mm)	Matrix	Flip angle
CE-MRA	FL3D	250	651/12	1.1 × 1.0 × 1.5	4/1.2	320 × 240	25
T2WI	HASTE	400	1350/92	1.4 × 1.1 × 4.0	4/0.4	384 × 256	60
T2WI	SPC	260	2000/126	1.0 × 1.0 × 1.0	1/0	256 × 256	150
T2WI	TRUFI	400	3.87/1.68	1.7 × 1.6 × 4.0	3–4/0–0.4 (cm)	256 × 144	60
MRS (1.5 T)	PRESS	20	1500/135	2.0 × 2.0 × 2.0		256 × 256	60

Note: *FL3D-FLASH* fast low angle shot 3D imaging, *HASTE* half Fourier single shot turbo spin echo, *SPC-SPACE* sampling perfection with application-optimized contrast using different flip angle evolutions, *TRUFI-True FISP* fast imaging with steady state precession, *PRESS* point resolved spectroscopy

Table 1.5 Various protocols applied in imaging different gynecological diseases [1, 2, 16]

Etiology	Key protocols	Special methods
Endometriosis	T2WI without fat-suppressed, T1WI	3D sequence
GTD	DWI, CE-MRA	
Pelvic floor dysfunction	SAG-T2WI, static and dynamic MR checking method	Valsalva maneuver, use vaginal gel
Cervical cancer	T2WI, DWI, DCE-MRI	Small FOV DWI
Endometrial cancer	T2WI, DWI, DCE-MRI	Sagittal DCE-MRI
Ovarian cancer	T2WI, DWI, DCE-MRI	
Müllerian duct anomalies	MRU, 3D sequence	MPR, the use of vaginal gel may be useful

Note: *GTD* gestational trophoblastic disease, *FOV* field of view, *DCE* dynamic contrast enhanced, *MRU* magnetic resonance urography, *MPR* multiplanar reconstruction

References

1. Wakefield JC, Downey K, Kyriazi S, deSouza NM. New MR techniques in gynecologic cancer. Am J Roentgenol. 2013;200:249–60.
2. Park SB. Functional MR imaging in gynecologic malignancies: current status and future perspectives. Abdom Radiol (NY). 2016;41(12):2509–23.
3. Sala E, Rockall A, Rangarajan D, Kubik-Huch RA. The role of dynamic contrast-enhanced and diffusion weighted magnetic resonance imaging in the female pelvis. Eur J Radiol. 2010;76(3):367–85.
4. Motoshima S, Irie H, Nakazono T, Kamura T, Kudo S. Diffusion-weighted MR imaging in gynecologic cancers. J Gynecol Oncol. 2011;22(4):275–87.
5. Otero-García MM, Mesa-Álvarez A, Nikolic O, et al. Role of MRI in staging and follow-up of endometrial and cervical cancer: pitfalls and mimickers. Insights Imaging. 2019;10(1):19.
6. Kim CY, Miller MJ Jr, Merkle EM. Time-resolved MR angiography as a useful sequence for assessment of ovarian vein reflux. AJR Am J Roentgenol. 2009;193(5):W458–63.
7. Naguib NN, Nour-Eldin NE, Hammerstingl RM, et al. Three-dimensional reconstructed contrast-enhanced MR angiography for internal iliac artery branch visualization before uterine artery embolization. J Vasc Interv Radiol. 2008;19(11):1569–75.
8. Kroencke TJ, Scheurig C, Kluner C, Taupitz M, Schnorr J, Hamm B. Uterine fibroids: contrast-enhanced MR angiography to predict ovarian artery supply—initial experience. Radiology. 2006;241(1):181–9.
9. Szpera-Goździewicz A, Gruca-Stryjak K, Bręborowicz GH, Ropacka-Lesiak M. Uterine arteriovenous malformation—diagnosis and management. Ginekol Pol. 2018;89(5):276–9.
10. Bookwalter CA, VanBuren WM, Neisen MJ, Bjarnason H. Imaging appearance and nonsurgical management of pelvic venous congestion syndrome. Radiographics. 2019;39(2):596–608.
11. Dick EA, Burnett C, Anstee A, et al. Time-resolved imaging of contrast kinetics three-dimensional (3D) magnetic resonance venog-

raphy in patients with pelvic congestion syndrome. Br J Radiol. 2010;83(994):882–7.
12. Troiano RN, McCarthy SM. Mullerian duct anomalies: imaging and clinical issues. Radiology. 2004;233(1):19–34.
13. Pan HX, Liu P, Duan H, Li PF, Chen RL, Tang L, Luo GN, Chen CL. Using 3D MRI can potentially enhance the ability of trained surgeons to more precisely diagnose Mullerian duct anomalies compared to MR alone. Eur J Obstet Gynecol Reprod Biol. 2018;228:313–8.
14. Maciel C, Bharwani N, Kubik-Huch RA, et al. MRI of female genital tract congenital anomalies: European Society of Urogenital Radiology (ESUR) guidelines. Eur Radiol. 2020;30(8):4272–83.
15. Ma FH, Qiang JW, Cai SQ, Zhao SH, Zhang GF, Rao YM. MR spectroscopy for differentiating benign from malignant solid adnexal tumors. AJR Am J Roentgenol. 2015;204(6):W724–30.
16. Law YM, Fielding JR. MRI of pelvic floor dysfunction: review. AJR Am J Roentgenol. 2008;191(6 Suppl):S45–53.

Part II

Uterine Tumors

2 Uterine Fibroids

He Zhang and Xiang Tao

2.1 Clinical History

Case 1

Female patient, 32 years old. She complained a mass in the pelvic cavity 1 week ago. Both tumor marker values and ROMA index were within the normal range. Ultrasonography displayed a mass with the diameter of 13 cm within the anterior wall of uterus. The final pathological result was uterine leiomyoma with bizarre nuclei with edematous degeneration. MRI images are shown in Fig. 2.1.

Case 2

Female patient, 46 years old. She has been diagnosed with uterine fibroids for nearly 20 years and complained of abdominal distension in recent 7 years. No abnormal vaginal bleeding or discharge. Tumor marker values were within the normal range. The patient underwent transabdominal hysterectomy and salpingectomy. The final pathological result was uterine myoma with edematous degeneration. MRI images are shown in Fig. 2.2.

Case 3

Female patient, 51 years old. The patient was diagnosed with uterine fibroid more than 10 years ago. The final pathological result was uterine cellular leiomyoma. MRI and pathological images are shown in Fig. 2.3.

H. Zhang (✉)
Department of Radiology, Obstetrics and Gynecology Hospital, Fudan University, Shanghai, People's Republic of China
e-mail: zhanghe1790@fckyy.org.cn

X. Tao
Department of Pathology, Obstetrics and Gynecology Hospital, Fudan University, Shanghai, People's Republic of China

G. Zhang (ed.), *MRI of Gynaecological Diseases*, https://doi.org/10.1007/978-981-99-3644-1_2

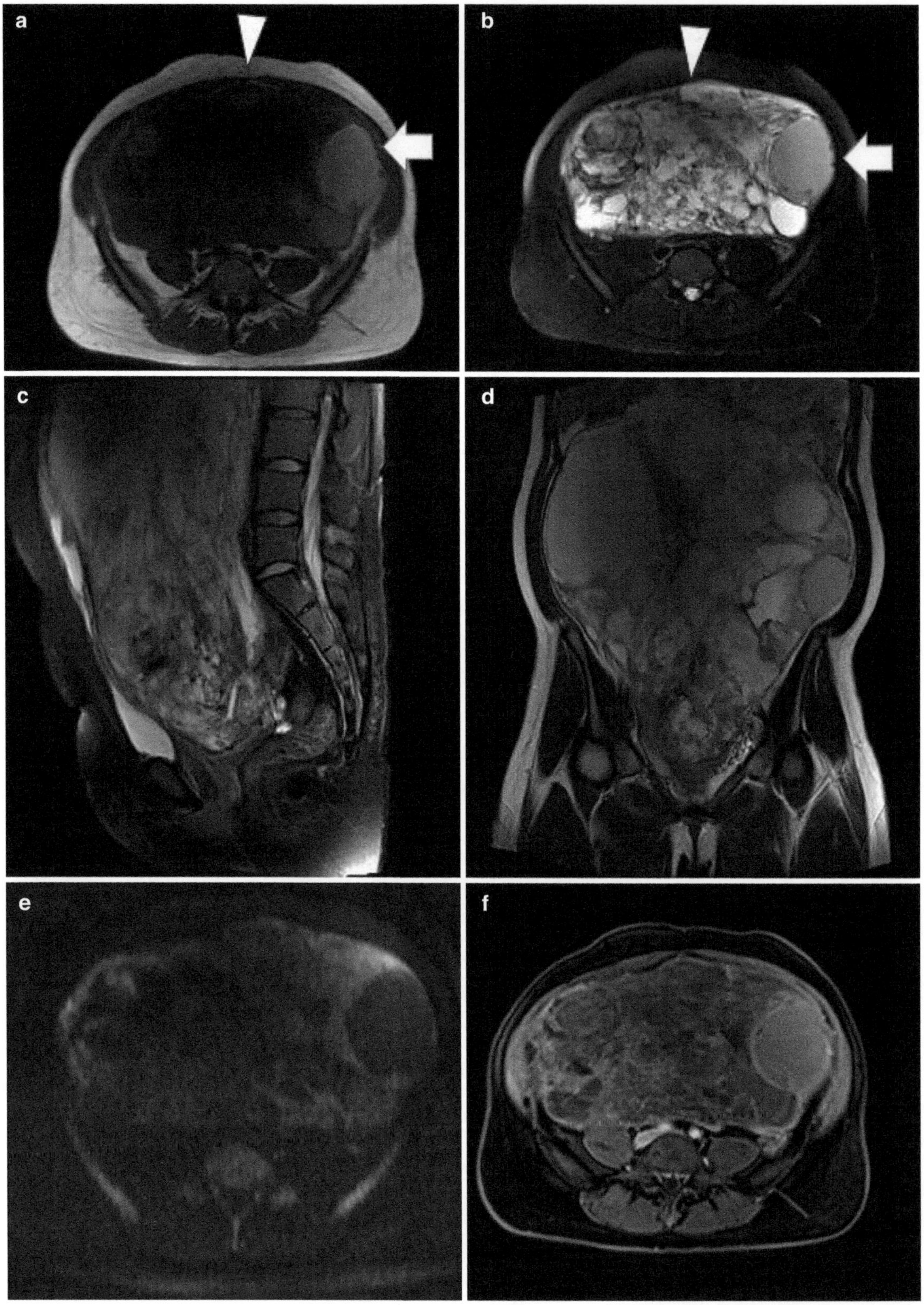

Fig. 2.1 **Case 1**. Uterine leiomyoma with bizarre nuclei with edematous degeneration. The huge mass mostly centered in the abdominal cavity with soft tissue signal intensity. The mass (arrowhead) mostly displayed as low to intermediate signal intensity on T1WI (**a**) and high signal intensity on fat-suppressed T2WI (**b**). Some cystic components showed high signal intensity on both T1WI and T2WI (arrow). Evidently, the mass had inhomogeneous signal intensity. The multilobular structure and irregular septation were seen on both sagittal (**c**) and coronal T2WI (**d**). The mass showed slightly high signal intensity on DWI (**e**) and moderate enhancement after contrast enhancement (**f**)

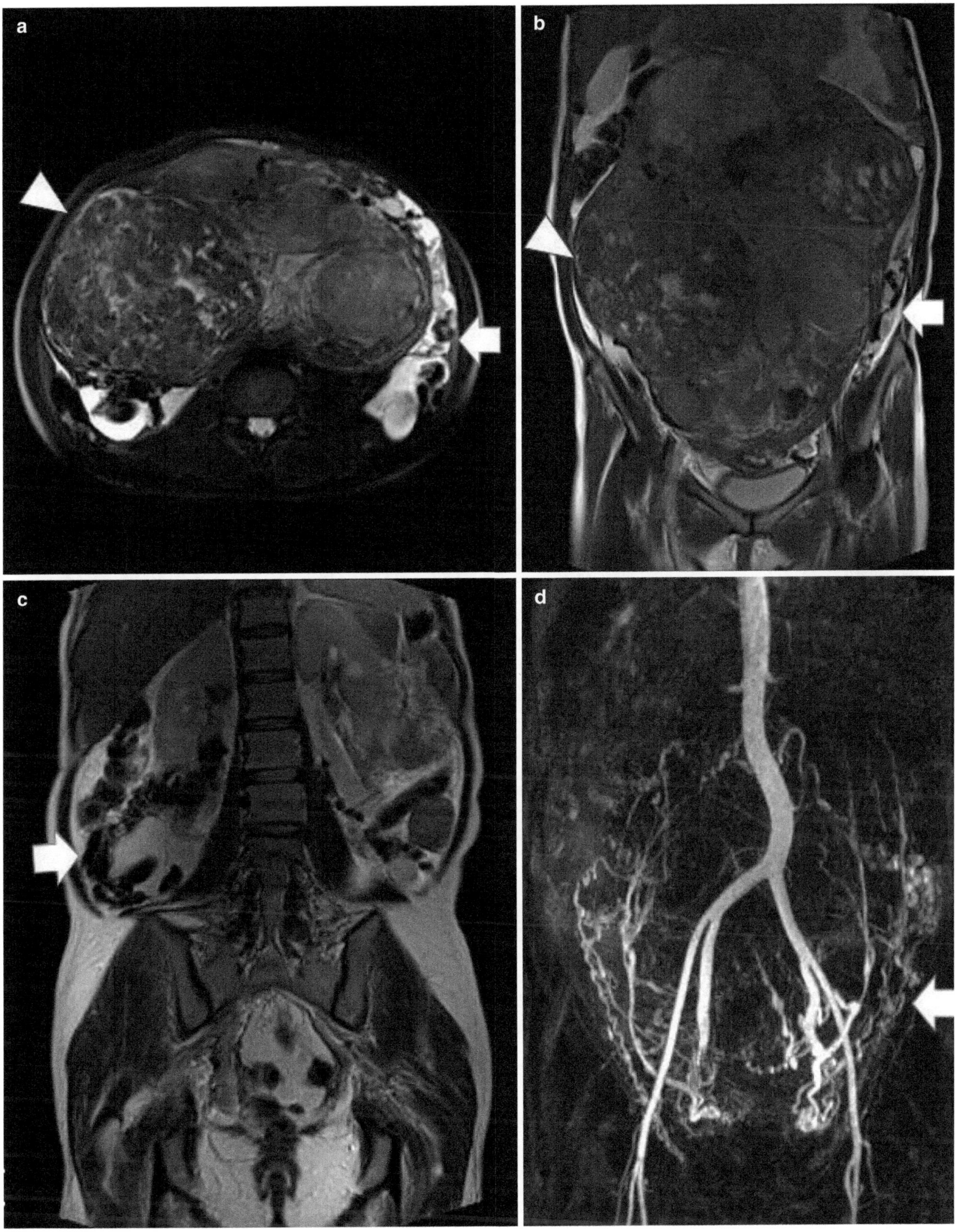

Fig. 2.2 Case 2. Uterine myoma with edematous degeneration. On axial fat-suppressed T2WI (**a**) and coronal T2WI (**b**), the mass occupied the whole abdominal cavity (arrowhead) with the surrounding collateral veins (arrows). The mass mainly displayed as heterogeneously intermediate to high signal intensity on T2WI. The collateral veins were more prominent on coronal T2WI (**c**) and contrast-enhanced MR angiography (MRA, **d**)

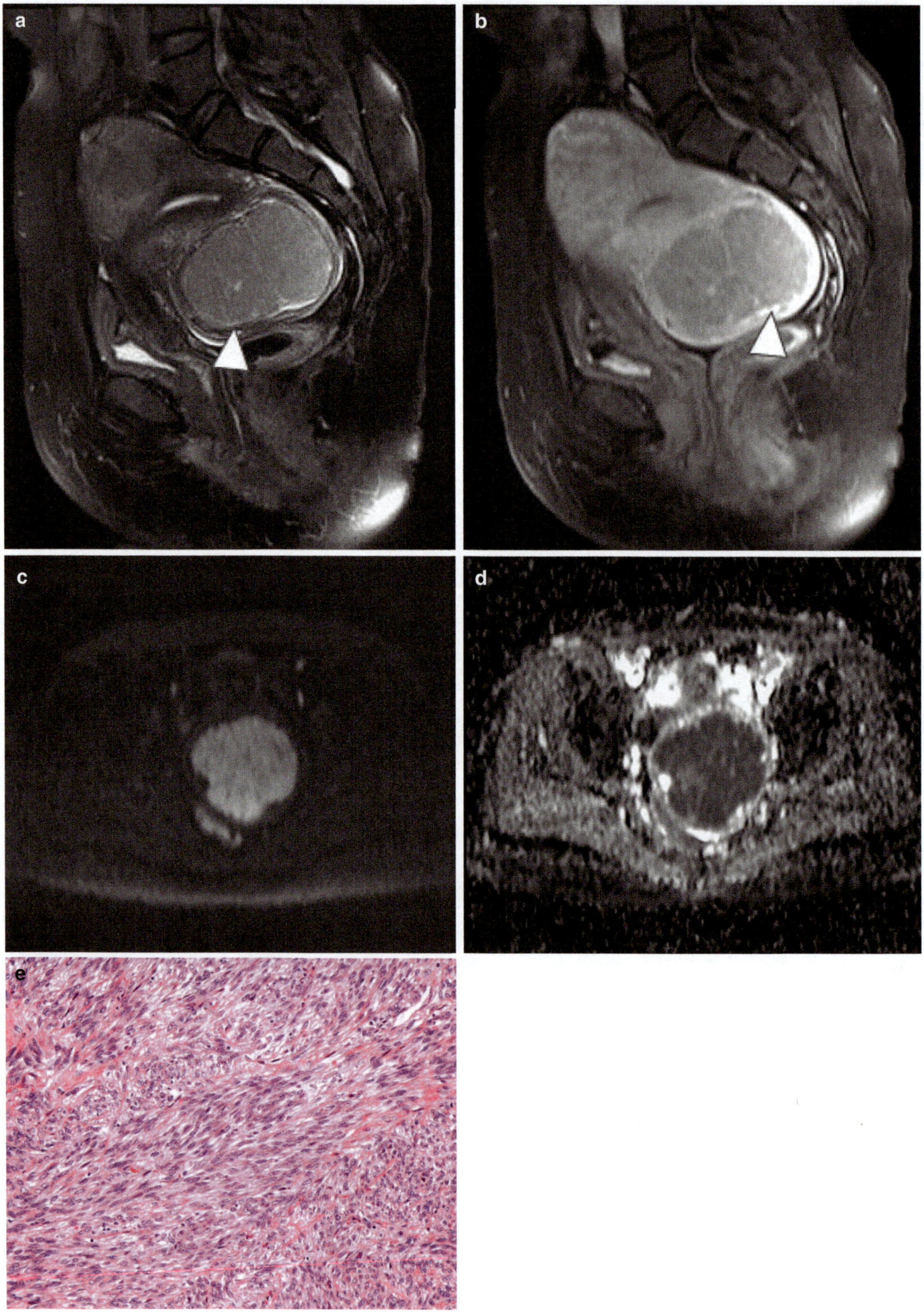

Fig. 2.3 **Case 3**. Uterine cellular leiomyoma. The well-circumscribed mass occupied beside the cervix with homogeneously intermediate signal on sagittal T2WI (**a**). On contrast-enhanced image (**b**), the mass showed peripheral enhancement (arrowhead). The mass displayed as high signal intensity on DWI (**c**) and low signal intensity on the corresponding ADC map (**d**). High-power microscope view showed the tumor cells were spindle-shaped, with bland and relatively uniform nuclei, and 1 or 2 small nucleoli were obvious. Vessels were sparse in the tumor (**e**, HE ×20)

2.2 Imaging Analysis

Uterine fibroids (leiomyomas or myomas) are the most common etiology in women of reproductive age [1, 2]. The prevalence rate varies based on the affected people. It is reported that nearly 80% of all women will have uterine fibroids, while many of them are asymptomatic. Clinical symptoms include abnormal uterine bleeding, dysmenorrhea, infertility, pregnancy loss, and so on. The FIGO classification system grades uterine fibroids into 8-scoring subtypes [3]. According to this classification system, clinicians could select the most suitable treatment options for patients with uterine fibroids at different anatomic sites. MRI, being a problem-solving modality method, will help both radiologists and clinicians to accurately characterize uterine fibroids and complications as well. Pathologically, uterine fibroids comprise of mitotically active leiomyoma, cellular leiomyoma, lipoleiomyoma, atypical leiomyoma (Fig. 2.1), and angiolipoleiomyoma, etc. In addition to histological variants, uterine fibroids could also develop tumor degeneration during the whole growth period. Microscopically, uterine fibroids have five types of degeneration (hyaline, cystic, myxoid/edematous, hemorrhagic, and calcific) (Fig. 2.2). Thus, all these changes result in the complex signals of uterine fibroids on MR images, and sometimes, radiologists need to determine both the origin and nature of tumor. Typically, uterine fibroids manifest as homogeneously intermediate signal intensity on T1WI and low signal intensity on T2WI; however, it will be obviously high signal intensity on T2WI due to the existence of edematous components [4, 5]. On contrast-enhanced images, owing to benign nature, tumor bodies always enhance like the way that normal uterine tissues do, and weak or lack of enhancement is found in degeneration components of uterine fibroids. Note that for uterine cellular leiomyoma subtype (Fig. 2.3), significant enhancement can be observed, the enhancement degree of which is much higher than normal uterus, making it difficult to differentiate from uterine leiomyosarcoma [6].

2.3 Differential Diagnosis

According to our experience, two key points can help to identify uterine fibroids and uterine leiomyosarcoma on MR images. First, malignancies always have tumoral necrosis or hemorrhage, which display as high signal intensity on T1WI images; second, on contrast-enhanced MR images, contrast agent in uterine leiomyosarcoma tissue will show more rapid flow-in and flow-out enhancement than normal uterine tissues. Differential diagnosis spectrum also needs to include uterine polyp, adenomyoma, and gastrointestinal stromal tumor (GIST) in the pelvis [7]. It is really difficult, sometimes, to determine the origin of tumor on imaging. For GIST, uterus is more evidently compressed into the contralateral side by the mass with intact uterine anatomical structure. After contrast enhancement, enhancement type of GIST varies and significant enhancement is common, because degeneration components are rare in GIST. Also, some ovarian masses (e.g., ovarian fibrothecoma) in adnexa area look like the subserosal fibroids for both similar signal and the way of enhancement on MR images (see "Ovarian Masses" Chaps. 12–31). Finally, the definite diagnosis is made by histopathological analysis combined with immunohistochemical results.

References

1. Nougaret S, Cunha TM, Benadla N, Neron M, Robbins JB. Benign uterine disease: the added role of imaging. Obstet Gynecol Clin N Am. 2021;48(1):193–214.
2. Florence AM, Fatehi M. Leiomyoma. In: StatPearls. Treasure Island, FL: StatPearls Publishing LLC; 2021.
3. Gomez E, Nguyen MT, Fursevich D, Macura K, Gupta A. MRI-based pictorial review of the FIGO classification system for uterine fibroids. Abdom Radiol (NY). 2021;46(5):2146–55.
4. Nougaret S, Sbarra M, Robbins J. Imaging spectrum of benign uterine disease and treatment options. Radiol Clin N Am. 2020;58(2):239–56.
5. Brown MA. MR imaging of benign uterine disease. Magn Reson Imaging Clin N Am. 2006;14(4):439–453, v.
6. Sato K, Yuasa N, Fujita M, Fukushima Y. Clinical application of diffusion-weighted imaging for preoperative differentiation between uterine leiomyoma and leiomyosarcoma. Am J Obstet Gynecol. 2014;210(4):368.e361–8.
7. Fujii S, Mukuda N, Ochiai R, Yunaga H, Murakami A, Gonda T, Kishimoto M, Yamaji D, Ishibashi M. MR imaging findings of unusual leiomyoma and malignant uterine myometrial tumors: what the radiologist should know. Jpn J Radiol. 2021;39(6):527–39.

3 Endometrial Stromal Sarcoma

He Zhang

3.1 Clinical History

Case 1
A 62-year-old woman with pathologically proven endometrial stromal sarcoma (low grade). She has been menopausal for almost 12 years and has no complaints of abnormal vaginal bleeding or discharge. She also reported of a uterine mass for a decade of years.

Case 2
A 54-year-old woman with pathologically proven endometrial stromal sarcoma (high grade). She was menopausal 4 years ago and complained of abnormal vaginal bleeding 1 month ago.

3.2 Imaging Analysis

Uterine sarcoma (US) is a rare etiology, accounting for 3% of all uterine malignancies [1]. WHO published the revised version for histological type of US. Endometrial stromal sarcoma (ESS) is the second most common carcinoma originating from endometrial stromal cell [2, 3]. It has three pathological subtypes: endometrial nodule, low-grade ESS (Fig. 3.1), and undifferentiated ESS. ESS approximately comprises of 0.2% of all uterine malignancies and 10–15% of all endometrial stromal tumors. Women in age between 40 and 55 years old are most common involved, with clinical symptoms including abdominal pain, abnormal vaginal bleeding, and irregular menstruation period. Nearly 25% of patients do not report any abnormal complaints. On clinic, ESS often invades parametrial tissue, and most often involves ovaries. On MRI, tumor often displays as polypoid mass with homogeneously intermediate signal intensity on T1WI and homogeneously high signal intensity on T2WI (Fig. 3.2). On contrast-enhanced images, tumor often shows inhomogeneously mild enhancement [4]. If low signal of uterine junctional zone is intact and continuous, it may represent that the myometrial layer is not involved. In contrast to endometrial cancer, ESS often has larger tumor size and more easily invades the myometrial layer. On DWI, the tumor will show relatively high signal compared to normal uterus [5].

H. Zhang (✉)
Department of Radiology, Obstetrics and Gynecology Hospital, Fudan University, Shanghai, People's Republic of China
e-mail: zhanghe1790@fckyy.org.cn

G. Zhang (ed.), *MRI of Gynaecological Diseases*, https://doi.org/10.1007/978-981-99-3644-1_3

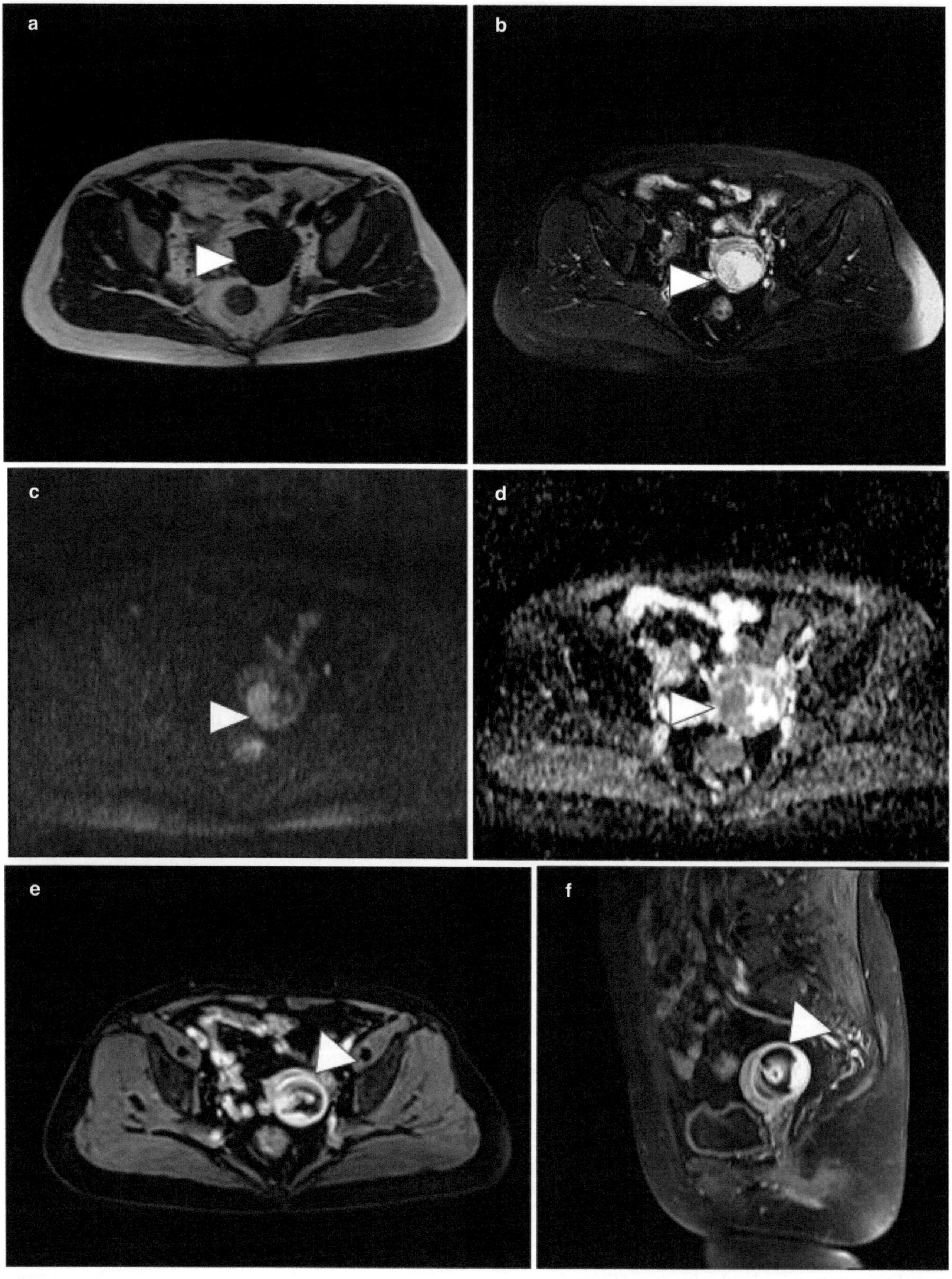

Fig. 3.1 **Case 1**. ESS (low grade). On T1WI, the uterus (arrowhead) enlarged slightly with no obvious abnormal signal detected (**a**); on T2WI, a cystic mass was seen centrally in the uterus (**b**). The mass (arrowhead) showed restricted diffusion signal on DWI (**c**) and the corresponding ADC map (**d**). On contrast-enhanced images, the mass showed avid enhancement with intact uterine junctional zone (**e, f**)

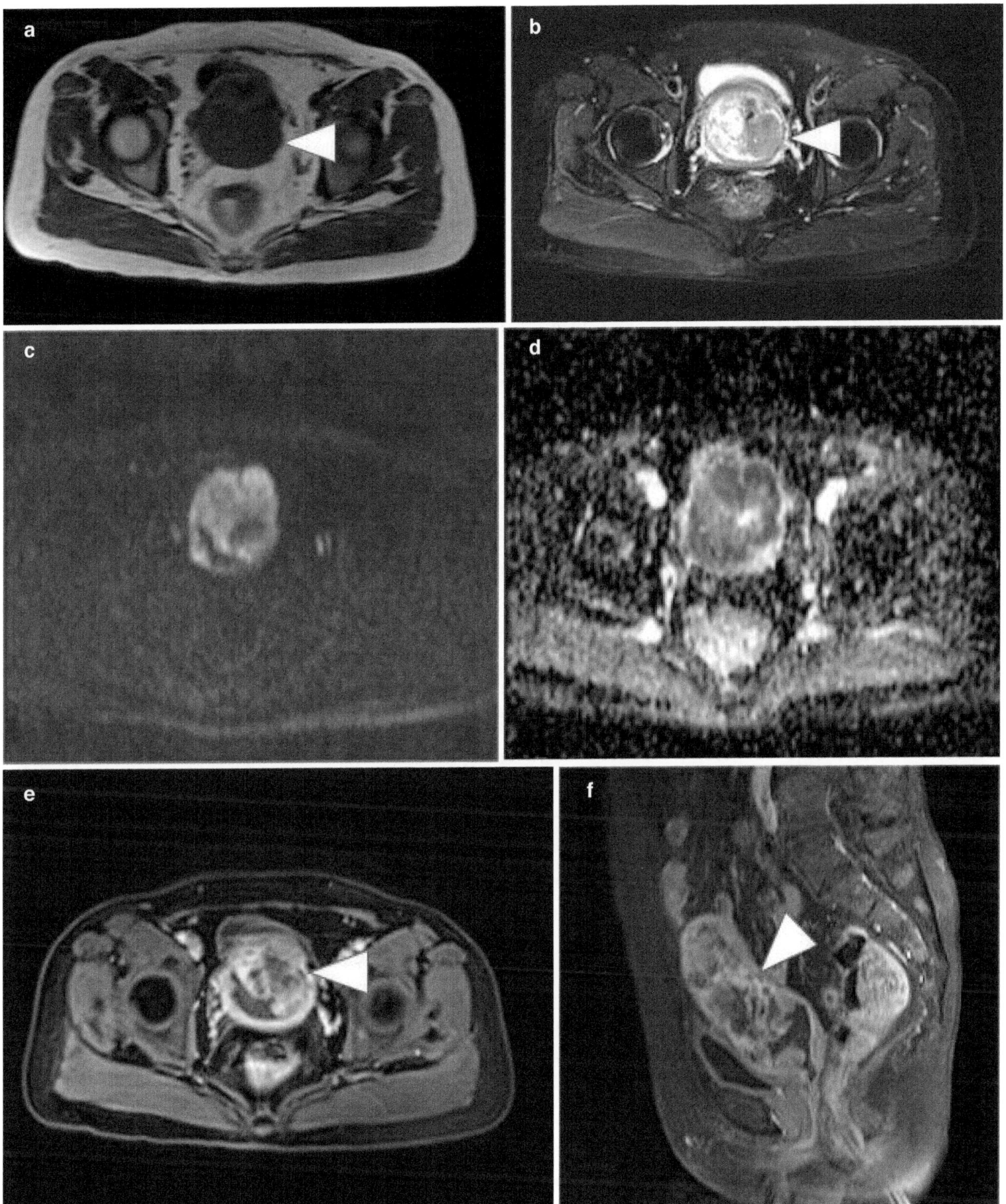

Fig. 3.2 **Case 2**. ESS (high grade). The heterogeneous mass (arrowhead) occupied the uterine cavity with mainly low signal on T1WI (**a**) and medium-high signal on T2WI (**b**). The mass showed restricted diffusion signal on DWI (**c**) and the corresponding ADC map (**d**). The mass enhanced obviously with superficial myometrial invasion reported in the histopathological diagnosis (**e**, **f**)

3.3 Differential Diagnosis

In contrast to uterine myoma, ESS more often has necrosis during tumor growth process. On delayed contrast-enhanced images, ESS often shows weaker enhancement than normal myometrial layer [6]. Uterine myomas often have degeneration changes, showing variable signals on MR images; however, after contrast enhancement, myomas always show similar enhancement type as that of normal uterus. Endometrial cancer is one of the most common tumors of female reproductive system, which develops from endometrium and infiltrates myometrium further. For some cases, the differential diagnosis between each other is difficult and needs to be confirmed by histopathological diagnosis.

References

1. D'Angelo E, Prat J. Uterine sarcomas: a review. Gynecol Oncol. 2010;116(1):131–9.
2. Chiang S, Oliva E. Recent developments in uterine mesenchymal neoplasms. Histopathology. 2013;62(1):124–37.
3. Shah SH, Jagannathan JP, Krajewski K, O'Regan KN, George S, Ramaiya NH. Uterine sarcomas: then and now. Am J Roentgenol. 2012;199(1):213–23.
4. Tirumani S, Ojili V, Shanbhogue A, Fasih N, Ryan J, Reinhold C. Current concepts in the imaging of uterine sarcoma. Abdom Imaging. 2013;38(2):397–411.
5. Fujii S, Kaneda S, Tsukamoto K, Kakite S, Kanasaki Y, Matsusue E, et al. Diffusion-weighted imaging of uterine endometrial stromal sarcoma: a report of 2 cases. J Comput Assist Tomogr. 2010;34(3):377–9.
6. Sohaib SA, Verma H, Attygalle AD, Ind TEJ. Imaging of uterine malignancies. Semin Ultrasound CT MRI. 2010;31(5):377–87.

Endometrial Carcinosarcoma

4

He Zhang

4.1 Imaging Analysis

Endometrial carcinosarcoma (ECS) is also known as "malignant mixed Müllerian tumor," which is the most common histological subtype of uterine sarcoma (US) [1, 2]. ECS accounts for approximately 50% of US, including tumors originating from both epithelial and stroma components. Current studies demonstrate that the majority of tumor develops from epithelial components, and therefore, both its clinical manifestations and prognosis mimic endometrial cancer. The update FIGO staging has classified ECS as one of the subtypes of endometrial cancer [3]. We retrospectively collected these cases from the old database, so we still discuss imaging findings based on previous pathological results. ECS usually occurs in menopause women and sometimes can also be found in young women. Some cases have medical records of pelvic radiotherapy history. Clinical history includes abnormal vaginal bleeding, abdominal distension, and enlargement of uterus. Serum CA125 level could help to monitor recurrence and follow up after treatment. For stage I patients, the 5-year survival rate is nearly 60%; while for stage IV patients, it is only about 9%. Overall, 5-year survival rate is approximately 35% [4, 5].

On MRI, tumor often appears as a large mass with a broad base attached to the uterus, protruding into uterine cavity and cervix. There are necrosis areas in the tumor body, displaying as low signal intensity on T1WI (Fig. 4.1) and high signal intensity on T2WI (Figs. 4.2–4.4). The tumor shows restricted diffusion on DWI (Fig. 4.5) and the corresponding ADC map (Fig. 4.6). On contrast-enhanced images (Figs. 4.7 and 4.8), the tumor shows weaker enhancement than normal endometrium, which is helpful to determine the myometrial invasion. For 1/3 of patients at the first medical visit, the tumors invade the adjacent structures. The most common involved site is ovaries, followed by vagina. Peritoneal involvement is rare. Lymph nodes enlargement are seen in nearly 20% of patients, mostly detected around iliac and aortic vessels. At this time, CT is the best modality to evaluate lymph nodes condition. Distant metastatic sites include lung, liver, and bone. Approximately 50–60% of cases will relapse depending on initial staging [6].

H. Zhang (✉)
Department of Radiology, Obstetrics and Gynecology Hospital, Fudan University, Shanghai, People's Republic of China
e-mail: zhanghe1790@fckyy.org.cn

G. Zhang (ed.), *MRI of Gynaecological Diseases*, https://doi.org/10.1007/978-981-99-3644-1_4

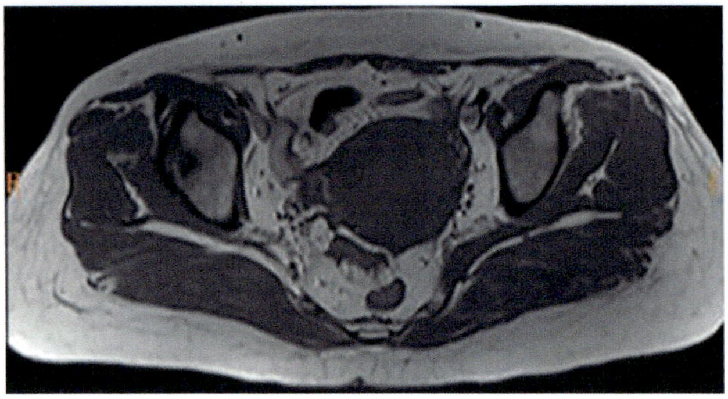

Fig. 4.1 A 54-year-old woman with ECS. The tumor located in the uterine cavity with isointense signal on T1WI

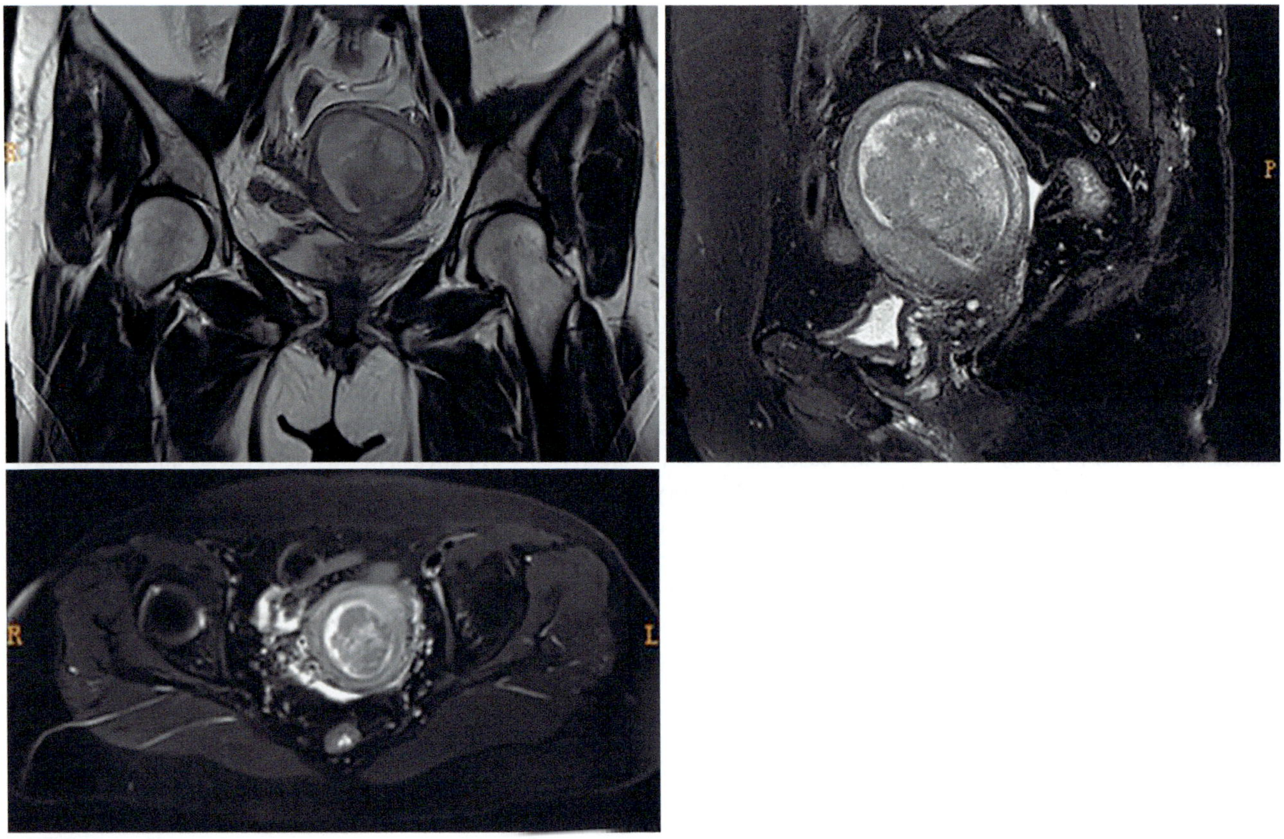

Figs. 4.2–4.4 A 54-year-old woman with ECS. The tumor located in the uterine cavity with isointense signal on T2WI; on fat-suppressed T2WI sequence, the lobulated mass centered into the uterine cavity

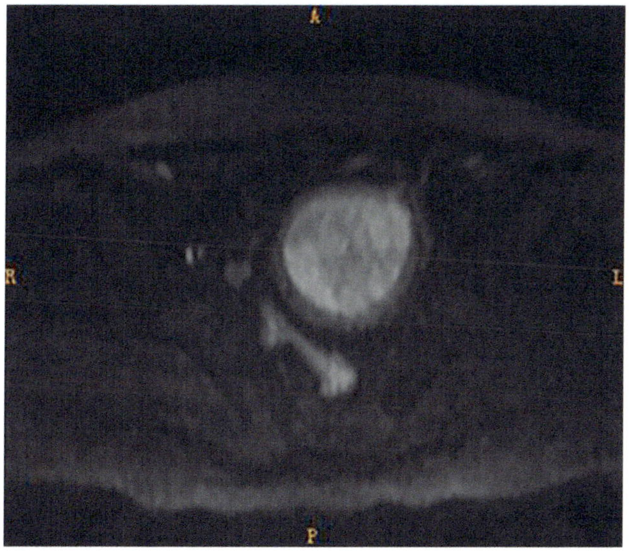

Fig. 4.5 A 54-year-old woman with ECS. On DWI, the mass displayed as homogeneously high signal

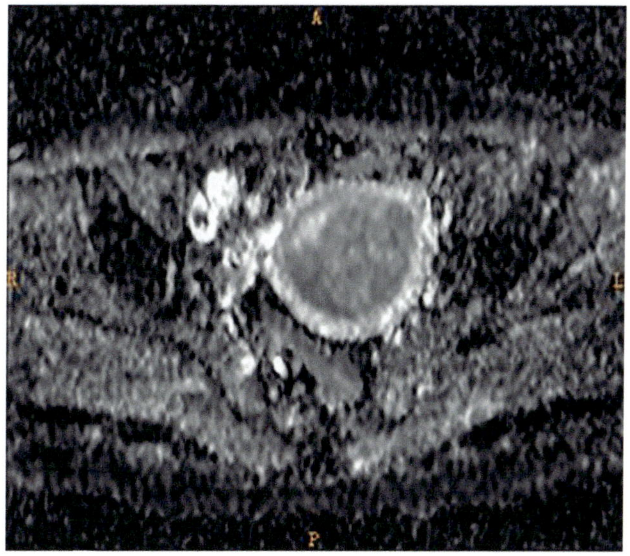

Fig. 4.6 A 54-year-old woman with ECS. On DWI, the mass displayed relatively low signal on the corresponding ADC map

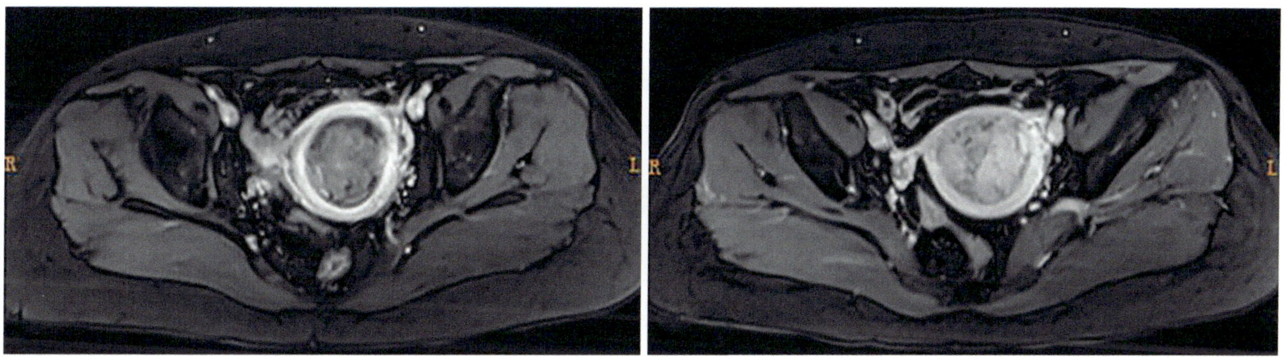

Figs. 4.7 and 4.8 A 54-year-old woman with ECS. The mass enhanced less significantly on early-stage and equivalently on late-stage contrast-enhanced images

4.2 Differential Diagnosis

It is difficult to differentiate ECS from endometrial cancer on imaging. For ECS, heterogeneous mass is more common, with focal abnormal tumoral enhancement. Compared with leiomyosarcoma of uterus, tumor hemorrhage and necrosis are uncommon.

References

1. Kato H, Kanematsu M, Furui T, Imai A, Hirose Y, Kondo H, et al. Carcinosarcoma of the uterus: radiologic–pathologic correlations with magnetic resonance imaging including diffusion-weighted imaging. Magn Reson Imaging. 2008;26(10):1446–50.
2. D'Angelo E, Prat J. Uterine sarcomas: a review. Gynecol Oncol. 2010;116(1):131–9.
3. Tanaka YO, Tsunoda H, Minami R, Yoshikawa H, Minami M. Carcinosarcoma of the uterus: MR findings. J Magn Reson Imaging. 2008;28(2):434–9.
4. Sohaib SA, Verma H, Attygalle AD, Ind TEJ. Imaging of uterine malignancies. Semin Ultrasound CT MRI. 2010;31(5):377–87.
5. Shah SH, Jagannathan JP, Krajewski K, O'Regan KN, George S, Ramaiya NH. Uterine sarcomas: then and now. Am J Roentgenol. 2012;199(1):213–23.
6. Schorge J, Williams JW. Williams gynecology. McGraw-Hill Companies, Incorporated; 2008.

5 Endometrial Adenosarcoma

He Zhang

5.1 Clinical History

Female patient, 26 years old. She complained of delayed menstruation and had no history of gynecological diseases. Ultrasonography showed a hypoechoic mass, having an unclear boundary with uterine body. The final pathological result was endometrial adenosarcoma.

5.2 Imaging Analysis

Endometrial adenosarcoma (EAS) is a rare, low malignant potential uterine tumor; pathologically, it is a kind of subtype between adenofibroma and carcinosarcoma [1]. It usually affects postmenopausal women. Clinical symptoms include abnormal vaginal bleeding, vaginal discharge, pelvic pain, and pelvic mass. Most of EAS origins from endometrium and less commonly from cervix or myometrium. Pelvic involvement is rare and, if present, can invade bilateral ovaries and the adjacent intestinal loop [2, 3]. Prognosis of EAS is significantly better than endometrial carcinosarcoma (ECS) except for lesions involving myometrium [4–6]. Recurrent lesions usually arise from vagina, pelvic, or abdominal cavity. Distant metastatic lesions are rare. On imaging, features of EAS are similar with ECS, characterized by a pedicled mass protruding into uterine cavity and cervix. On MRI, EAS often manifests as multilobular, cystic mass mimicking gestational mass (Figs. 5.1 and 5.2). High signal of EAS on T2WI represents necrotic components and glandular tissue (Figs. 5.3 and 5.4). Main treatment methods include hysterectomy, chemotherapy, and radiation therapy. Nearly 1/3 of patients will relapse within 5 years after the initial treatment [7].

H. Zhang (✉)
Department of Radiology, Obstetrics and Gynecology Hospital,
Fudan University, Shanghai, People's Republic of China
e-mail: zhanghe1790@fckyy.org.cn

G. Zhang (ed.), *MRI of Gynaecological Diseases*, https://doi.org/10.1007/978-981-99-3644-1_5

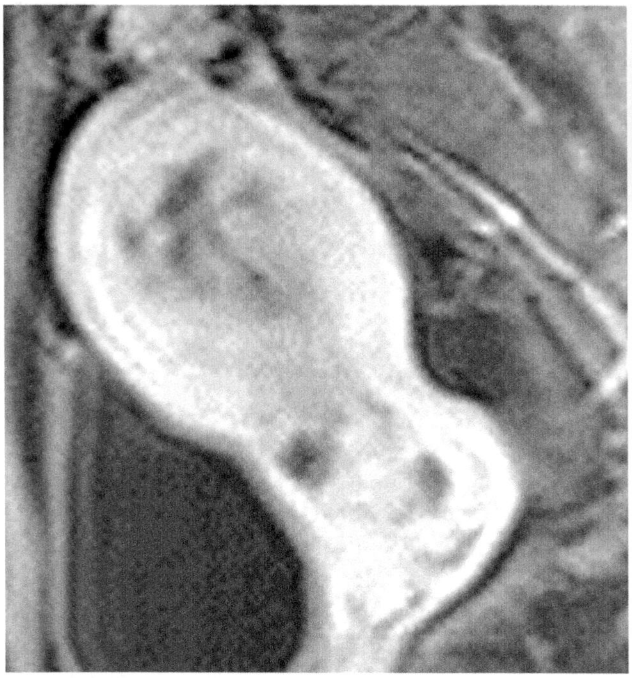
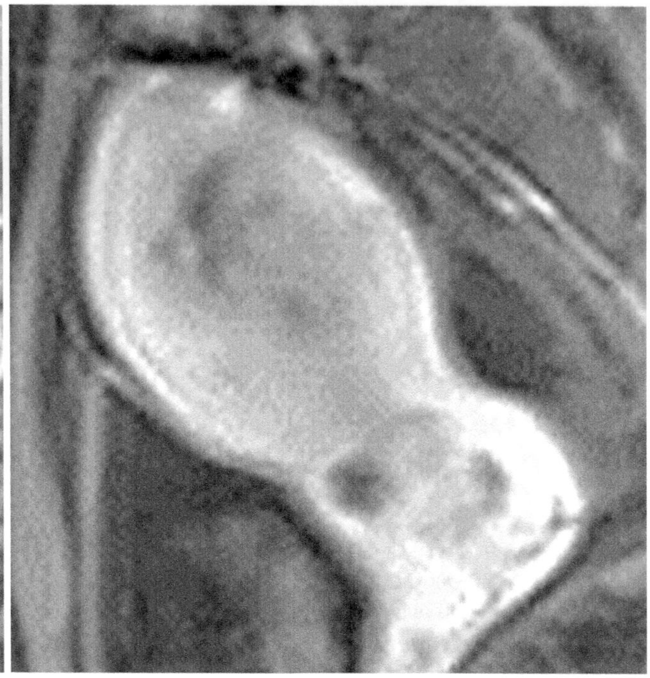

Figs. 5.1 and 5.2 The tumor body showed relatively weak enhancement than normal myometrium on the both early and delayed contrast-enhanced images

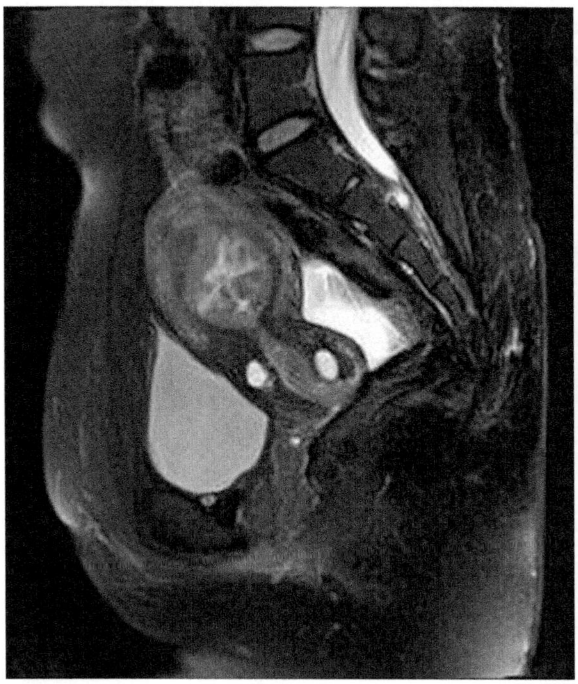
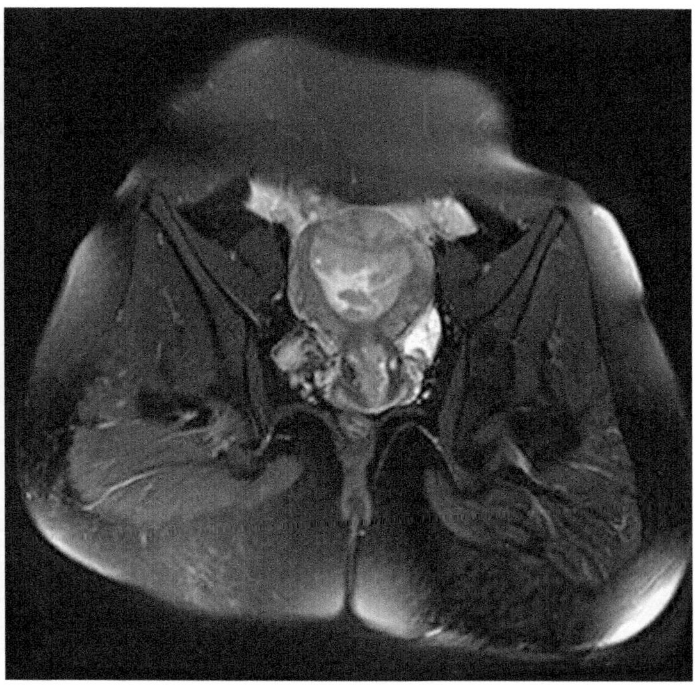

Figs. 5.3 and 5.4 On sagittal and coronal T2WI, the tumor involved both uterine cavity and cervix, and the uterine junctional zone seemed intact

References

1. D'Angelo E, Prat J. Uterine sarcomas: a review. Gynecol Oncol. 2010;116(1):131–9.
2. Chiang S, Oliva E. Recent developments in uterine mesenchymal neoplasms. Histopathology. 2013;62(1):124–37.
3. Schorge J, Williams JW. Williams gynecology. McGraw-Hill Companies, Incorporated; 2008.
4. Lu Z, Chen H, Shi S. CT and MRI findings of endometrical carcinosarcoma of uterine. J Clin Radiol (Chinese). 2012;31(9):1352–5.
5. He Zhang GZ, Tian XM, Zhang H. Magnetic resonance and diffusion-weighted imaging in categorization of uterine sarcomas: correlation with pathological findings. Clin Imaging. 2014;38(6):836–44.
6. Genever AV, Abdi S. Can MRI predict the diagnosis of endometrial carcinosarcoma? Clin Radiol. 2011;66(7):621–4.
7. Qiu LL, Yu RS, Chen Y, Zhang Q. Sarcomas of abdominal organs: computed tomography and magnetic resonance imaging findings. Semin Ultrasound CT MRI. 2011;32(5):405–21.

Leiomyosarcoma of Uterus

6

He Zhang

6.1 Imaging Analysis

Leiomyosarcoma (LS) of uterus is the second most common uterine sarcoma, accounting for approximately 40% of all uterine sarcomas. Current studies support that LS of uterus is primary sarcoma, only less than 5% of them develop from malignant transformation of benign uterine fibroids. Pathologically, morphological features include apoptosis and necrosis, and cellular polymorphism can be used to differentiate LS from uterine fibroids and other small round cell tumors. Clinical symptoms are nonspecific, including abnormal vaginal bleeding, pelvic pain, and pelvic mass. The peak age of onset is the fourth to fifth decades, and only 15% of patients are younger than 40 years old. Previous radiotherapy history is the independent risk factor for LS of uterus [1, 2]. On MRI, imaging features vary based on its size and presence of necrotic components. In general, signal characteristics of LS show similarly to those of uterine fibroids, displaying as isointensity signal on both T1WI (Fig. 6.1) and T2WI (Fig. 6.2). Intratumoral hemorrhagic foci manifest as high signal on T1WI. Contrast-enhanced MR images (Fig. 6.3) show earlier enhancement than normal myometrium which can help to determine the location of the tumor (myometrium, endometrium or subserous) [3–5].

H. Zhang (✉)
Department of Radiology, Obstetrics and Gynecology Hospital,
Fudan University, Shanghai, People's Republic of China
e-mail: zhanghe1790@fckyy.org.cn

G. Zhang (ed.), *MRI of Gynaecological Diseases*, https://doi.org/10.1007/978-981-99-3644-1_6

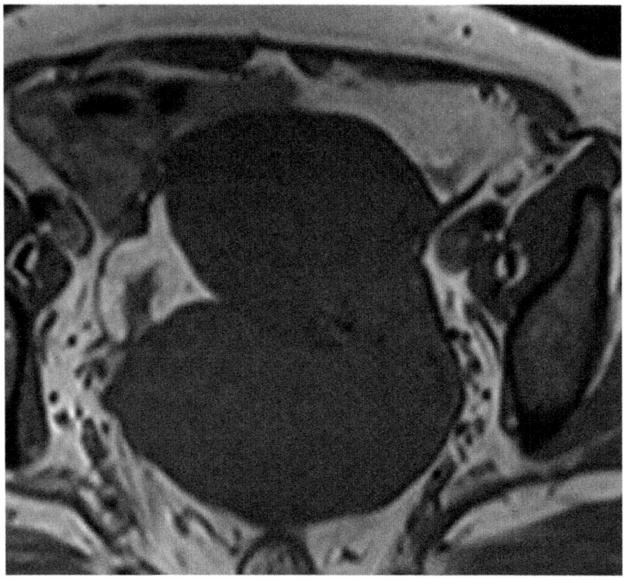

Fig. 6.1 Leiomyosarcoma of uterus. The mass located in the rectouterine pouch with homogeneous signal on T1WI

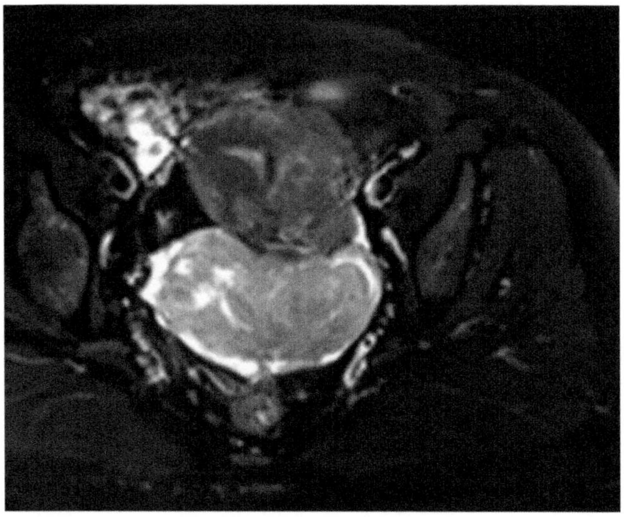

Fig. 6.2 Leiomyosarcoma of uterus. The mass located in the rectouterine pouch with intermediate to high signal on T2WI

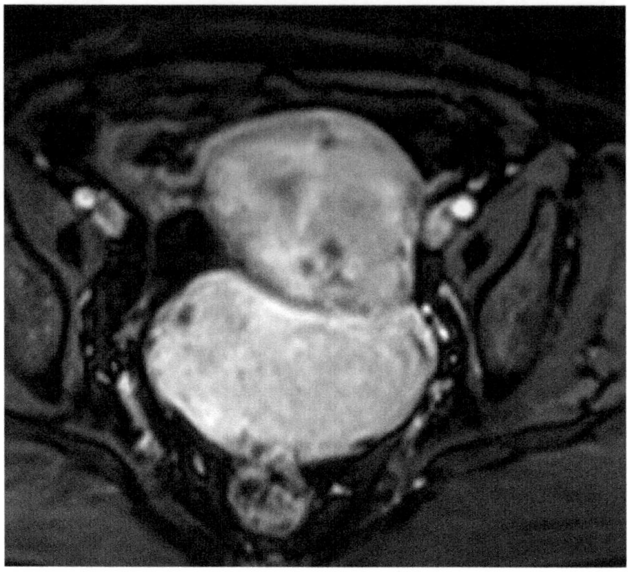

Fig. 6.3 Leiomyosarcoma of uterus. On DWI, the mass showed enhanced homogeneously on contrast-enhanced images

6.2 Differential Diagnosis

Compared with uterine fibroids, LS of uterus often have larger size and grow more rapidly with existence of both intratumoral hemorrhagic and necrotic components. These biological characteristics will be exactly reflected on MRI, indicating the diagnosis of LS. Ill-defined boundary of LS is also considered as important characteristic for differentiating LS of uterus from uterine fibroids. In recent study, researchers reported the cut-off value of 0.905×10^{-3} mm^2/s on ADC map obtained from diffusion weighted imaging (DWI) (Fig. 6.4) and improved the diagnostic sensitivity to 98% for LS of uterus in 156 cases (51 sarcomas and 105 leiomyomas) from three independent medical centers [6–9].

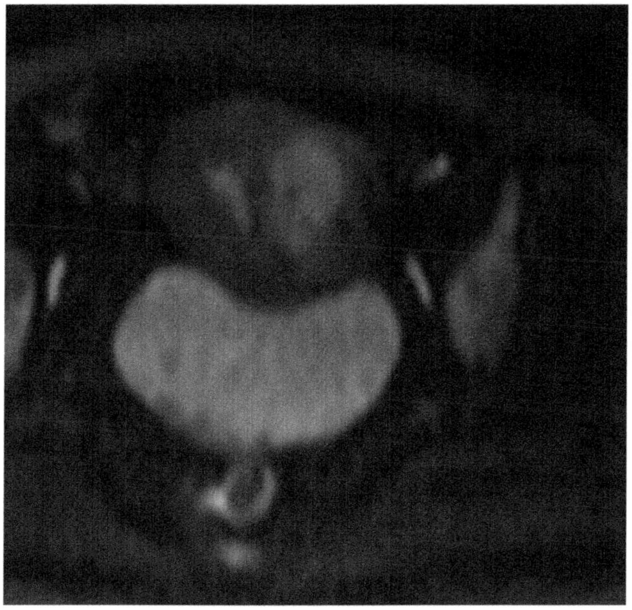

Fig. 6.4 Leiomyosarcoma of uterus. On DWI, the mass showed restricted diffusion signal

References

1. D'Angelo E, Prat J. Uterine sarcomas: a review. Gynecol Oncol. 2010;116(1):131–9.
2. Prat J. FIGO staging for uterine sarcomas. Int J Gynecol Obstet. 2009;104(3):177–8.
3. He Zhang GZ, Tian XM, Zhang H. Magnetic resonance and diffusion-weighted imaging in categorization of uterine sarcomas: correlation with pathological findings. Clin Imaging. 2014;38(6):836–44.
4. Sala EWS, Senior E, Lomas D. MRI of malignant neoplasms of the uterine corpus and cervix. Am J Roentgenol. 2007;188(6):1577–87.
5. Tanaka YO, Nishida M, Tsunoda H, Okamoto Y, Yoshikawa H. Smooth muscle tumors of uncertain malignant potential and leiomyosarcomas of the uterus: MR findings. J Magn Reson Imaging. 2004;20(6):998–1007.
6. Namimoto T, Yamashita Y, Awai K, Nakaura T, Yanaga Y, Hirai T, et al. Combined use of T2-weighted and diffusion-weighted 3-T MR imaging for differentiating uterine sarcomas from benign leiomyomas. Eur Radiol. 2009;19(11):2756–64.
7. Xie J. MRI findings of uterine sarcoma. Guangxie Medicine (Chinese). 2012;34(5):560–1.
8. Giuntoli RLI, Lessard-Anderson CR, Gerardi MA, Kushnir CL, Cliby WA, Metzinger DS, et al. Comparison of current staging systems and a novel staging system for uterine leiomyosarcoma. Int J Gynecol Cancer. 2013;23(5):869–76. https://doi.org/10.1097/IGC.0b013e3182916a1e.
9. Moghadam R, Lathi RB, Shahmohamady B, Saberi NS, Nezhat CH, Nezhat F, et al. Predictive value of magnetic resonance imaging in differentiating between leiomyoma and adenomyosis. J Soc Laparoendosc Surg. 2006;10(2):216–9.

7 Uterine Lymphoma

He Zhang

7.1 Clinical History

A 64-year-old woman, menopause 16 years ago, complained of lower abdominal distention without any inducement 6 months ago, and she did not seek medical treatment. Ultrasonography indicated intrauterine space-occupying lesion. There was no abnormal vaginal bleeding and discharge. She underwent total hysterectomy, bilateral salpingo-oophorectomy, partial greater omentum resection, and resection of intestinal lesions. Postoperative pathology: uterine lymphoma.

7.2 Imaging Analysis

Primary genital tract lymphoma is extremely rare, of which the B-cell phenotype is the predominant type with better prognosis than T-cell lymphoma [1]. There are four subtypes of lymphoma involving the ovary: diffuse large B-cell lymphoma, Burkitt's lymphoma (BL), lymphoblastic lymphoma, or anaplastic large cell lymphoma [2]. It is difficult to distinguish primary and secondary lymphoma based solely on imaging findings, while the treatment and prognosis are different [3, 4]. In this case, the tumor displayed as homogeneously solid mass without any necrosis or fat/liquid component within it. On contrast-enhanced MRI images, the tumor showed mild or moderate enhancement compared with normal myometrium [5, 6]. It was noticed that no obvious pelvic fluid was found. Our case was consistent with Ferrozzi's report [7], that primary genital tract lymphoma appeared as solid mass with isointense signals on both T1WI (Fig. 7.1) and T2WI (Figs. 7.2 and 7.3). On contrast-enhanced images (Fig. 7.4), the tumor always displays mild or moderate enhancement, indicating its difference from other malignant ovarian tumors. In a word, owing to the rare incidence and atypical imaging features, primary genital tract lymphoma is a great challenge for radiologists to obtain a correct diagnosis before surgery. MRI has excellent soft tissue resolution, and can clearly delineate tumor margin and extent, providing reliable information for both radiologists and clinicians. Ovarian fibroma, thecoma, germ cell tumors, and metastatic tumors all should be considered as the differential diagnoses. The final diagnosis should be established on the histopathological results in relation with clinical history.

H. Zhang (✉)
Department of Radiology, Obstetrics and Gynecology Hospital, Fudan University, Shanghai, People's Republic of China
e-mail: zhanghe1790@fckyy.org.cn

G. Zhang (ed.), *MRI of Gynaecological Diseases*, https://doi.org/10.1007/978-981-99-3644-1_7

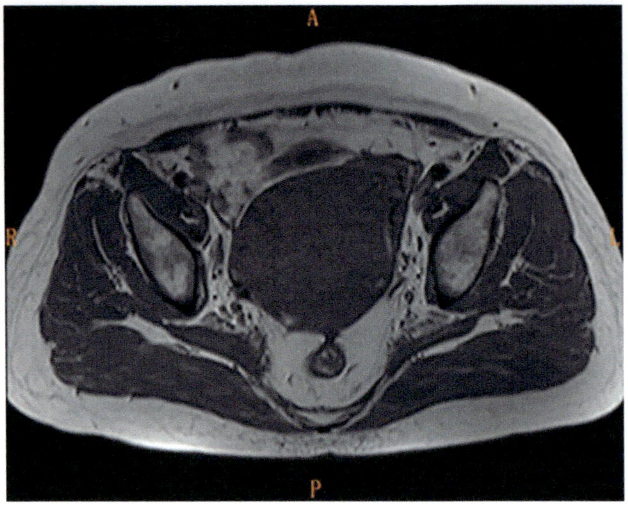

Fig. 7.1 The uterus enlarged wholly with the thickness of uterine junctional zone, appearing as homogeneous intermediate signal on axial T1WI

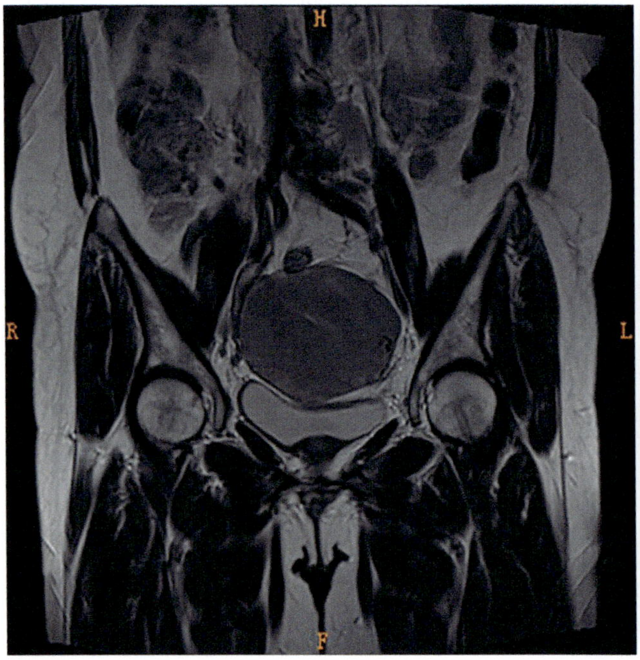

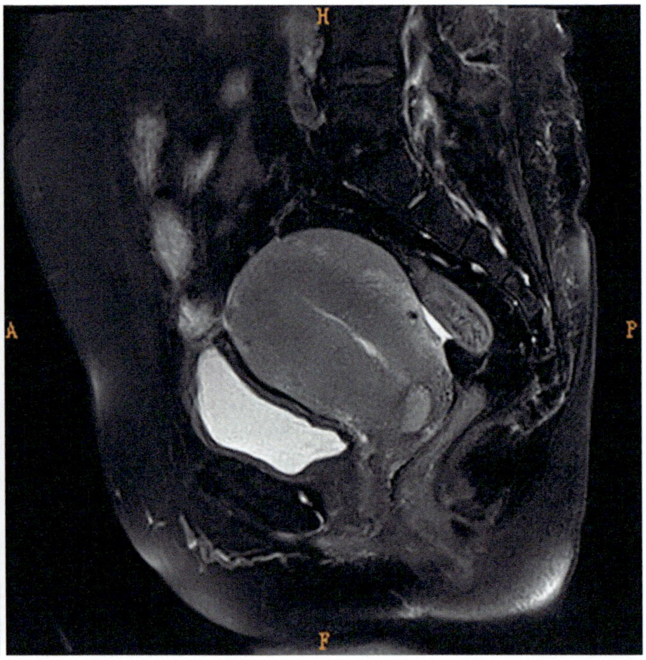

Figs. 7.2 and 7.3 The uterus enlarged wholly with the thickness of uterine junctional zone, appearing as homogeneous intermediate signal on coronal T2WI. The endometrium showed no abnormal signal on sagittal T2WI

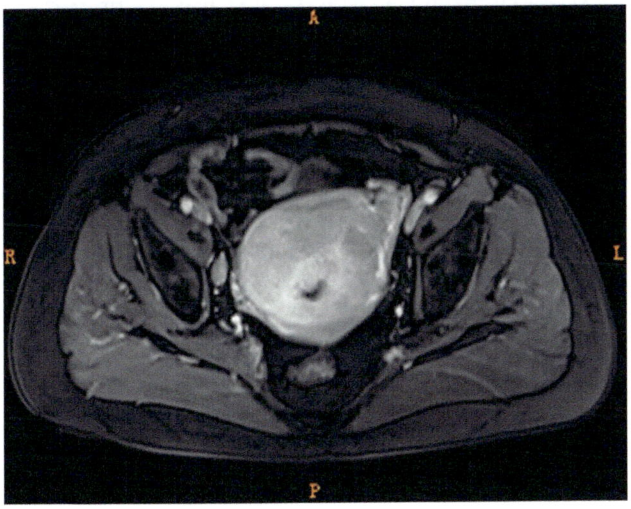

Fig. 7.4 The tumor showed mild enhancement after contrast enhancement

7.3 Differential Diagnosis

Considering the differential diagnosis, some ovarian solid masses, such as ovarian sex cord-stromal tumors and germ cell tumors, must be included for the possible differential diagnosis [8]. Thecoma or fibrothecoma is the most common benign ovarian solid tumors encountered on clinic. The characteristic signals of ovarian thecoma are always low signals on any MRI sequences because there is little of water molecule among fibrous components, making it easily differentiated from other ovarian tumors. For young patients, germ cell tumors are another common ovarian disease with elevated AFP level, which may provide a useful clue for the correct diagnosis. For bilateral solid ovarian masses, metastatic tumors should also be excluded and careful review of clinical history is necessary to make a proper diagnosis (Figs. 7.5 and 7.6).

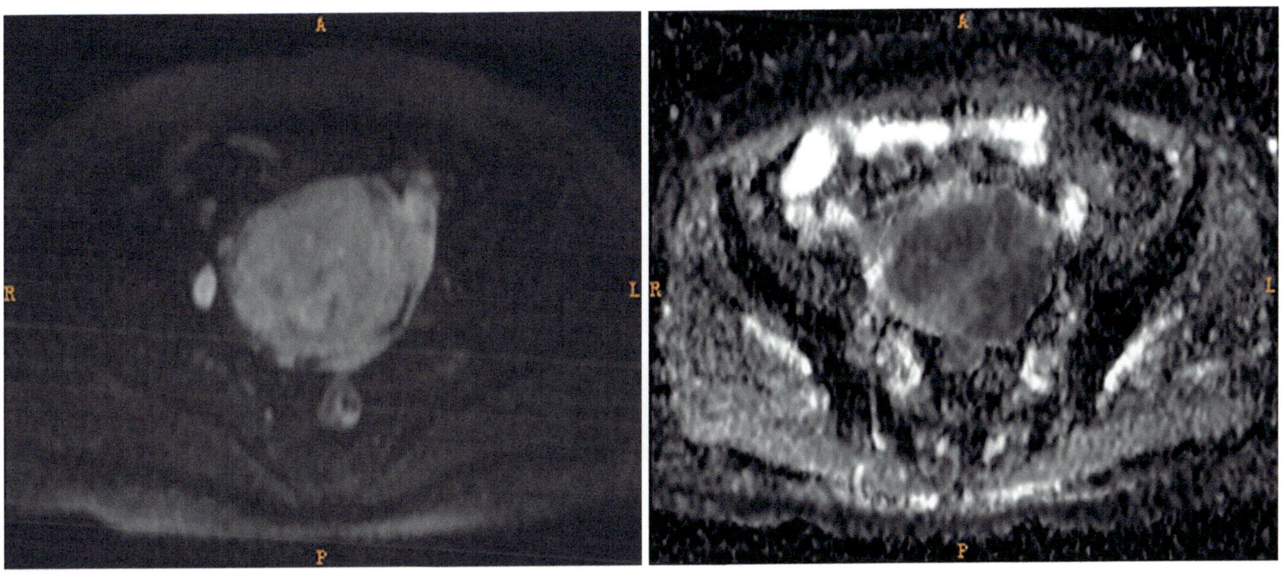

Figs. 7.5 and 7.6 On DWI, the uterus showed homogeneous high signal, and the enlarged lymph node adjacent to the right iliac vessels also showed high signal. The tumor showed homogeneous low signal on the corresponding ADC map

References

1. Yadav BS, George P, Sharma SC, Gorsi U, McClennan E, Martino MA, et al. Primary non-Hodgkin lymphoma of the ovary. Semin Oncol. 2014;41(3):e19–30.
2. Mandato VD, Palermo R, Falbo A, Capodanno I, Capodanno F, Gelli MC, et al. Primary diffuse large B-cell lymphoma of the uterus: case report and review. Anticancer Res. 2014;34(8):4377–90.
3. Samama M, van Poelgeest M. Primary malignant lymphoma of the uterus: a case report and review of the literature. Case Rep Oncol. 2011;4(3):560–3.
4. Crawshaw J, Sohaib SA, Wotherspoon A, Shepherd JH. Primary non-Hodgkin's lymphoma of the ovaries: imaging findings. Br J Radiol. 2007;80(956):e155–e8.
5. Ahmad AK, Hui P, Litkouhi B, Azodi M, Rutherford T, McCarthy S, et al. Institutional review of primary non-Hodgkin lymphoma of the female genital tract: a 33-year experience. Int J Gynecol Cancer. 2014;24(7):1250–5.
6. Bianchi P, Torcia F, Vitali M, Cozza G, Matteoli M, Giovanale V. An atypical presentation of sporadic ovarian Burkitt's lymphoma: case report and review of the literature. J Ovarian Res. 2013;6(1):46.
7. Ferrozzi FTG, Bovac D, Zuccoli G. Non-Hodgkin lymphomas of the ovaries: MR findings. J Comput Assist Tomogr. 2000;24(3):416–20.
8. Jung SE, Lee JM, Rha SE, Byun JY, Jung JI, Hahn ST. CT and MR imaging of ovarian tumors with emphasis on differential diagnosis. Radiographics. 2002;22(6):1305–25.

8 Cervical Cancer

Xuan Yin

8.1 Clinical History

The 37-year-old female patient complained of a small amount of vaginal bleeding with discharge, obvious after sexual intercourse. Ultrasonography indicated that there was a low echo area in the cervix, with clear boundary, irregular shape, and rich blood flow signals. Gynecological examination showed that the cervix was 4 cm in diameter with cauliflower surface and contact bleeding. She underwent cervical biopsy under colposcope. Pathological findings: (cervical tissue) invasive squamous cell carcinoma. Physical examination after admission revealed a cervical soft mass with a diameter of 5 cm and contact bleeding.

On MRI, abnormal mass was observed in the cervix, with a size of 5 cm × 4.2 cm × 4.3 cm, showing slightly high signal intensity on T2WI (Figs. 8.1 and 8.2). The mass showed high signal on DWI (Fig. 8.3) and low signal on the corresponding ADC map (Fig. 8.4). Early enhancement was observed after contrast enhancement (Figs. 8.5 and 8.6). The upper edge of the lesion exceeded endocervix, and the boundary between lower edge of the lesion and vaginal fornix was unclear. The posterior fornix disappeared, and the stroma on both sides became thinner.

Operation was performed on the seventh day after admission. Intraoperatively, the tumor was located in the posterior lip of cervix with a diameter of 5 cm. Extensive total abdominal hysterectomy, bilateral salpingectomy, pelvic lymph node dissection, and bilateral ovarian suspension were performed. Postoperative pathological findings: invasive squamous cell carcinoma of the cervix, keratinizing. Infiltrate deep fibromuscular layer of the cervix to the lateral wall. The upper margin infiltrated the inner membrane and muscular layer of uterus, and the lower margin infiltrated the mucosa and stroma of vaginal wall. Squamous cell carcinoma in situ was seen at 6°–11° of vaginal wall margin. There was no tumor involvement in bilateral parametrium. No metastasis was found in 17 lymph nodes. Immunohistochemical findings: CK7 (+), CK-h (+) and P16 (+), about (+), Ki-67 (+60%), P53 (−), CD31 (−), D240 (−). The patient was discharged 18 days after surgery.

X. Yin (✉)
Department of Radiology, Obstetrics and Gynecology Hospital, Fudan University, Shanghai, People's Republic of China

G. Zhang (ed.), *MRI of Gynaecological Diseases*, https://doi.org/10.1007/978-981-99-3644-1_8

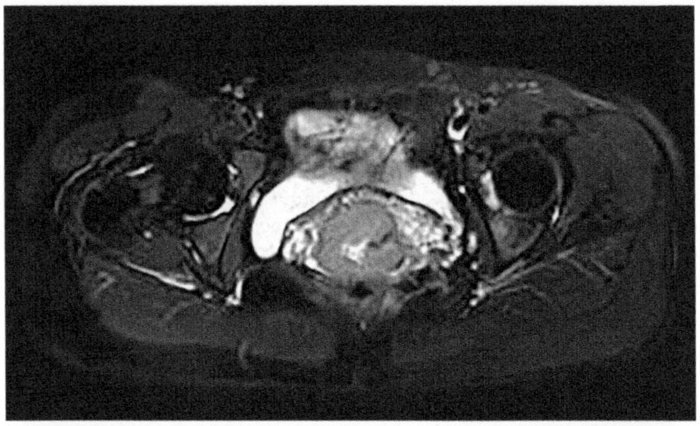

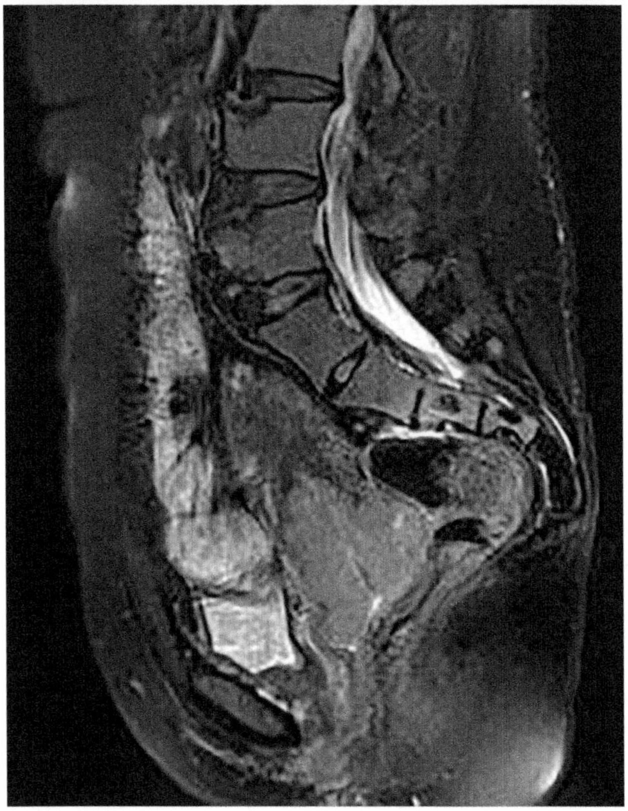

Figs. 8.1 and 8.2 Axial T2-weighted image: the cervix showed a soft tissue mass with slightly high signal intensity. Sagittal T2-weighted image: the upper edge of the lesion exceeded the cervical opening, and the lower edge was not demarcated from the vaginal fornix

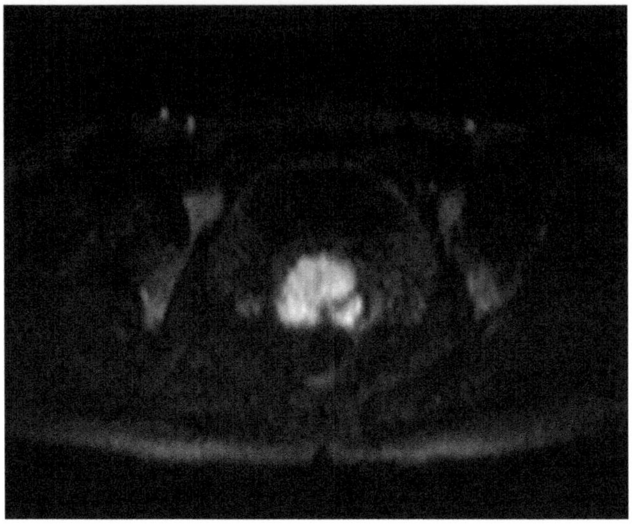

Fig. 8.3 High signal on DWI and low signal on the corresponding ADC map

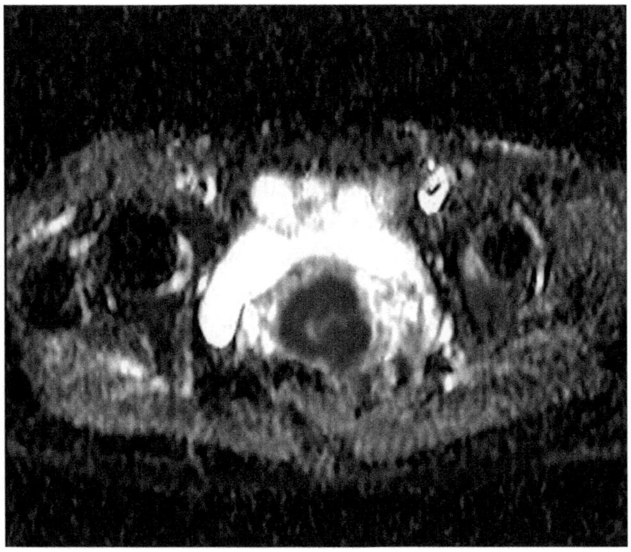

Fig. 8.4 High signal on DWI and low signal on the corresponding ADC map

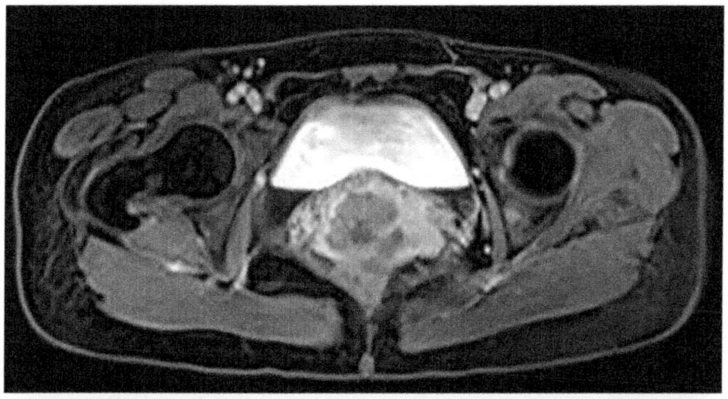

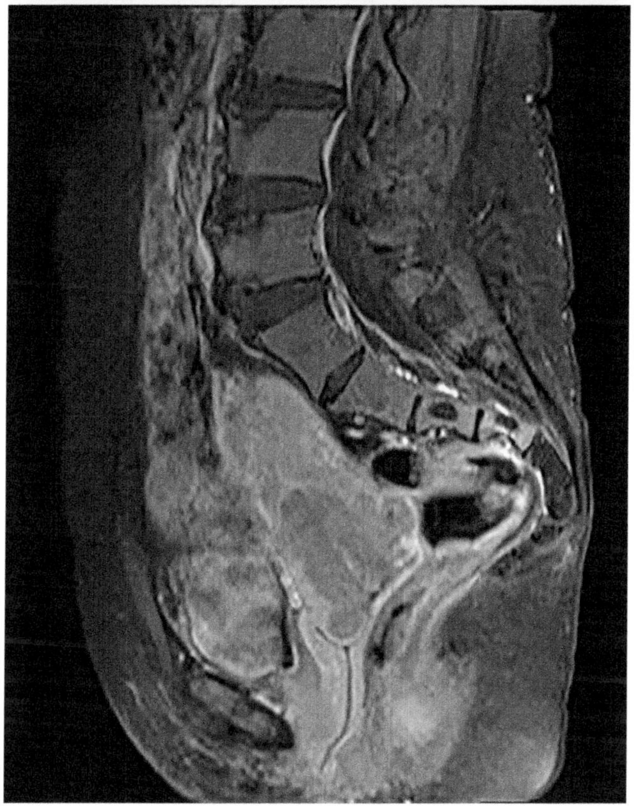

Figs. 8.5 and 8.6 Axial contrast-enhanced fat-suppressed T1-weighted image: the lesion was solid and significantly enhanced, with thinning of the bilateral stroma. Sagittal contrast-enhanced fat-suppressed T1-weighted image: the posterior fornix of the vagina was unclear, and the posterior wall of the vagina was significantly enhanced

8.2 Imaging Analysis

Cervical cancer is one of the most common gynecological malignant tumors in women [1]. In recent years, the mortality rate of cervical cancer has decreased significantly, but the incidence rate of women of childbearing age has increased. Risk factors include early age of first sexual intercourse, sexual behavior disorders, multiparity, smoking, human papillomavirus (HPV) infection, and herpes simplex virus II infection. HPV infection is the main risk factor for cervical cancer.

Most cervical cancers occur in the transformation zone at the junction between squamous and columnar cervical epithelium. This transformation zone is located at the external cervical orifice. The transformation zone of elderly people moves up to the cervical canal. Cervical cancer is mostly squamous cell carcinoma, accounting for about 85%, and adenocarcinoma for about 15% [2]. Squamous cell carcinoma is more common on the surface of cervical canal, while adenocarcinoma is more common in the cervical canal. According to the growth pattern and morphology of the tumor, cervical cancer can be divided into exogenous type, endogenous type, ulcerative type, and cervical canal type [3]. Irregular vaginal bleeding, vaginal discharge, and pelvic pain are the main clinical symptoms of cervical cancer.

On MRI, normal cervical tissue shows low signal intensity in the outer muscle layer, obvious low signal intensity in the intramuscular layer, and obvious high signal intensity in the mucosa layer on T2WI. Cervical cancer can be presented as a mass resembling round or irregular shape, with isointense signal on T1WI and hyperintense signal on T2WI. Most of the lesions on contrast-enhanced images show moderate heterogeneous enhancement, with no enhancement in the central necrotic area. Cervical cancer mainly shows high signal intensity on DWI, which is in sharp contrast to the normal structure around the tumor. The mean ADC value of malignant cervical lesion is $0.82 \times 10^{-3} \pm 0.1$ SD mm^2/s, while the mean ADC value in the control group is 1.56×10^{-3} mm^2/s. ADC value of 1.07×10^{-3} mm^2/s is a cut-off value between normal cervical tissue and malignant cervical lesion.

Compared with the hypointense signal of normal cervical stroma and hyperintense signal of parauterine adipose tissue, it can clearly show the depth of tumor invasion to the cervix. MRI can also show parauterine and pelvic wall invasion, as well as adjacent organs involvement and lymphadenopathy [4]. When high-signal tumor tissue is found in the cervix on T2WI and the inner edge of the low-signal ring in the normal cervical stroma is smooth without interruption, cervical cancer does not invade the stroma. When the cervical stroma low signal ring is partially or completely replaced by the high signal, and the cervical outer margin is smooth and the boundary between it and the parauterine fat space is clear and sharp, it indicates that the cervical stroma is invaded, but there is no parauterine invasion. When the outer margin of the cervix is irregular, rough, and uneven, or there is a high-signal strip like shadow with irregular edge in the parauterine tissue, it can be estimated as parauterine invasion. Pelvic wall invasion is characterized by loss of fat space between tumor tissue and pelvic wall, coarse and irregular edges of pelvic wall muscles, or high signal foci of tumor tissue in pelvic wall muscles (obturator internus, piriformis, levator ani muscle). Vaginal involvement is characterized by a mass protruding into the vagina or by replacement of the normal low signal of vaginal wall with a high signal focus on T2WI. Cervical cancer transcends endocervix and protrudes into the uterine cavity or disappears in the normal three-layer structure of the uterine body on T2WI and is replaced by tumor tissue with high signal focus, which can be estimated as invasion of the uterine body. Cystorectal involvement is characterized by segmental thickening of bladder wall and rectum wall. Contrast-enhanced examination can help confirm the diagnosis if bladder or rectum wall shows the same signal changes as tumor tissue. Lymph nodes with a short diameter >1 cm and annular enhancement can be regarded as lymphatic metastasis [5].

8.3 Differential Diagnosis

Cervical cancer should be differentiated from cervical invasion of vaginal cancer and cervical canal endometrial cancer differentiation. When vaginal cancer invades the cervix, it is shown as a solid mass in the fornix, which is connected with the cervix, while endometrial cancer invades the cervix displays as a mass whose main body is in the uterine cavity and local infiltration of the cervix, which needs to be carefully identified.

References

1. Parkin DM, Bray F, Ferlay J, et al. Global cancer statistics, 2002. CA Cancer J Clin. 2005;55:74–108.
2. Kaur H, Silverman PM, Iyer RB, et al. Diagnosis, staging, and surveillance of cervical carcinoma. AJR Am J Roentgenol. 2003;180(6):1621–31.
3. Okamoto Y, Tanaka YO, Nishida M, et al. MR imaging of the uterine cervix: imaging-pathologic correlation. Radiographics. 2003;23(2):425–45.
4. Balleyguier C, Saha E, Da Cunha T, et al. Staging of uterine cervical cancer with MRI: guidelines of the European Society of Urogenital Radiology. Eur Radiol. 2011;21(5):1102–10.
5. Manfredi R, Gui B, Giovanzana A, et al. Localized cervical cancer (stage <IIB): accuracy of MRI imaging in planning less extensive surgery. Radiol Med. 2009;114(6):960–75.

9 Endometrial Carcinoma

Jia Liu

Endometrial carcinoma (EC) is one of the most common gynecological cancer in the developed country. The incidence rate has been increasing these years. In our country, EC accounts for approximately 7% and 20–30% of female malignancies and female reproductive tract malignancies, respectively. The mean age of diagnosis is 60 years old. It usually occurs in postmenopausal women, although 20–25% of ECs are diagnosed before menopause [1]. EC of early stage has a good prognosis. Once metastasis or recurrence occurs, the prognosis is significantly worse and the median survival time is significantly shortened [2]. The incidence of EC is related to obesity, hypertension, nulliparous, exogenous estrogen application, and diabetes. Prognosis of EC patients depends on multiple different factors, most of which such as histological type and grade, age of the patient, size of the tumor, depth of myometrium invasion, and lymphovascular spaces invasion [3]. Magnetic resonance imaging (MRI) has high soft tissue resolution and has proven to be the most important imaging modality for assessment of the tumor's relationship to surrounding structures.

9.1 Imaging Analysis

When MRI is applied for EC, the examination indicators mainly include tumor size, shape and extent, endometrial thickness, signal of tumor, integrity of cervical stromal ring and junctional zone, bilateral adnexa area, pelvic and retroperitoneal lymph node conditions, etc. The American College of Radiology (ACR) recommends that MR evaluation should be the first choice of imaging technique for preoperative assessment of patients with EC [4].

On MRI, EC appears isointense relative to the myometrium on T1-weighted image. On T2-weighted image, tumor may demonstrate heterogeneous signal intensity but is most commonly hyperintense relative to the myometrium. The signal intensity of tumor increased on DWI images with high *b* value when compared with the surrounding normal tissues. Correspondently, the restricted water diffusion of tumors generated a low signal intensity on ADC maps. The DWI images should always be reviewed with their corresponding ADC maps and dynamic contrast enhancement (DCE) images, to avoid T2-shining through effect, necrotic and hemorrhagic areas, vessels, and motion artifacts.

On MRI, the key imaging sequence of EC is T2WI of high resolution. This is importantly done by choosing a sagittal T2WI of uterus. Then two T2WI sequences angled perpendicularly of the uterus are routinely performed (Fig. 9.1). To avoid volume averaging of the uterine cavity caused by uterine tilt, they improved assessment of myometrial invasion. And it improved the diagnostic accuracy of EC with myometrial invasion. The signal intensity of the junctional zone is an important sign to determine whether EC is infiltrating the superficial myometrium (Fig. 9.2). Depth of myometrial invasion (less or $\geq$ than 50%) divides superficial from deep myometrial invasion (Figs. 9.1 and 9.3). Despite the superiority of MRI in evaluating myometrial invasion in EC patients, the presence of fibroids (Fig. 9.4), adenomyosis, and large endometrial tumors expanding the endometrial cavity may limit proper evaluation [5]. Thus, complementary problem-solving modalities should be performed complementary to T2WI. The guideline published by the European Society of Urogenitourinary Radiology for EC staging recommends DCE-MRI for the complementary diagnosis of myometrial invasion [6]. The difference of blood perfusion between EC and normal myometrium can be reflected by DCE-MRI, which demonstrate hypointense relative to the myometrium. This is helpful to discriminate the depth of myometrial invasion. The best time to demonstrate tumor-to-myometrial contrast is generally seen on delayed (2–4 min after administration of contrast agent) images. DWI has high sensitivity and specificity in detecting deep myometrial invasion, and more importantly, it can reliably rule out deep

J. Liu (✉)
Department of Radiology, Obstetrics and Gynecology Hospital, Fudan University, Shanghai, People's Republic of China

G. Zhang (ed.), *MRI of Gynaecological Diseases*, https://doi.org/10.1007/978-981-99-3644-1_9

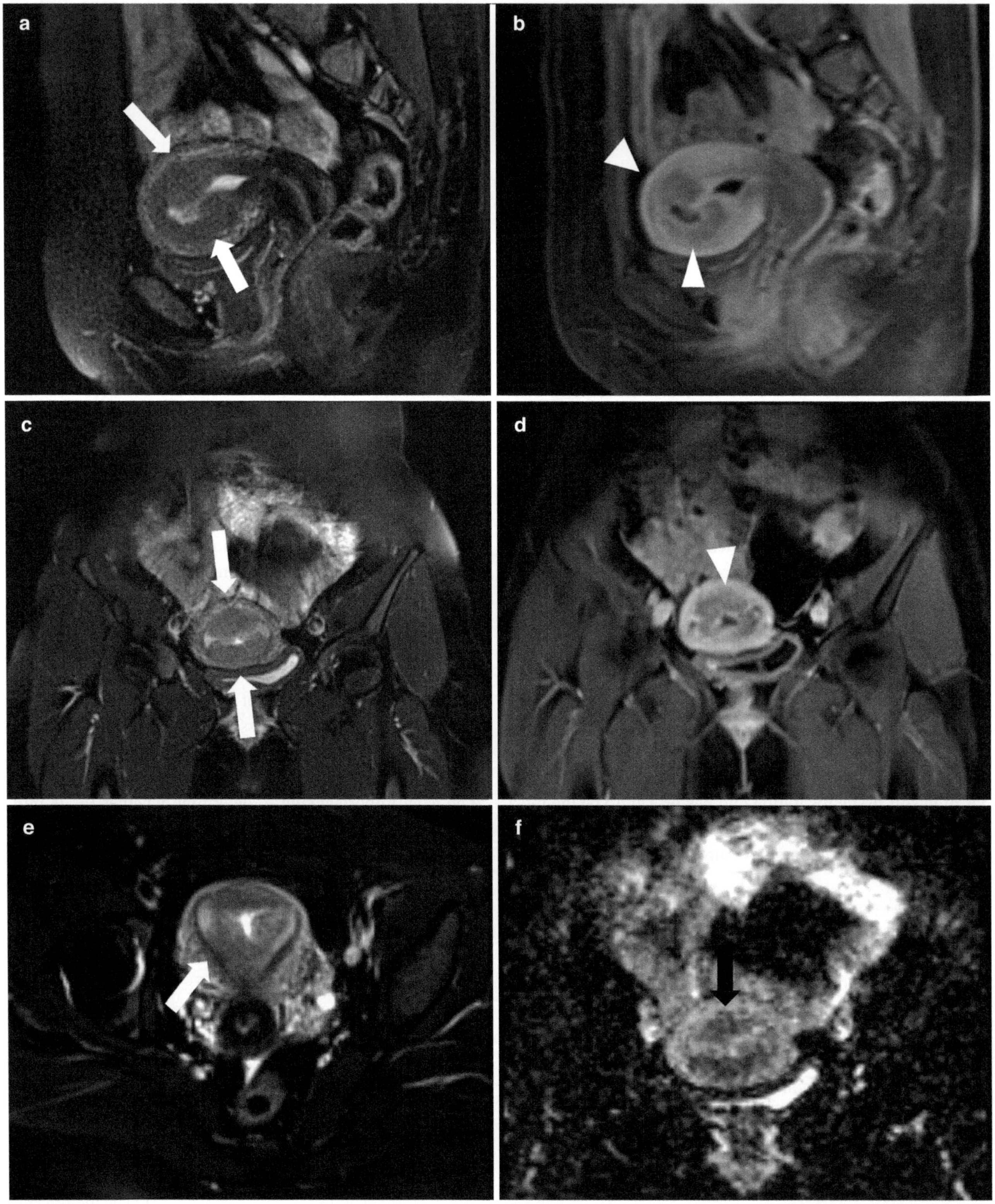

Fig. 9.1 Endometrial carcinoma with deep myometrial invasion in a 38-year-old woman. (**a**) Sagittal T2WI images with fat suppression and two T2-weighted sequences angled perpendicularly of the uterus (**c**, **e**) showed a thickened junctional zone of uterus. No obvious intrauterine mass was observed. (**b**, **d**) Sagittal and coronal contrast-enhanced T1WI images showed relatively low signal intensity in myometrium. (**f**) The lesion showed low signal intensity (black arrow) on ADC map. Gross specimen showed endometrium thickness of 0.1 cm diffusely thickened of myometrium. No obvious lesion was observed in the uterine cavity. Histopathological results showed endometrial carcinoma of grade I, invading the deep myometrium

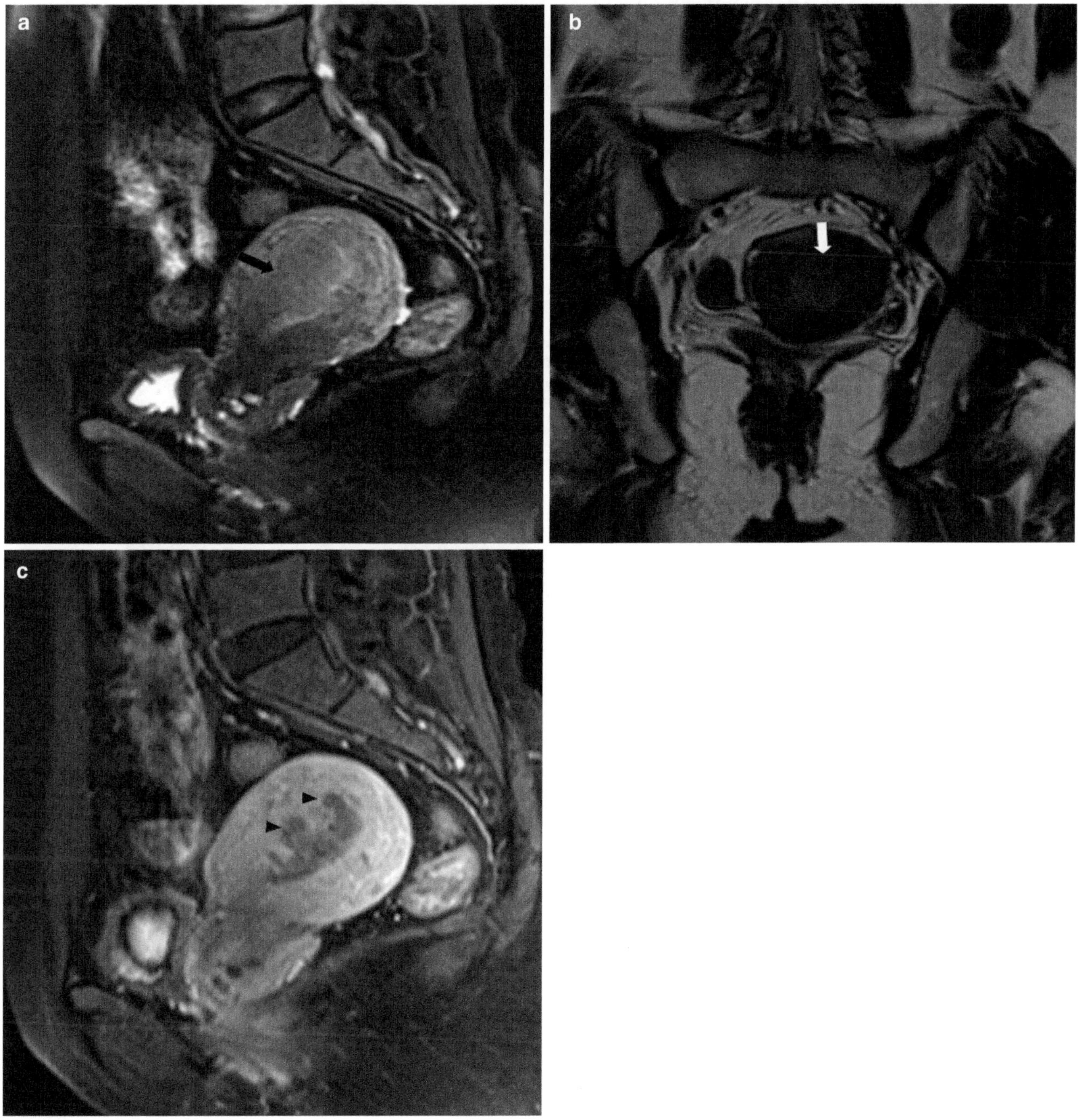

Fig. 9.2 Endometrial carcinoma with superficial myometrial invasion in a 49-year-old woman. (**a**, **b**) Sagittal and coronal T2WI images showed intrauterine mass, lacking contrast with the anterior wall of the uterus (black arrow, white arrow). (**c**) In the delayed phase after contrast enhancement, homogeneous enhancement of the myometrium was observed on T2WI images, while the lesion was mild to moderate enhanced, with superficial myometrial invasion of the anterior wall of the uterus (black arrowhead)

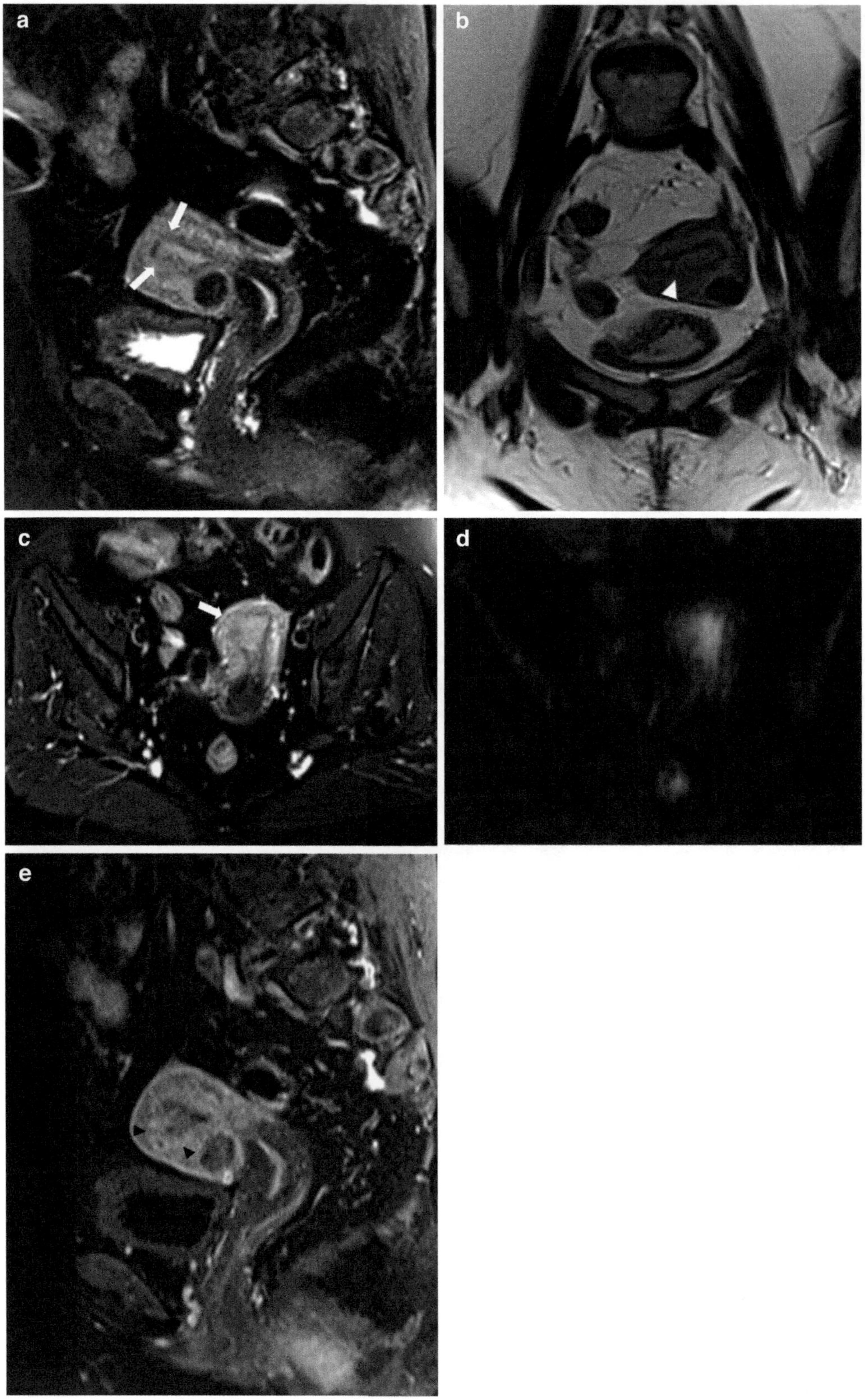

Fig. 9.3 Endometrial carcinoma with deep myometrial invasion in a 67-year-old woman. (**a**, **b**) Sagittal T2WI image with fat suppression and coronal T2WI image showed a moderate hyperintense lesion in the uterine cavity, and the junctional zone of anterior myometrium is obscure (white arrow, white arrowhead). (**c**) Axial T2WI with fat suppression image showed the junctional zone is obscure (white arrow). (**d**) On the DWI sequence, the intrauterine tumor is moderate hyperintense. (**e**) Sagittal contrast-enhanced T1WI image showed a hypointense intrauterine lesion surrounded by a relatively hyperintense myometrium. Deep myometrial invasion of anterior myometrium is demonstrated and confirmed by histopathology (black arrowhead)

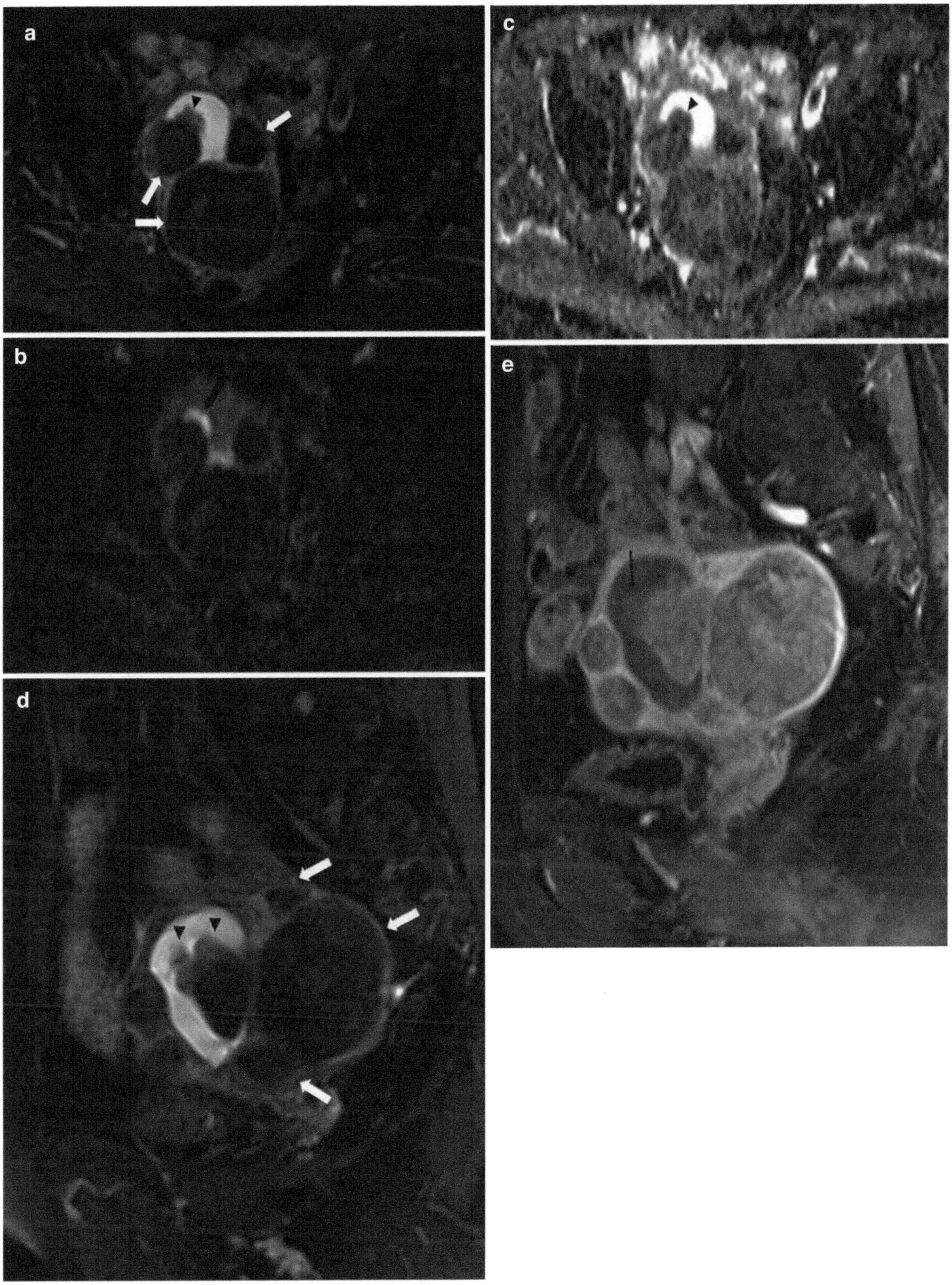

Fig. 9.4 Endometrial serous carcinoma in a 75-year-old woman with multiple intramural myomas. (**a**, **d**) Axial and sagittal T2WI images with fat suppression showed multiple intramural myomas of the uterus (white arrow). Lobulated moderate hyperintense lesion (black arrowhead) was seen in the dilated uterine cavity accompanied by effusion. (**b**, **c**) The lesion showed high signal intensity (black arrow) on DWI and significantly decreased signal intensity on the corresponding ADC map (black arrowhead). (**e**) Sagittal contrast-enhanced T1WI image showed a hypointense intrauterine lesion (long black arrow) and a relatively hyperintense myometrium with multiple intramural myomas

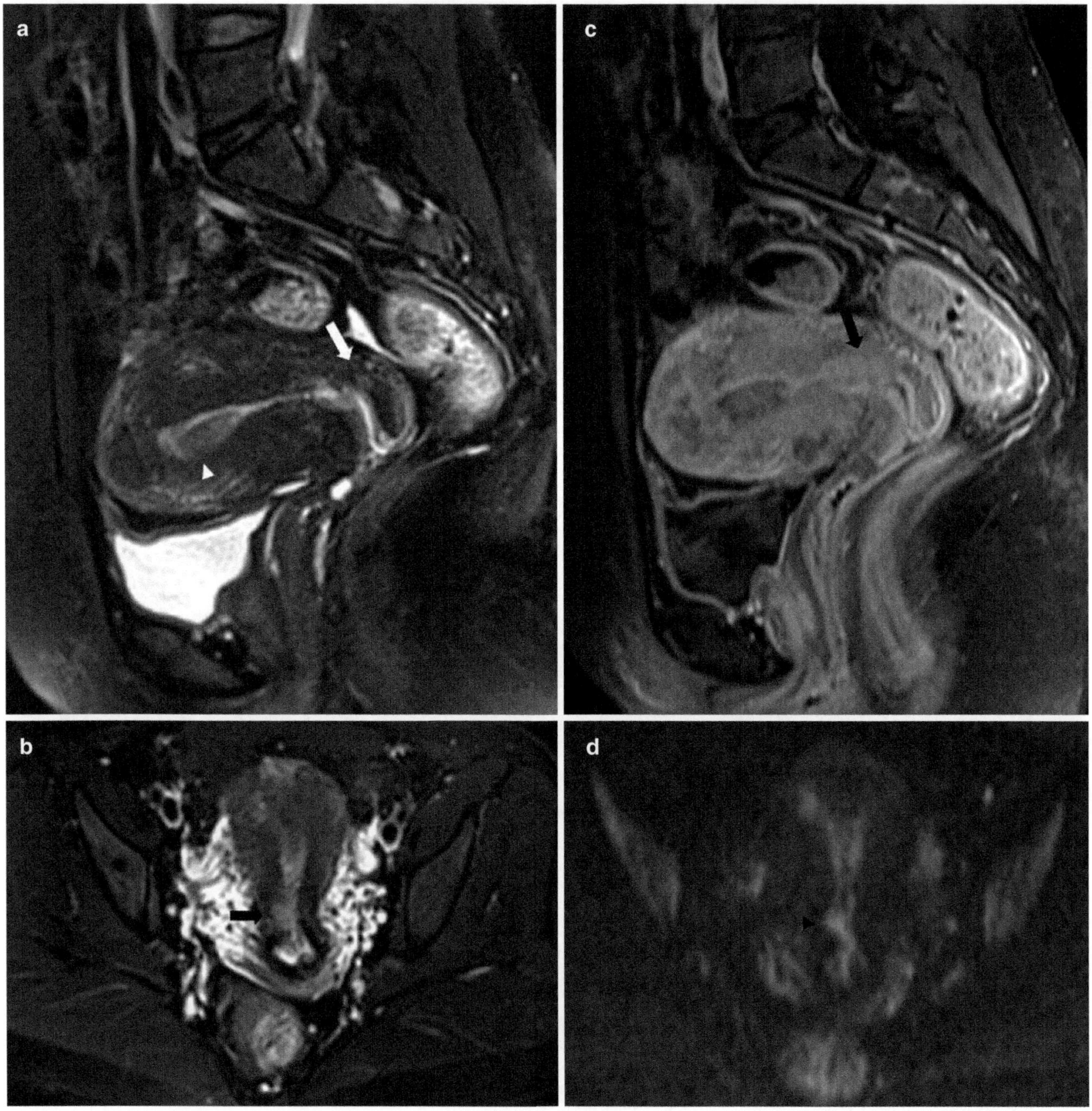

Fig. 9.5 Endometrial carcinoma with superficial myometrial and cervical invasion in a 42-year-old woman. (**a**) Sagittal T2WI image with fat suppression showed slightly high signal intensity in uterine cavity (white arrowhead) and a moderate hyperintense lesion (white arrow) in cervical canal. (**b**) Axial T2WI image with fat suppression showed a moderate hyperintense lesion in cervical canal, and the cervical stromal ring was obscure (black arrow). (**c**) Sagittal contrast-enhanced T1WI image showed cervical stromal invasion without a clear distinction between epithelium and stroma. (**d**) The lesion showed high signal intensity (black arrowhead) on DWI

myometrial invasion [7]. The combination of DCE and DWI can better improve the diagnostic accuracy.

In terms of cervical stroma invasion (Figs. 9.5 and 9.6), the optimal contrast timing for diagnosing is 3–4 min after contrast enhancement, allowing the best discrimination between tumor tissue and the cervical stroma [8]. Cervical stroma invasion can better assess by scanning thin oblique axial image perpendicular to the long axis of the cervical canal. The detection of metastatic lymph nodes relies heavily on the size of the lymph node. Using a 1 cm cut-off for the

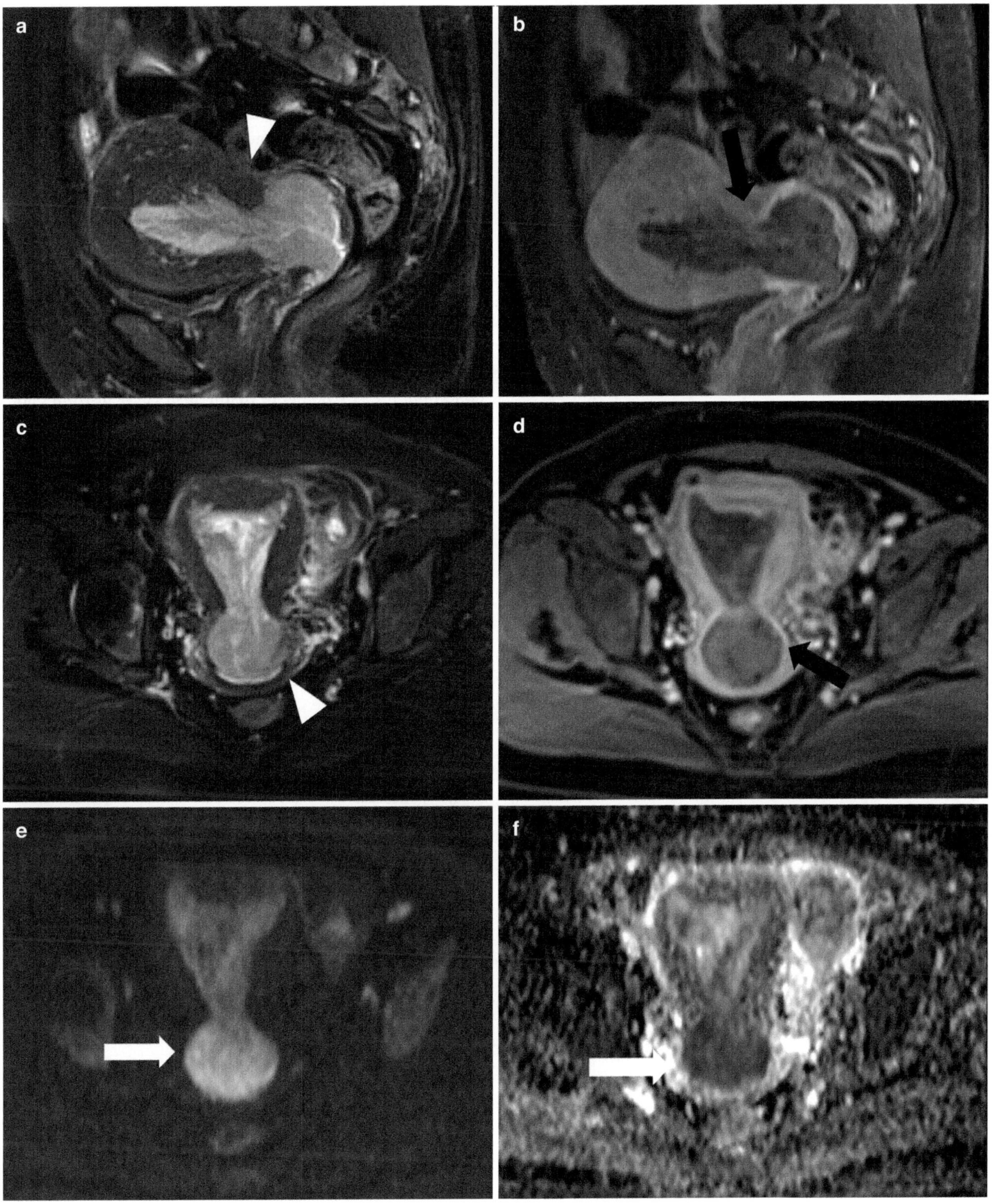

Fig. 9.6 Endometrial carcinoma with cervical involvement in a 52-year-old woman. (**a**, **c**) Sagittal and axial T2WI images with fat suppression showed slightly high signal intensity in uterine cavity and cervical canal (white arrowhead), which was markedly dilated. The junctional zone and the cervical stromal ring were obscure. (**b**, **d**) Sagittal and axial contrast-enhanced T1WI image showed superficial myometrial and cervical stromal invasion without a clear distinction between epithelium and stroma (black arrow). (**e**, **f**) The lesion showed high signal intensity on DWI and low signal intensity on the corresponding ADC map (white arrow). Histopathological results showed endometrial carcinoma of grade I, with deep myometrial infiltration of the lower segment of the uterus. The lesion penetrated down into the 1/3 superficial fibromuscular layer of the cervical canal

short axis of the enlarged lymph node in endometrial cancer, MRI specificity for the detection of metastatic nodes increases up to 97.8%, but with allowable sensitivity of 24–73%. Nodal evaluation by MRI can still be limited because lymph nodes can be of normal size in case of micrometastasis. Using other criteria to assess nodal involvement such as nodal margins and shape in conventional MRI has not yet shown to improve sensitivity of metastatic nodal detection [9–11]. DWI can improve the detection of pelvic metastatic lymph nodes in gynecological malignancies, especially those patients with massive pelvic effusion and lack of pelvic adipose tissue [7]. MRI specificity for the detection of metastatic nodes resulted in better sensitivity (25% vs. 83%) but similar specificity (98% vs. 99%) [12].

9.2 Differential Diagnosis

EC needs to be differentiated from endometrial polyps, submucosal myoma, endometrial hyperplasia or atypical hyperplasia, and some kinds of cervical adenocarcinoma (Fig. 9.7). Endometrial polyps are generally found in women aged between 40–50 years old. On MR imaging, they demonstrate intermediate signal intensity on T1-weighted images and high linear low intensity on T2-weighted images. They sometimes distend the endometrial cavity [13, 14]. There is no high signal intensity on DWI. A submucosal myoma usually manifests as a mass with signal intensity that is iso- to hypointense relative to the normal myometrium on T1WI and hypointense on T2WI and diffusion weighted images. As talk attaching to the myometrium often could be seen on MRI. On DCE-MRI, the signal intensity of the tumor was similar to that of myometrium [15, 16]. Endometrial hyperplasia or atypical hyperplasia usually demonstrated endometrium thickening with signal heterogeneity and hypointense on diffusion weighted images with no myometrial invasion. Contrast-enhanced MR images show a significantly heterogeneous enhancement. It is difficult to determine tumor origin when the primary lesion site is predominantly located in the lower uterine segment and endocervix on MRI. In this condition, the key points of distinguish cervical from endometrial primary cancer mainly are (1) the center of the tumor is located in the cervical canal or the uterine cavity; (2) a longitudinal shape is more frequently observed in EC, while a round or oval shape is more commonly found in cervical cancer [17]; and (3) cervical cancers are hypervascular tumors and usually show earlier enhancement compared to the myometrium, and endometrial cancers are usually hypovascular tumors and do not enhance on the early phase of contrast agent administration [18].

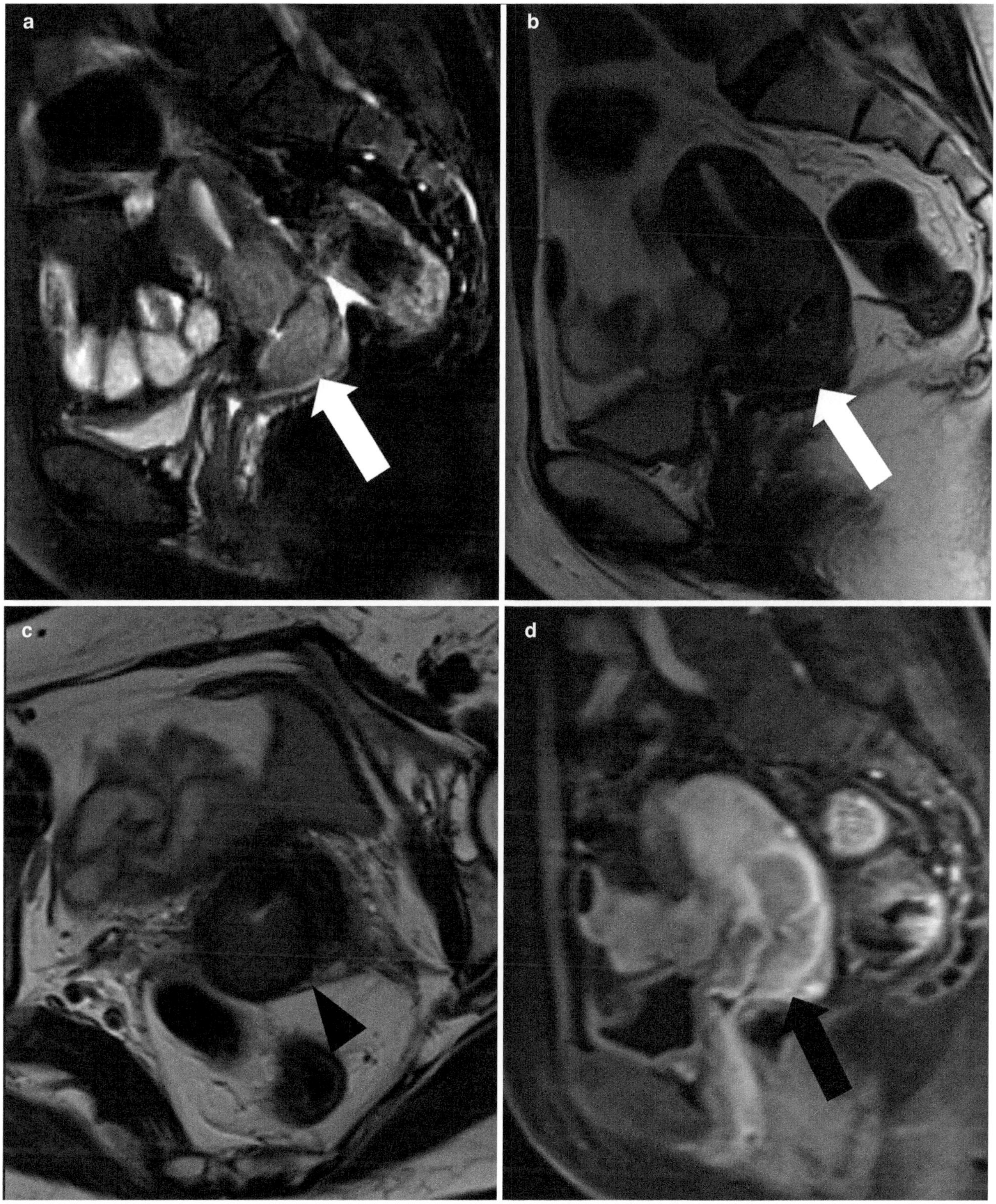

Fig. 9.7 Cervical adenosquamous carcinoma with uterine involvement in a 56-year-old woman. (**a**, **b**) Sagittal T2WI images with and without fat suppression showed moderate hyperintense lesion (white arrow) in the cervix and the lower segment of uterus. (**c**) The small FOV oblique axial T2WI image which is perpendicular to the long axis of cervix showed a moderate hyperintense lesion with no parametrial tissue involved (black arrowhead). (**d**) Sagittal contrast-enhanced T1WI image showed a hypointense lesion (long black arrow) of cervix and uterus. Histopathological results showed infiltrating adenosquamous carcinoma of the cervix. The neoplasm involves the endometrium upward and infiltrated the myometrium of uterus

References

1. Li M, Wu S, Xie Y, et al. Cervical invasion, lymphovascular space invasion, and ovarian metastasis as predictors of lymph node metastasis and poor outcome on stages I to III endometrial cancers: a single-center retrospective study. World J Surg Oncol. 2019;17(1):193–4.
2. Mcalpine JN, Temkin SM, Mackay HJ. Endometrial cancer: not your grandmother's cancer. Cancer. 2016;122(18):2787–98.
3. Rizzo S, Femia M, Buscarino V, et al. Endometrial cancer: an overview of novelties in treatment and related imaging keypoints for local staging. Cancer Imaging. 2018;18(1):45.
4. Lee JH, Dubinsky T, Javitt MC, et al. ACR appropriateness Criteria® pretreatment evaluation and follow-up of endometrial cancer of the uterus. Ultrasound Q. 2011;27(2):139–45.
5. Scoutt LM, McCarthy SM, Flynn SD, et al. Clinical stage I endometrial carcinoma: pitfalls in preoperative assessment with MR imaging. Work in progress. Radiology. 1995;194:567–72.
6. Beets-tanr GH, Lambregts DMJ, Maas M, et al. Magnetic resonance imaging for clinical management of rectal cancer: updated recommendations from the 2016 European Society of Gastrointestinal and Abdominal Radiology (ESGAR) consensus meeting. Eur Radiol. 2018;28(4):1465–75.
7. Andreano A, Rechichi G, Rebora P, et al. MR DWI for preoperative staging of myometrial invasion in EC. Eur Radiol. 2014;24:1327–38.
8. Haldorsen IS, Salvesen HB, et al. What is the best preoperative imaging for endometrium cancer? Curr Oncol Rep. 2016;18:25–9.
9. Bipat S, Glas AS, van der Velden J, et al. Computed tomography and magnetic resonance imaging in staging of uterine cervical carcinoma: a systematic review. Gynecol Oncol. 2003;91:59–66.
10. Rockall AG, Sohaib SA, Harisinghani MG, et al. Diagnostic performance of nanoparticle-enhanced magnetic resonance imaging in the diagnosis of lymph node metastases in patients with endometrial and cervical cancer. J Clin Oncol. 2004;23:2813–21.
11. Choi HJ, Kim SH, Seo S-S, et al. MRI for pretreatment lymph node staging in uterine cervical cancer. Am J Roentgenol. 2006;187:W538–43.
12. Lin G, Ho KC, Wang JJ, et al. Detection of lymph node metastasis in cervical and uterine cancers by diffusion-weighted magnetic resonance imaging at 3T. J Magn Reson Imaging. 2008;28:128–35.
13. Takeuchi M, Matsuzaki K, Uehara H, Yoshida S, Nishitani H, Shimazu H. Pathologies of the uterine endometrial cavity: usual and unusual manifestations and pitfalls on magnetic resonance imaging. Eur Radiol. 2005;15:2244–55.
14. Grasel RP, Outwater EK, Siegelman ES, et al. Endometrial polyps: MR imaging features and distinction from endometrial carcinoma. Radiology. 2000;214:47–52.
15. Tamai K, Koyama T, Saga T, Morisawa N, Fujimoto K, Mikami Y, Togashi K. Unusual appearances of uterine leiomyomas: the utility of diffusion-weighted MR imaging for differentiating uterine sarcomas from benign leiomyomas. Eur Radiol. 2008;18:723–30.
16. Ueda H, Togashi K, Konishi I, et al. Unusual appearances of uterine leiomyomas: MR imaging findings and their histopathologic backgrounds. Radiographics. 1999;19:S131–45.
17. Lin YC, Lin G, Chen YR, Yen TC, Wang CC, Ng KK. Role of magnetic resonance imaging and apparent diffusion coefficient at 3T in distinguishing between adenocarcinoma of the uterine cervix and endometrium. Chang Gung Med J. 2011;34:93–100.
18. He H, Bhosale P, Wei W, et al. MRI is highly specific in determining primary cervical versus endometrial cancer when biopsy results are inconclusive. Clin Radiol. 2013;68:1107–13.

Part III

Vulvar and Vaginal Lesions

10 Vulvar and Vaginal Cancer

Xuan Yin

10.1 Clinical History

The patient was a 66-year-old woman, who had pruritus of vulva for nearly 3 years and found vulvar vegetations for more than 1 year. The patient has menopausal for 15 years, no irregular vaginal bleeding after menopause, and vulvar itching for 3 years. A previous vulva biopsy revealed papillary hyperplasia of squamous epithelium with hyperkeratosis in the skin tissue of the right labia minora. The pain of vulvar itching had become worse.

Gynecological examination showed white induration with a diameter of 2 cm on the right inner side of labia majora, with ulceration and tenderness on the surface. The vaginal and urethral orifices were not involved.

MRI: Abnormal mass was observed in the right vulva, with a size of about 1.5 cm × 1.0 cm, and the boundary was not smooth. Isointense signal on T1WI (Fig. 10.1), slightly high signal intensity on T2WI (Fig. 10.2), significantly enhanced after contrast enhancement (Figs. 10.3 and 10.4). Subcutaneous soft tissue edema was observed (Fig. 10.2).

Fourteen days after admission, extensive vulvar resection and bilateral inguinal lymph node dissection under laparoscopy were performed. The labia majora and minora, clitoris, vaginal vestibule, and perineum were removed.

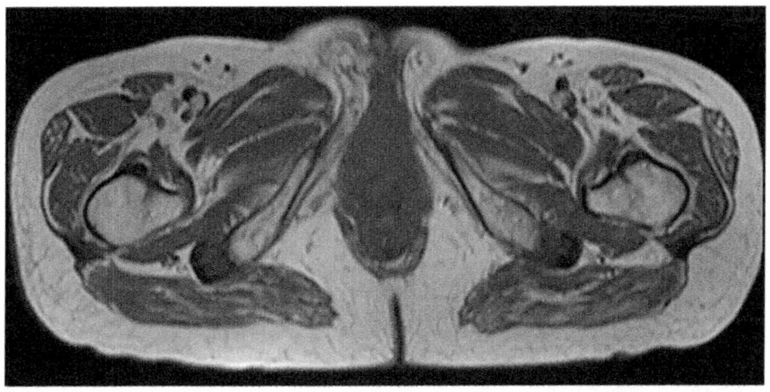

Fig. 10.1 Axial T1WI demonstrated lobulated mass with intermediate signal in the right pudendal area

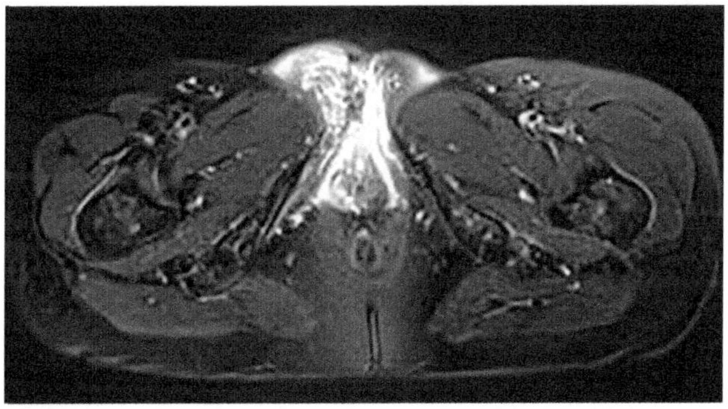

Fig. 10.2 The mass showed slightly high signal intensity on axial T2WI. Peripheral subcutaneous soft tissue edema was seen

X. Yin (✉)
Department of Radiology, Obstetrics and Gynecology Hospital, Fudan University, Shanghai, People's Republic of China

G. Zhang (ed.), *MRI of Gynaecological Diseases*, https://doi.org/10.1007/978-981-99-3644-1_10

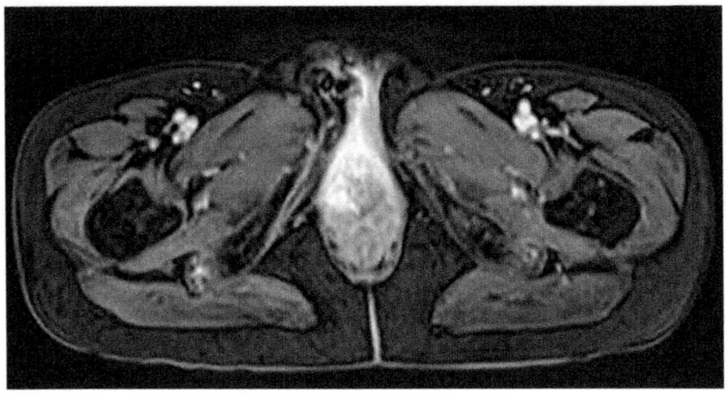

Fig. 10.3 Contrast-enhanced images showed solid lesion with obvious enhancement

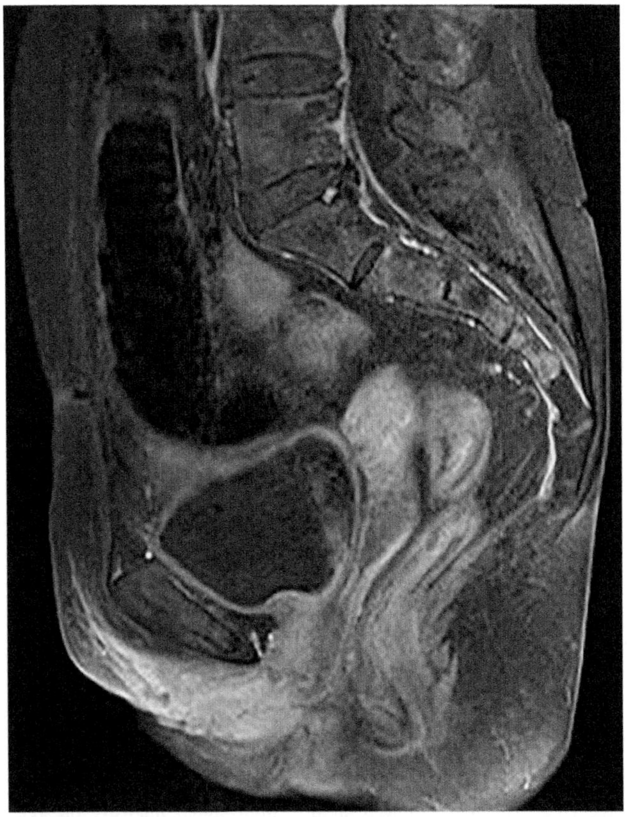

Fig. 10.4 Contrast-enhanced images showed solid lesion with obvious enhancement

Postoperative pathological result: highly differentiated squamous cell carcinoma (vulvar neoplasm).

10.2 Imaging Analysis

Vulvar squamous cell carcinoma is an uncommon malignant tumor that accounts for 5–8% of gynecologic malignancies [1]. It occurs mostly in women aged 65–70 years old. Patients with vulvar cancer have no obvious specific manifestations. It is usually found with a defect in the vulva. Onset time is more than 6 months.

Based on association with human papillomavirus (HPV), squamous cell carcinoma (SCC) includes two subtypes: HPV-associated and HPV-independent. Approximately 50% of squamous cell carcinomas occur in premenopausal women and are often associated with HPV, which leads to vulvar intraepithelial neoplasia. In approximately 40% of cases, occurring in women aged 70–80 years old, it is usually not associated with HPV but is associated with one or more causes such as differentiated vulvar intraepithelial neoplasia, mossy sclerosis, and squamous cell hyperplasia. HPV-independent vulvar SCC has a worse prognosis and a higher recurrence rate and is more likely to progress rapidly.

HPV has been implicated as a causative agent. As more young people become infected with HPV, particularly subtypes 16 and 18, the incidence of vulvar cancer is increasing.

The most common site of vulvar cancer is the labium (80%), followed by the clitoris (10%) and perineum (10%). Most of them are unilateral, a few are bilateral, and occasionally occur in multiple parts. Disease area has white, dark brown, and red to wait for fester, defect, and skin thickening change more [2]. The main type was exogenous and local infiltration. Most are diagnosed with pruritus, pain, burning, and dyspareunia. Vulvar cancer could be detected early because it is on the surface of the body. However, because it is easy to confuse with prodromal disease and ignore some common symptoms, there are still a considerable number of cases diagnosed until the middle and late stage of the disease [3, 4]. It brings some difficulty to the treatment. Vulvar cancer often arises from preexisting skin conditions [1, 5].

Lymphatic metastasis is the main cause of vulvar carcinoma. Many studies have shown that an important prognostic factor for vulvar cancer is lymph node status.

Detailed examination of preoperative MRI plays a crucial role in subsequent treatment design, and MRI can assess subtle involvement of adjacent organs and pelvic lateral walls.

Imaging findings show a solid mass of vulva with low signal intensity on T1WI and intermediate to high signal intensity on T2WI and significantly enhanced after contrast enhancement. Commonly vulvar carcinomas involve the labia majora or labia minora (70%), mons pubis, and perineum. Imaging is used to detect shallow or deep inguinal lymph nodes and pelvic lymph node involvement.

The lesion size of vulvar cancer is not an independent prognostic factor, while the status of inguinal lymph nodes is closely related to the prognosis of patients. Vulvar cancer spreads mainly through the lymphatic system to superficial and deep inguinal lymph nodes, followed by pelvic lymph node involvement. Pelvic lymph node metastases are considered distant metastases. In the absence of ipsilateral inguinal lymph node involvement, pelvic lymph nodes are rarely involved. MRI findings of lymph node metastases from vulvar carcinoma include lymph node short axis greater than

1 cm, irregular contour, necrosis, loss of fatty hilum, short axis/long axis ratio of 0.75 or greater, and lymph node signal intensity similar to that of the primary tumor [6].

In advanced stage, vulvar cancer masses can invade the urethra, vagina, bladder, and rectum, or be fixed in the pelvis, or even distant metastasis to the liver.

10.3 Differential Diagnosis

It is mainly differentiated from other vulvar tumors. Bartholin cyst and invasive angiomyxoma are common. Bartholin cyst is mostly located on the outer lower part of the vaginal wall. It appears as a well-defined cystic mass. There is no obvious enhancement after contrast enhancement. The invasive angiomyxoma originates from the mesenchymal tissue and tends to occur in the perineum and pelvic cavity of menopausal women. It is a cystic or multilocular mass that moves to the surrounding organs without direct invasion.

References

1. Rouzier R, Haddad B, Atallah D, et al. Surgery for vulvar cancer. Clin Obstet Gynecol. 2005;48(4):869–78.
2. Fuh KC, Berek JS. Current management of vulvar cancer. Hematol Oncol Clin North Am. 2012;26(1):45–62.
3. Fonseca-Moutinho JA. Recurrent vulvar cancer. Clin Obstet Gynecol. 2005;48(4):879–83.
4. Platz CE, Benda JA. Female genital tract cancer. Cancer. 1995;75(1 Suppl):270–94.
5. van der Velden J, van Lindert AC, Gimbrere CH, et al. Epidemiologic data on vulvar cancer: comparison of hospital with population based data. Gynecol Oncol. 1996;62(3):379–83.
6. Hacker NF. Revised FIGO staging for carcinoma of the vulva. Int J Gynaecol Obstet. 2009;105:105–6.

11 Leiomyoma of Vulva

Xuan Yin

11.1 Clinical History

A 59-year-old female patient had a 1.5 cm diameter vulvar mass 2 years ago without any medical history. The mass caused discomfort at the perineum in sitting and walking. There was no erythema, swelling, itching, or pain. She went to our outpatient department 1 month ago. Vulvar examination showed a right labia majora firm multilobulate pedicled mass with a diameter of 6 cm, soft and without tenderness.

MRI: Abnormal mass was observed in the right labia majora with a clear boundary. The size of the tumor was about 6.7 cm × 2.7 cm × 3.3 cm. The intermediate signal was observed on T1WI (Fig. 11.1), and intermediate to high signal intensity was observed on T2WI (Fig. 11.2). Significant homogeneous enhancement was observed after contrast enhancement (Figs. 11.3 and 11.4).

She underwent surgical excision of the mass 6 days after admission. The mass was about 7 cm in size, soft, and well-defined. The mass passed up to the pubic bone and down to the area around the anus. Postoperative pathology: (vulvar mass) leiomyoma. Immunohistochemical results: AE1/AE3 (−), Caldesmon (+), SMA (Blood vessel walls +), Desmin (+), Myogenin (−), MyoD1 (−), S-100 (+), CD34 (+), and Ki-67 (1%+).

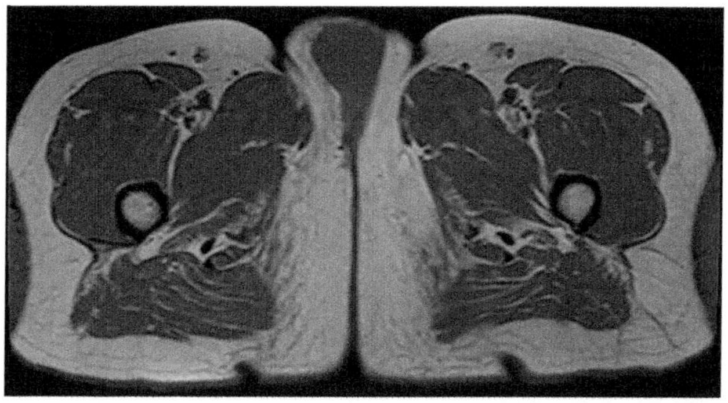

Fig. 11.1 Axial T1-weighted image: on the right labia majora, there was an intermediate signal mass with a clear boundary

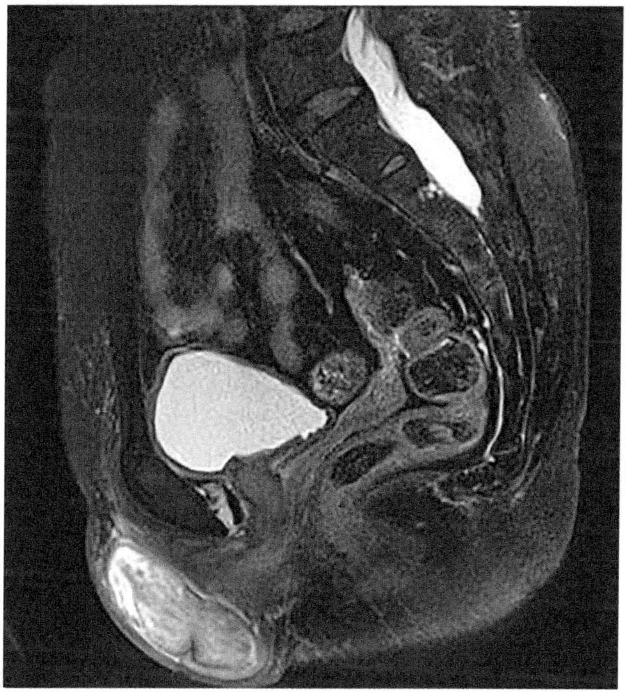

Fig. 11.2 Axial T2-weighted image: intermediate to high signal intensity was observed on T2WI with the visible capsule

X. Yin (✉)
Department of Radiology, Obstetrics and Gynecology Hospital, Fudan University, Shanghai, People's Republic of China

G. Zhang (ed.), *MRI of Gynaecological Diseases*, https://doi.org/10.1007/978-981-99-3644-1_11

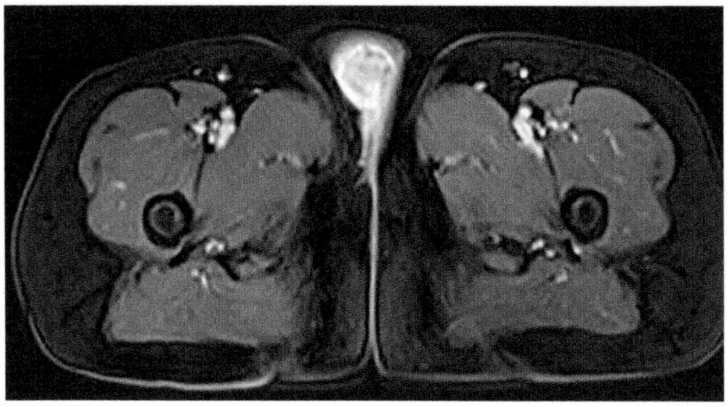

Fig. 11.3 Axial and sagittal contrast-enhanced fat-suppressed T1-weighted images: the lesion showed significant homogeneous enhancement and clear boundary after contrast enhancement

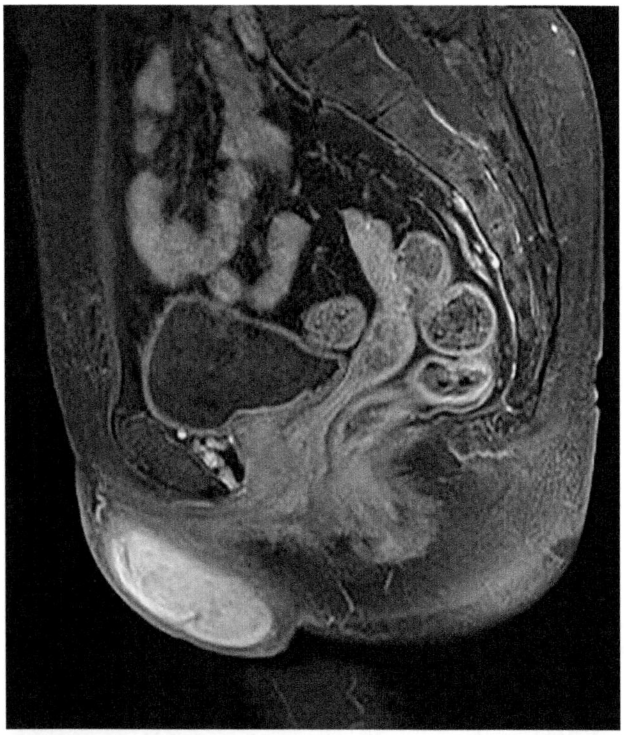

Fig. 11.4 Axial and sagittal contrast-enhanced fat-suppressed T1-weighted images: the lesion showed significant homogeneous enhancement and clear boundary after contrast enhancement

11.2 Imaging Analysis

Vulvar leiomyomas are developed from the vascular smooth muscle of the vulva, the erectile tissue, or the smooth muscle of the teres ligament. It is a rare benign tumor made up of smooth muscle cells [1]. Its etiology is poorly understood, but estrogens and progesterone are likely involved. Immunohistochemical findings reveal estrogen and/or progesterone receptors. It can occur at all ages, more often seen in young women.

Clinical presentation varies, generally asymptomatic. The main manifestation is local painless vulvar mass. Sometimes there are symptoms of pain, itching, and erythema. If the tumor is too large, the patient can feel uncomfortable at the perineum in sitting and walking and even affect movement. If the mass is close to the urethral opening, it can lead to dysuria, frequent urination, and other symptoms [2, 3].

The common location is the Bartholin gland region, also seen in the labia majora, labia minora, and clitoris. Physical examination may reveal a mass located under the labia or labial frenulum. Generally, the tumor is a single well-circumscribed firm mass with broad base and partial mobility. Occasionally, palpation also reveals a peduncle in a superficial mass or simply a swelling in a deeper mass. The lesions are spherical, lobulated, or dumbbell-shaped. Tumors vary in size and texture depending on the amount of fibrous tissue and the presence or absence of deformation. The microscopic appearance on pathological examination is similar to that of uterine fibroids. Surgical monobloc excision of the mass is the main treatment. There are few recurrences with a good prognosis. Long-term follow-up of all cases is advisable [4].

On MRI shows a vulvar mass with clear and smooth boundaries. Hypointense signal on T1WI and isointense signal on T2WI mimicking that of smooth muscle. The mass is significantly homogeneously enhanced after contrast enhancement [5].

Vulvar leiomyoma should be alert to the possibility of malignant transformation if the following factors exist: (1) The tumor diameter is greater than 5 cm. (2) The tumor is ill-defined. (3) Mitotic phase is >5 high magnification fields. (4) The presence of excess cells indicates active hyperplasia with the possibility of leiomyosarcoma. Therefore, attention should be paid to inguinal lymph nodes in preoperative imaging.

11.3 Differential Diagnosis

It needs to be differentiated from other vulvar masses, such as Bartholin's gland cysts and aggressive angiomyxoma (AAM). The vulva Bartholin's gland cysts are cystic masses with well-defined boundaries and no obvious enhancement after contrast enhancement. AAM usually occurs in patients of reproductive age. AAM has an isointense signal on T1-weighted images and higher signal intensity on T2-weighted images because there is loose or maybe myxoid stroma in it.

References

1. Kurdi S, Arafat AS, Almegbel M, Aladham M. Leiomyoma of the vulva: a diagnostic challenge case report. Case Rep Obstet Gynecol. 2016;2016:8780764.
2. Ziouziou I, Bennani H, Zouaidia F, El Ghaouti M, Haddan A, Mahassini N, Karmouni T, El Khader K, Koutani A, Iben Attya Andaloussi A. Retroperitoneal leiomyoma: a case report. Prog Urol. 2014;24(5):262–5.
3. Zhao T, Liu X, Lu Y. Myxoid epithelial leiomyoma of the vulva: a case report and literature review. Case Rep Obstet Gynecol. 2015;2015:894830. Epub 2015 Jun 22.
4. Levy RA, Winham WM, Bryant CS, et al. Smooth muscle neoplasms of the vulva masquerading as Bartholin gland duct cysts. Proc (Bayl Univ Med Cent). 2014;27:25–7.
5. Owen C, Armstrong AY. Clinical management of leiomyoma. Obstet Gynecol Clin N Am. 2015;42:67–85.

Part IV

Benign Tumors of the Ovary

12 Ovarian Serous Cystadenoma

Mengwei Zhang

12.1 Clinical History

Female patient, 67 years old, had experienced menopausal 14 years ago, lower abdominal distention for 1 month, and no abnormal vaginal bleeding and discharge. Ultrasound examination revealed a hypoechoic space-occupying lesion in the pelvic cavity, and she underwent laparotomy of left ovarian cystectomy.

Postoperative pathological result: serous cystadenoma of the left ovary.

12.2 Imaging Analysis

Ovarian serous cystadenoma originates from ovarian surface epithelium and differentiates into oviductal epithelium, accounting for 25% of benign ovarian tumors [1, 2]. It can occur from childhood to postmenopause, mostly at reproductive age, with an average age of 36 years old. Most patients have no special symptoms, and when the tumor is large, there may be lower abdominal distension, abdominal pain, or compression symptoms, such as frequent urination and urgency. In a small number of cases, symptoms of acute abdomen, including abdominal pain, peritoneal irritation and fever, are caused by torsion of the tumor pedicle or infection, hemorrhage, and necrosis. On clinical physical examination, abdominal distension is common, and a smooth, mobile cystic mass may be palpable in the parauterine area.

The bilateral incidence rate of ovarian serous cystadenoma is about 12–23%, mostly less than 10 cm in diameter and mostly round-like [2, 3]. Unilocular is common, while bilocular and multilocular are rare. The cystic fluid has a thin, watery, and clear fluid appearance. On pre-contrast CT, it has low density near water, and about 15% of the tumor cyst wall showed sand-like calcification [1, 3]. On MRI, it shows homogeneous low signal intensity on T1WI (Fig. 12.1), high signal intensity on T2WI (Figs. 12.2 and 12.3), and low signal intensity on DWI. The cyst wall is thin and uniform, with a few small papillary projections, and enhanced sequence shows clearer outline of cyst wall (Fig. 12.4) [4, 5].

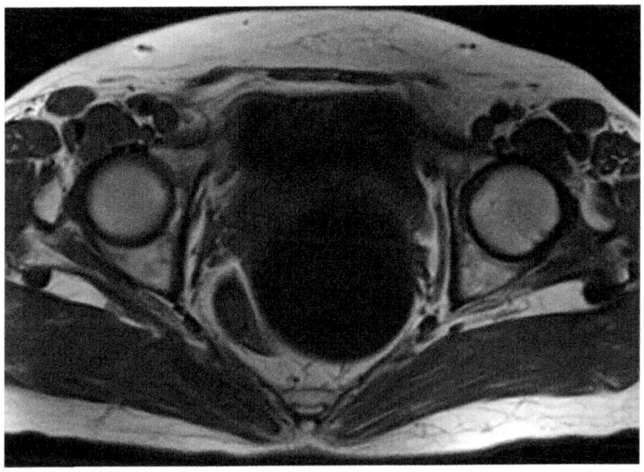

Fig. 12.1 Round-like abnormal signal in the pelvic cavity showing homogeneous hypointense on axial T1WI

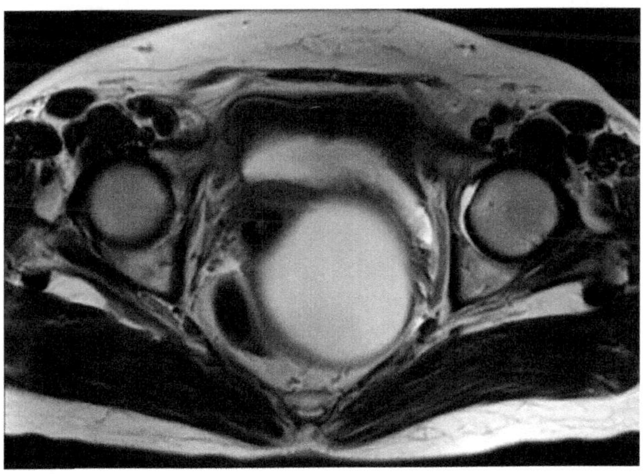

Fig. 12.2 The cystic mass showed homogeneous watery hyperintensity on axial T2WI

M. Zhang (✉)
Department of Radiology, Obstetrics and Gynecology Hospital, Fudan University, Shanghai, People's Republic of China

G. Zhang (ed.), *MRI of Gynaecological Diseases*, https://doi.org/10.1007/978-981-99-3644-1_12

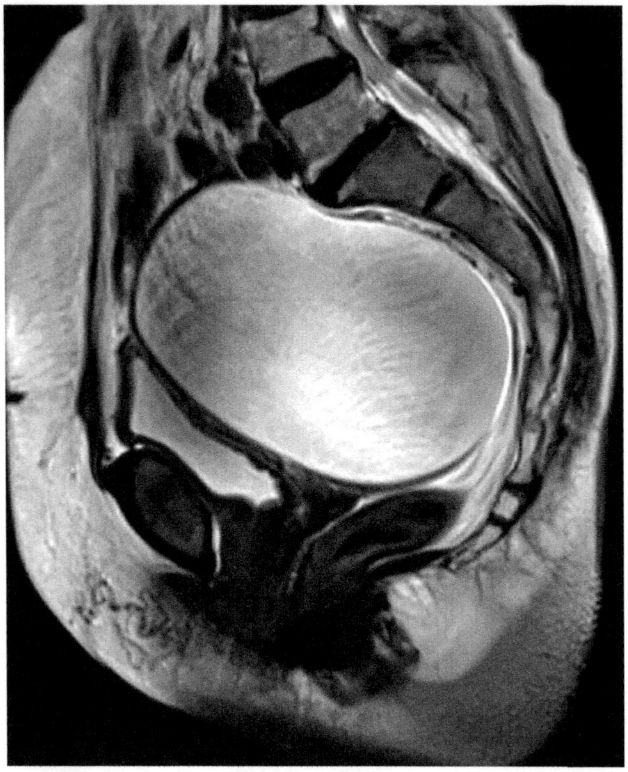

Fig. 12.3 The cystic mass was round-like on sagittal T2WI, with homogeneous watery hyperintensity inside. Bladder showed compression

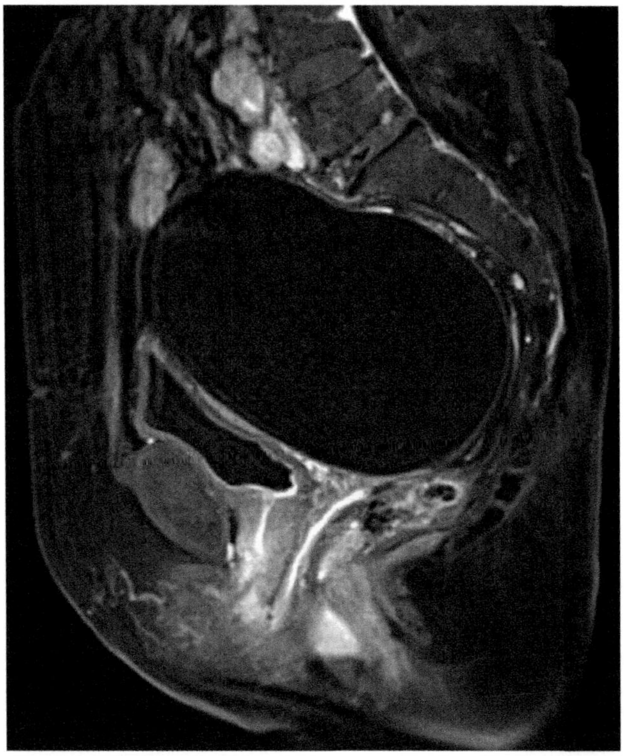

Fig. 12.4 The cyst wall of the mass enhanced on sagittal contrast-enhanced sequence, the wall was uniform and thin

12.3 Differential Diagnosis

It is mainly differentiated from pelvic cystic tumor-like lesions, including mesosalpinx cyst, ovarian physiological cyst, pelvic encapsulated effusion, pelvic lymphatic cyst, and neurogenic bladder. The wall of mesosalpinx cyst is thin, and cyst fluid has a watery density without obvious enhancement. Ovarian physiological cysts are small in size, and a few large physiological cysts (nearly 5 cm) are difficult to differentiate from serous cystadenoma by imaging methods. When suspected of physiological cysts, short-term follow-up observation is feasible; physiological cysts can be reduced or disappeared. Pelvic encapsulated effusion is irregular in shape, with indentation on the margin. Pelvic lymphatic cyst is located in the inner wall of pelvic cavity, that is small in size, and is prone to compression deformation. Most of them have a clinical history of pelvic surgery. The key to distinguish from neurogenic bladder is to find the bladder, which is significantly reduced in volume after urinary catheterization.

References

1. Buy JN, Ghossain MA, Sciot C, et al. Epithelial tumors of the ovary: CT findings and correlation with US. Radiology. 1991;178:811–8.
2. Imaoka I, Wada A, Kaji Y, et al. Developing an MRI strategy for diagnosis of ovarian masses. Radiographics. 2006;26:1421–48.
3. Fukuda T, Ikeuchi M, Hashimoto H, et al. Computed tomography of ovarian masses. J Comput Assist Tomogr. 1986;10(6):990–6.
4. Bazot M, Daraï E, Nassar-Slaba J, et al. Value of magnetic resonance imaging for the diagnosis of ovarian tumors: a review. J Comput Assist Tomogr. 2008;3:712–23.
5. Stevens SK, Hricak H, Stern JL, et al. Ovarian lesions: detection and characterization with gadolinium-enhanced MRI at 1.5T. Radiology. 1991;181:481–8.

13 Ovarian Mucinous Cystadenoma

Mengwei Zhang

13.1 Clinical History

Female patient, 62 years old, had menopause 9 years ago, presented with a pelvic mass of more than 1 month on health checkup. One month ago, she felt a movable abdominal mass, and ultrasound examination showed anechoic area in the pelvic cavity, 133 mm × 87 mm × 101 mm in size, with internal septation. Ultrasonography diagnosis: pelvic multilocular cystic mass with possible ovarian origin. CA125: 10.28 U/mL, CA199: 12.24 U/mL. Physical examination on admission: a mass of the size of about 4 months pregnancy can be palpable above the uterus, with hard texture, no obvious boundary, and good mobility.

She underwent laparoscopic total hysterectomy and bilateral salpingo-oophorectomy. Intraoperative findings: the uterus was in the anterior position, with a size of 4 cm × 4 cm × 3 cm and regular shape. The left ovary presented with cystic enlargement, with a size of 13 cm × 13 cm × 12 cm, the surface was smooth, and the appearance of the left fallopian tube was normal. No abnormality was found in the right ovary and fallopian tube. No abnormality was found in the bladder and rectouterine pouch.

Postoperative pathological result: (1) left ovarian multilocular mucinous cystadenoma, with local mucinous epithelial hyperplasia; (2) uterine leiomyoma with calcification.

13.2 Imaging Analysis

Mucinous tumor is the second most common ovarian tumor, second only to serous tumor. On the basis of clinical and pathological characteristics, mucinous tumors are classified as benign, borderline, and malignant, of which 80% are benign [1, 2]. It is more common in women between 30 and 50 years old. Compared with serous cystadenoma, only 2–5% are bilateral, and most of the lesions are unilateral. Pathologically, the tumor is often huge, and the cyst can fill the entire abdominal cavity. The capsule is smooth, and it is often divided into multilocular compartments. Numerous daughter chambers are gathered into a honeycomb shape, and the cyst cavity is filled with milky white viscous secretions or thin and translucent mucus. Microscopically, the epithelium of the cystic wall is high columnar, the apex of the cell contains mucous vacuoles, and the nucleus is at the bottom of the cell [3].

Typical ovarian mucinous cystadenoma is a huge multilocular cystic mass with thin cystic wall and septation (≤3 mm). The cystic fluid contains gelatinous substances or liquids of various viscosity, so MRI signals are complex and variable, showing high, low, equal signals on T2WI, and different signals are in adjacent chambers, showing low, equal, and high signals on T1WI due to different protein content. There is no obvious solid component in it [4]. A few mucinous cystadenomas present as unilocular cystic, and the signals are like that of water. This case was multilocular cystic, with thin cystic wall, and the signals of daughter chambers were homogeneous. It showed low signal on T1WI (Figs. 13.1–13.2) and high signal on T2WI (Figs. 13.3–13.6); after contrast enhancement, the cystic fluid was not enhanced (Figs. 13.7–13.9), which was consistent with the typical manifestations of mucinous cystadenoma, so the diagnosis was not difficult.

Mucinous cystadenoma should be distinguished from borderline mucinous cystadenoma, mucinous adenocarcinoma, and multilocular cystic serous tumors. Mucinous adenocarcinoma may be manifested as multilocular cystic mass with more solid components, and significantly irregular cystic wall and septation, which is not difficult to distinguish from mucinous cystadenoma. Borderline mucinous tumors have no interstitial infiltration and few solid components. Pathological and imaging manifestations are between benign and malignant tumors, but they have potential malignancy, can be implanted and metastasized, and are prone to recurrence. The treatment is different from that of benign tumors,

M. Zhang (✉)
Department of Radiology, Obstetrics and Gynecology Hospital, Fudan University, Shanghai, People's Republic of China

G. Zhang (ed.), *MRI of Gynaecological Diseases*, https://doi.org/10.1007/978-981-99-3644-1_13

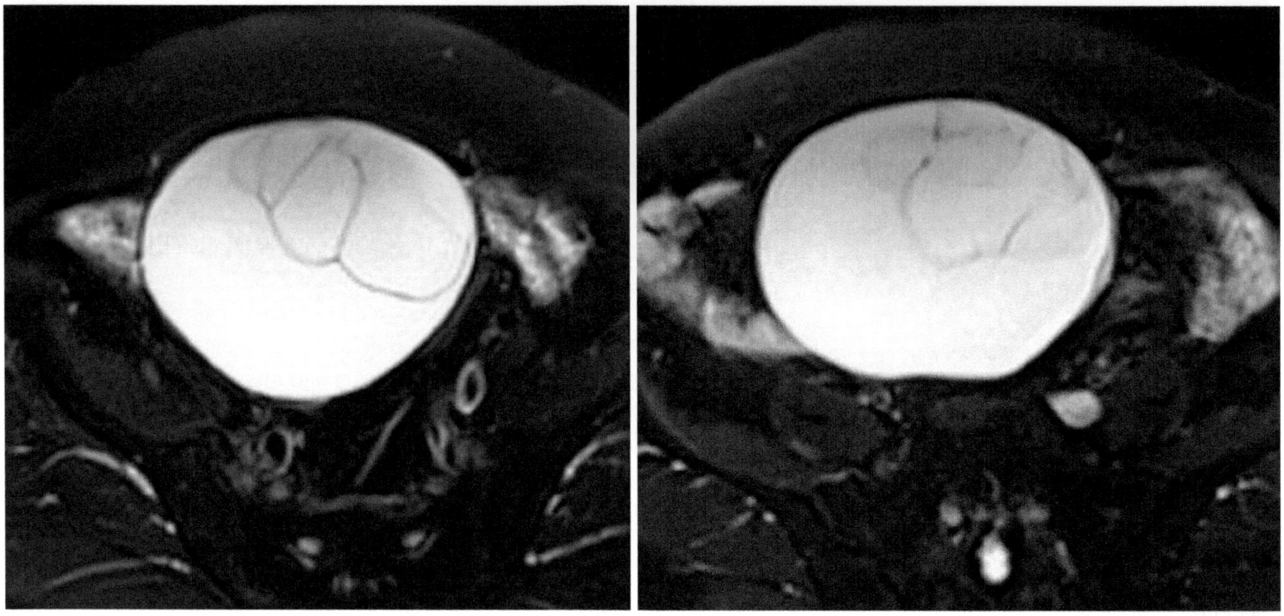

Figs. 13.1–13.2 Axial T1WI: the cystic fluid showed low signal on T1WI

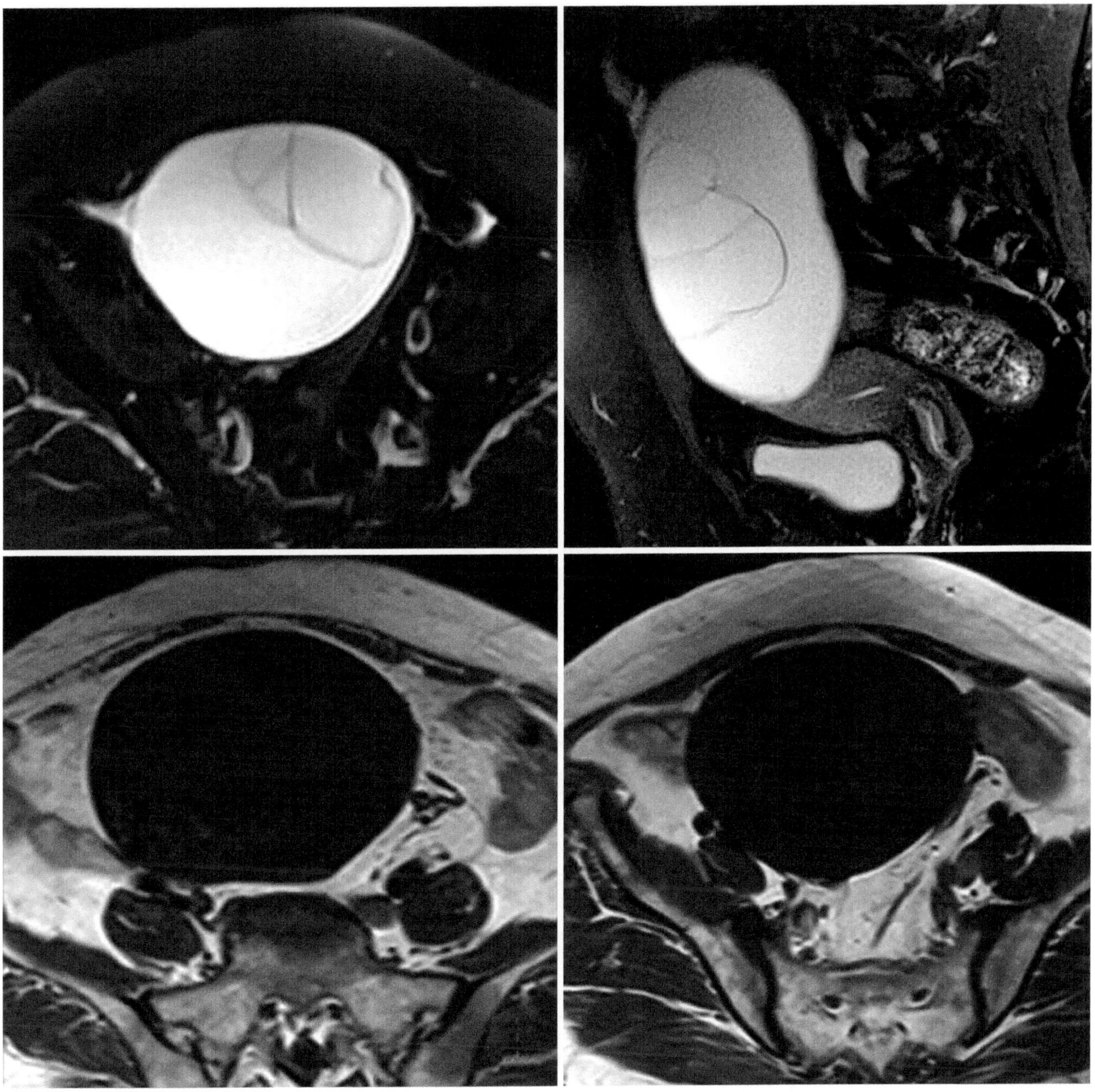

Figs. 13.3–13.6 Axial and sagittal fat-suppressed T2WI: a multilocular cystic space-occupying lesion was found above the uterus and ovary in shape, with regular boundaries, and multiple thin septa were visible inside. The cystic fluid showed high signal on T2WI

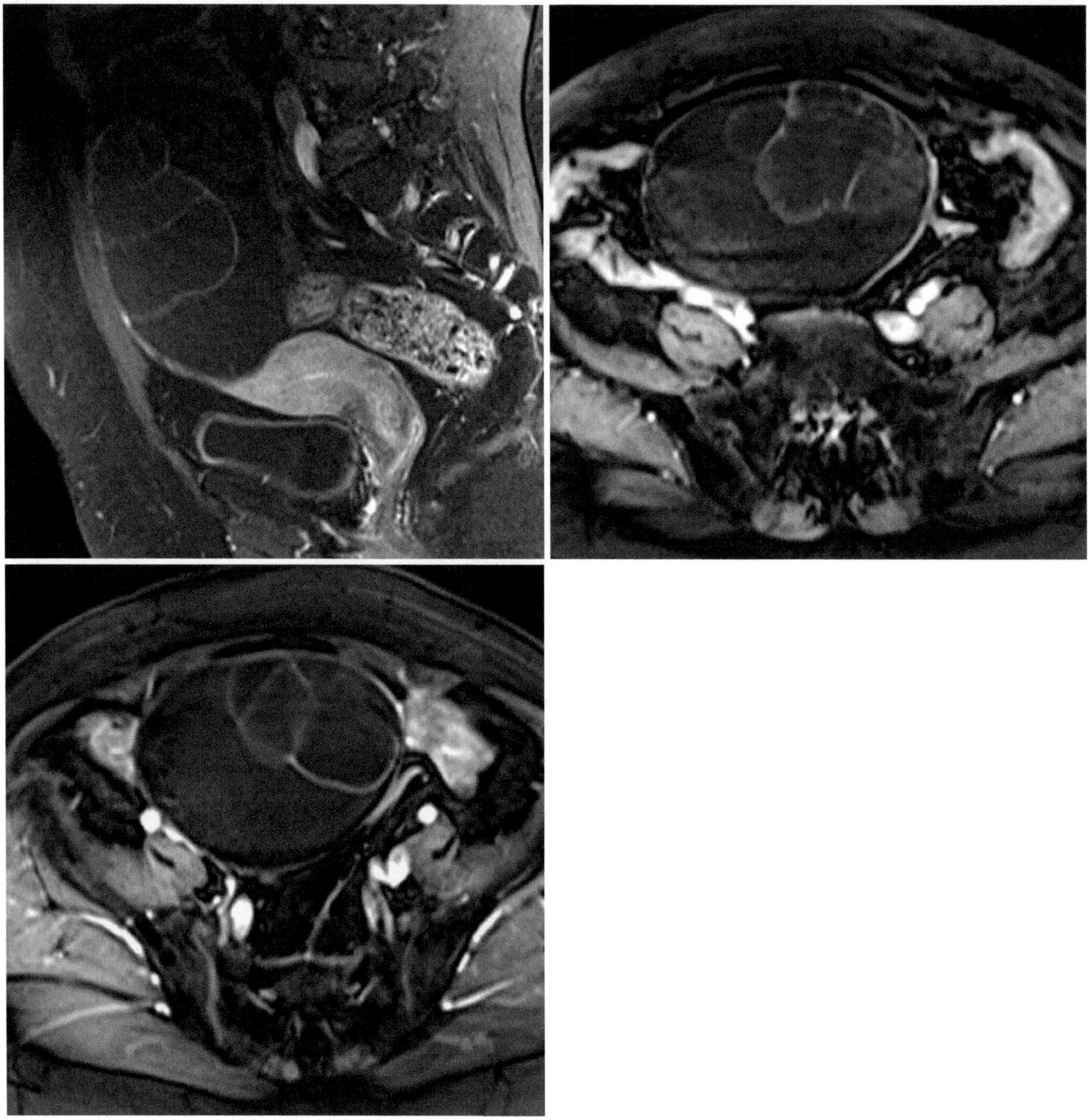

Figs. 13.7–13.9 Axial and sagittal contrast-enhanced T1WI: after contrast enhancement, the septa and capsule were enhanced, and no significant enhancement was shown in cystic fluid

so it is of great significance to distinguish the two. Shuhui et al. [5] analyzed and compared the MRI features of 23 benign and 19 borderline mucinous tumors, and the results showed that honeycomb loculi, high signal cystic fluid on T1WI, low signal cystic fluid on T2WI, irregular thickening of cystic wall or septa (≥5 mm), vegetations, or papillary projections (≥5 mm) tended to be borderline mucinous tumors. However, the signal of the cystic fluid was more homogeneous, and the cystic wall and septa were thinner (<5 mm) tended to be mucinous cystadenoma. Serous cystadenoma can also be manifested as multilocular cystic, cystic fluid signal is relatively homogeneous, but papillary mural nodules are less common. Therefore, when a multilocular cystic mass is present in the pelvic cavity, the cystic wall, septation, loculi, and cystic fluid signal should be carefully evaluated for identification.

References

1. Buy JN. Gynecological imaging. Springer Berlin Heidelberg; 2013.
2. Jung SE, Lee JM, Rha SE, et al. CT and MR imaging of ovarian tumors with emphasis on differential diagnosis. Radiographics. 2002;22:1305–25.
3. Luyken C, Blümcke I, Fimmers R, et al. Supratentorial gangliogliomas: histopathologic grading and tumor recurrence in 184 patients with a median follow-up of 8 years. Cancer. 2004;101(1):146–55.
4. Imaoka I, Wada A, Kaji Y, et al. Developing an MR imaging strategy for diagnosis of ovarian masses. Radiographics. 2006;26:1431–48.
5. Shuhui Z, Jinwei Q, Guofu Z, et al. MRI features in differentiation borderline from benign mucinous ovarian cystadenoma. Chin J Radiol. 2012;46(4):327–31.

14 Ovarian Transitional Cell Tumor

Mengwei Zhang

14.1 Clinical History

Female patient, 62 years old, had experienced menopause for 12 years ago, lower abdominal distention for 2 month, and no abnormal vaginal bleeding and discharge. Gynecological examination revealed a pelvic mass. Serum CA125: 125.24 U/mL. She underwent laparotomy of total hysterectomy, bilateral salpingo-oophorectomy, greater omentum resection, and debulking surgery.

Postoperative pathological result: left ovarian transitional cell tumor, grade III

14.2 Imaging Analysis

Ovarian transitional cell tumor, also known as Brenner tumor, originates from the superficial epithelium of ovary. It is a rare tumor, accounting for about 2% of all ovarian tumors, 99% is benign, and borderline and malignant are rare. Most tumors are small, ranging from 0.5 to 2 cm, and a few can reach 10 cm. Benign ovarian transitional cell tumor is unilocular or multilocular cystic and difficult to differentiate from serous or mucinous cystadenoma [1]. Borderline transitional cell tumor is mostly cystic tumor with inner wall or septa papillary projections. Malignant transitional cell tumor is mostly solid, sometimes with cystic cavities, and presents with solid and cystic. Microscopically, there are scattered transitional cell nests in the dense fibrous stroma [2]. In 15–30% cases of transitional cell tumor, both ovaries are accompanied by another tumor, and the most common tumors are cystadenoma, teratoma or cystadenocarcinoma [3]. 23% are complicated with other gynecological malignancies. Patients aged 40–70 years old are asymptomatic, but a few have lower abdominal pain or abnormal vaginal bleeding, and a hard mass may be palpable during gynecological examination. Most tumors are solid or solid and cystic, and few are cystic. When solid and cystic (Fig. 14.1), the cystic part was unilocular or multilocular; with clear boundary, the solid part of tumor has uniform density. After contrast enhancement, the tumor shows homogeneous mild to moderate enhancement, without hemorrhage or necrotic areas (Fig. 14.2). The characteristic CT manifestations are extensive amorphous calcification within the solid part of tumor, which is seen in 54% of the cases, mainly as a result of degenerative changes in the stroma. Therefore, it is commonly differentiated from other solid tumors [4–6]. Ovarian transitional cell tumor is characterized by hypointense in the solid region on T2WI (Fig. 14.3), similar to fibroma, but signal intensity of the former is homogeneous, while the latter is often accompanied by edema and cystic change [6].

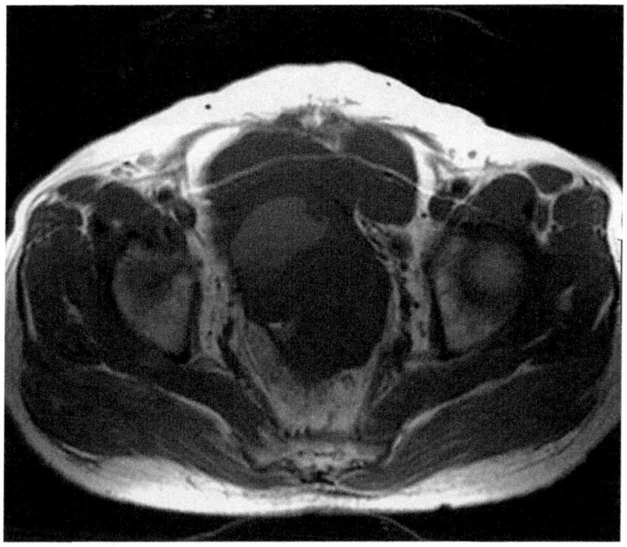

Fig. 14.1 Lobulated abnormal signal in the pelvic cavity, low signal intensity on T1WI, slightly higher signal locally

M. Zhang (✉)
Department of Radiology, Obstetrics and Gynecology Hospital, Fudan University, Shanghai, People's Republic of China

G. Zhang (ed.), *MRI of Gynaecological Diseases*, https://doi.org/10.1007/978-981-99-3644-1_14

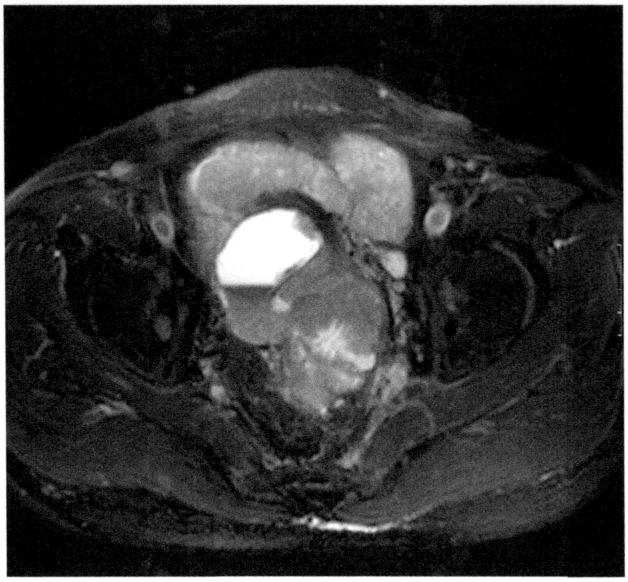

Fig. 14.2 After contrast enhancement, the tumor was moderately enhanced, and there was no enhancement in the cystic area

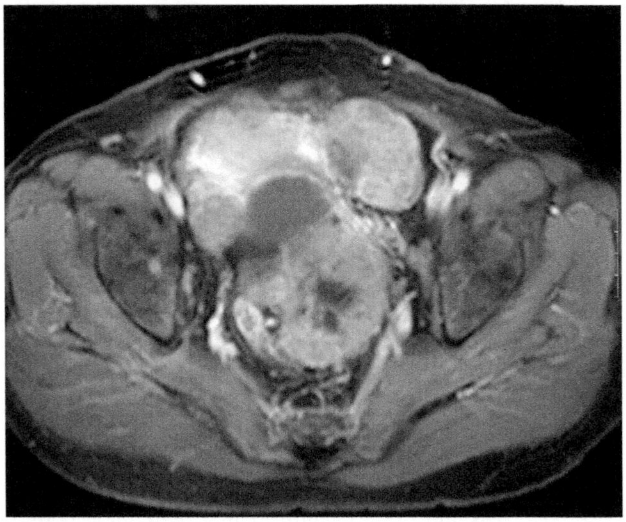

Fig. 14.3 On T2WI, the tumor showed low to moderate signal intensity, with round-like cystic high signal inside

14.3 Differential Diagnosis

It is mainly differentiated from ovarian sex cord-stromal tumors, including fibroma, thecoma, and granulosa cell tumor. Ovarian fibroma is a benign tumor, with calcification inside the tumor commonly. It shows extremely low signal intensity on T2WI, but edema often occurs when the tumor is large, and there is no significant or only mild enhancement after contrast enhancement. The area of theca cell enrichment of thecoma is cloud-like or nodular and shows high signal intensity on T2WI. After contrast enhancement, this area is significantly enhanced, which is easy to distinguish from transitional cell tumor. Elevated estrogen levels can be seen in granulosa cell tumor and thecoma. Granulosa cell tumor is a round-like mass, the cystic part is mostly honeycomb-like, and the solid part is slightly hyperintense on T2WI, with moderate enhancement after contrast enhancement. However, calcification is common in the solid part of transitional cell tumor, which is often accompanied by small patchy cystic changes. The solid part is slightly hypointense on T2WI, with moderate enhancement after contrast enhancement.

References

1. Borah T, Mahanta RK, Bora BD, et al. Brenner tumor of ovary: an incidental finding. J Midlife Health. 2011;2(1):40–1.
2. Verma A, Chander B, Verma S, et al. Malignant Brenner tumor of ovary. J Obstet Gynaecol India. 2014;64(2):148–9.
3. Terada T, Tateoka K. Ovarian cystic tumor composed of Brenner tumor and struma ovarii. Int J Clin Exp Pathol. 2012;5(3):274–7.
4. Ingin RJ, Andola SK, Zubair AA. Transitional cell carcinoma of the ovary: case series and review of literature. J Clin Diagn Res. 2014;8(8):FD07–8.
5. Won JM, Byung HK, Sung KK, et al. Brenner tumor of the ovary: CT and MRI findings. J Comput Assist Tomogr. 2000;24(1):72–6.
6. Oh SN, Rha SE, Jung SE, et al. Transitional cell tumor of the ovary: computed tomographic and magnetic resonance imaging features with pathological correlation. J Comput Assist Tomogr. 2009;33(1):106–12.

15 Ovarian Fibroma

Shuhui Zhao

15.1 Clinical History

Female patient, 63 years old, had been menopause for 9 years. Half a month ago, the patient came to our hospital because of waist soreness. Ultrasound examination showed a solid hypoechoic mass in the left adnexa area; the mass was 37 mm × 23 mm in size, with unclear boundary. CDFI showed no obvious blood flow signal. Serum tumor markers were normal. She underwent laparoscopic left salpingo-oophorectomy. Postoperative pathological result: spindle cell tumor of left ovary, consistent with fibroma.

15.2 Imaging Analysis

Ovarian fibroma is benign ovarian neoplasm classified as sex cord-stromal tumor. As the most common sex cord-stromal tumor, fibromas account for 4% of all ovarian neoplasms [1–3]. Fibromas can present at any age, although the mean age of occurrence is in the late 40s. It is usually a unilateral disease. Fibromas range in size from small to large lesions with a median diameter of 13 cm [3]. Morphologically, fibromas demonstrate as a well-defined oval, lobulated, round, or bilobed solid mass. Larger lesions are more likely to show the presence of cystic component. Calcification is present in 10% cases. Microscopically, fibromas are composed of whorled fascicles of cytologically bland spindle cells embedded in collagenous stroma [3]. Patients are most often asymptomatic. Fibroma is usually an incidental finding. Ovarian fibromas may present with ascites and pleural effusion, known as the Meigs syndrome. Typically, ascites and pleural effusion disappear with removal of tumor. Fibromas can mimic malignancy when present in Meigs syndrome [3–7].

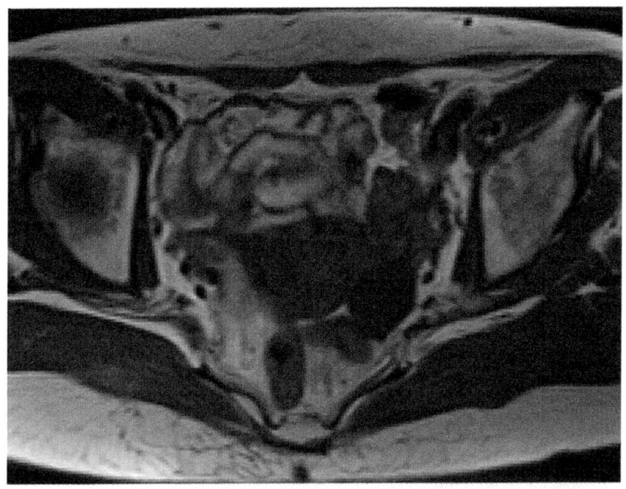

Fig. 15.1 Axial T1-weighted image showed an oval lesion of low signal intensity in the left adnexa area

Because fibromas have abundant collagen and fibrous contents, these tumors show relatively diagnostic imaging findings. The mass appears as a hypointense lesion on T1-weighted MR image (Fig. 15.1) with very low signal intensity on T2-weighted image (Figs. 15.2 and 15.3). Ovarian fibromas have mild and delayed enhancement after contrast enhancement (Fig. 15.4). Scattered high-signal-intensity areas in the mass indicate edema or cystic degeneration. The remaining ovary on the same side as the fibroma is commonly detected on MRI, especially in premenopausal women [1–3].

S. Zhao (✉)
Department of Radiology, Xinhua Hospital, Medical College of Shanghai Jiao Tong University,
Shanghai, People's Republic of China

G. Zhang (ed.), *MRI of Gynaecological Diseases*, https://doi.org/10.1007/978-981-99-3644-1_15

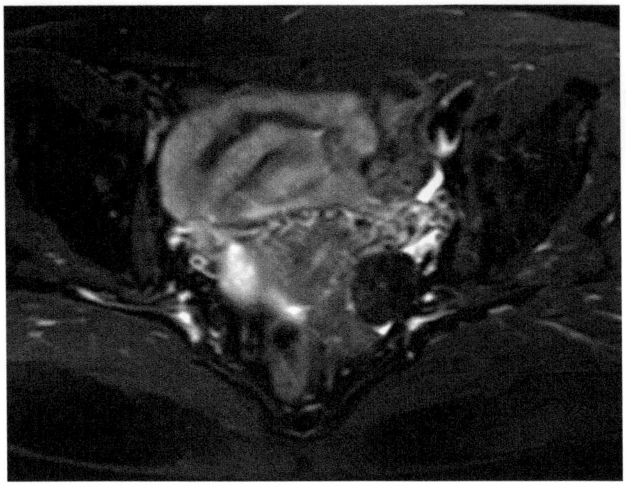

Fig. 15.2 T2-weighted with fat suppression image showed the mass had significantly low signal intensity

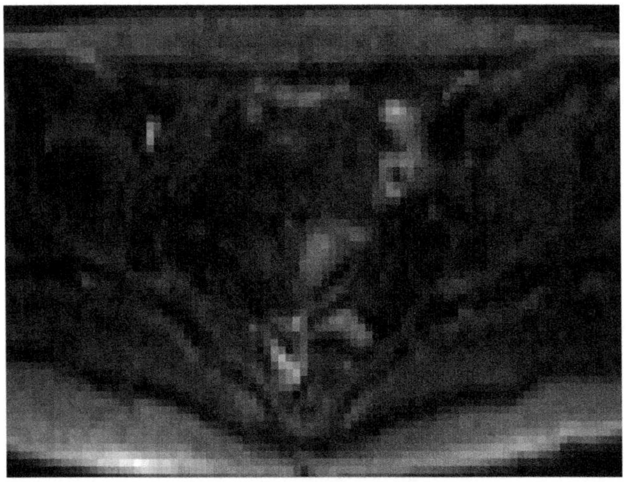

Fig. 15.3 The mass showed low signal intensity on DWI

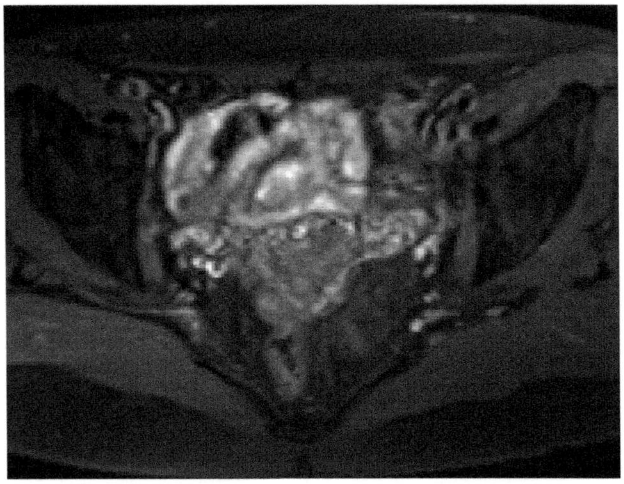

Fig. 15.4 T1-weighted contrast-enhanced image showed the mass was slightly enhanced

15.3 Differential Diagnosis

The main differential diagnosis of a solid adnexal mass with T2 hypointensity includes a uterine pedunculated leiomyoma, ovarian fibroma, and ovarian Brenner tumor. Bridging vessel sign (vessels connect uterus and mass) helps establish uterine origin of a pelvic mass. A separate ovary will often be seen in subserosal leiomyoma case. Fibromas enhance significantly less than uterine leiomyoma [3–7]. Brenner tumor is often a small mass. When benign, Brenner tumor tends to be homogeneous on imaging examination. They have moderate enhancement after contrast enhancement. Brenner tumor is often an incidental finding when operated for other ovarian etiology [3].

References

1. Jung SE, Rha SE, Lee JM, Park SY, Oh SN, Cho KS, et al. CT and MRI findings of sex cord-stromal tumor of the ovary. Am J Roentgenol. 2005;185(1):207–15.
2. Shinagare AB, Meylaerts LJ, Laury AR, Mortele KJ. MRI features of ovarian fibroma and fibrothecoma with histopathologic correlation. Am J Roentgenol. 2012;198(3):W296–303.
3. Shaaban AM. Diagnostic imaging: gynecology. Philadelphia, PA: Elsevier; 2015.
4. Montoriol P-F, Mons A, Ines DD, Bourdel N, Tixier L, Garcier JM. Fibrous tumors of the ovary: aetiologies and MRI features. Clin Radiol. 2013;68(12):1276–83.
5. Chung BM, Park SB, Lee JB, Park HJ, Kim YS, Oh YJ. Magnetic resonance imaging features of ovarian fibroma, fibrothecoma, and thecoma. Abdom Imaging. 2015;40(5):1263–72.
6. Kato H, Kanematsu M, Ono H, Yano R, Furui T, Morishige K, et al. Ovarian fibromas: MR imaging findings with emphasis on intratumoral cyst formation. Eur J Radiol. 2013;82(9):e417–21.
7. Oh SN, Rha SE, Byun JY, Lee YJ, Jung SE, Jung CK, Kim MR, et al. MRI features of ovarian fibromas: emphasis on their relationship to the ovary. Clin Radiol. 2008;63(5):529–35.

16 Struma Ovarii

Fenghua Ma

16.1 Clinical History

Female patient, 53 years old, who was found to have a pelvic mass for 15 years. Fifteen years ago, she was found to have a pelvic mass with a diameter of 2–3 cm due to heavy menstrual bleeding. The medical treatment was ineffective, and she underwent no treatment later. In 2010, she went to another hospital, and ultrasound examination showed a left pelvic cyst with a diameter of 8 cm. Surgery was recommended by gynecologist. However, she did not undergo surgery. Two months ago, she felt that the mass was significantly enlarged, accompanied by lower abdomen heaviness, frequent urination, and no urination pain. She went to the outpatient clinic of our hospital 20 days ago. Gynecological examination revealed that the uterine body was with the size of about 2 months pregnant, and a 15 cm mass was palpated in the left posterior area of the uterus. Examination of serum tumor markers: CA125: 19.4 U/mL, CA199: 64.6 U/mL. Physical examination on admission: a soft cystic mass with a diameter of 15 cm was found in the left adnexa area.

MRI examination: There was multilocular cystic mass in the left adnexa area, loculi >10, oval in shape, regular boundary, 13 cm × 12 cm × 9 cm in size, with low and slightly high signal intensity on T1WI (Figs. 16.1–16.2) and low and high signal intensity on T2WI (Figs. 16.3–16.8). The septal enhancement was shown after contrast enhancement (Figs. 16.9–16.12). There was no obvious effusion in the pelvic cavity and no obvious enlarged lymph nodes.

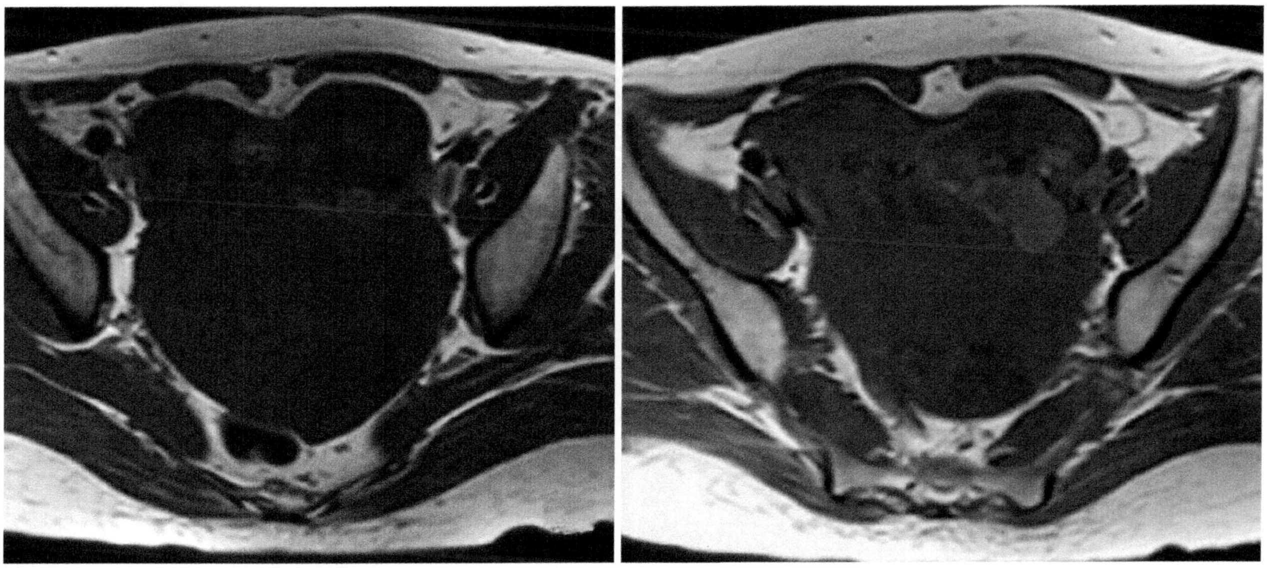

Figs. 16.1–16.2 Pre-contrast T1WI: a multilocular cystic mass was found in the left adnexa area, mainly hypointense signal intensity, and a small patchy of slightly hyperintense was seen locally

F. Ma (✉)
Department of Radiology, Obstetrics and Gynecology Hospital, Fudan University, Shanghai, People's Republic of China

G. Zhang (ed.), *MRI of Gynaecological Diseases*, https://doi.org/10.1007/978-981-99-3644-1_16

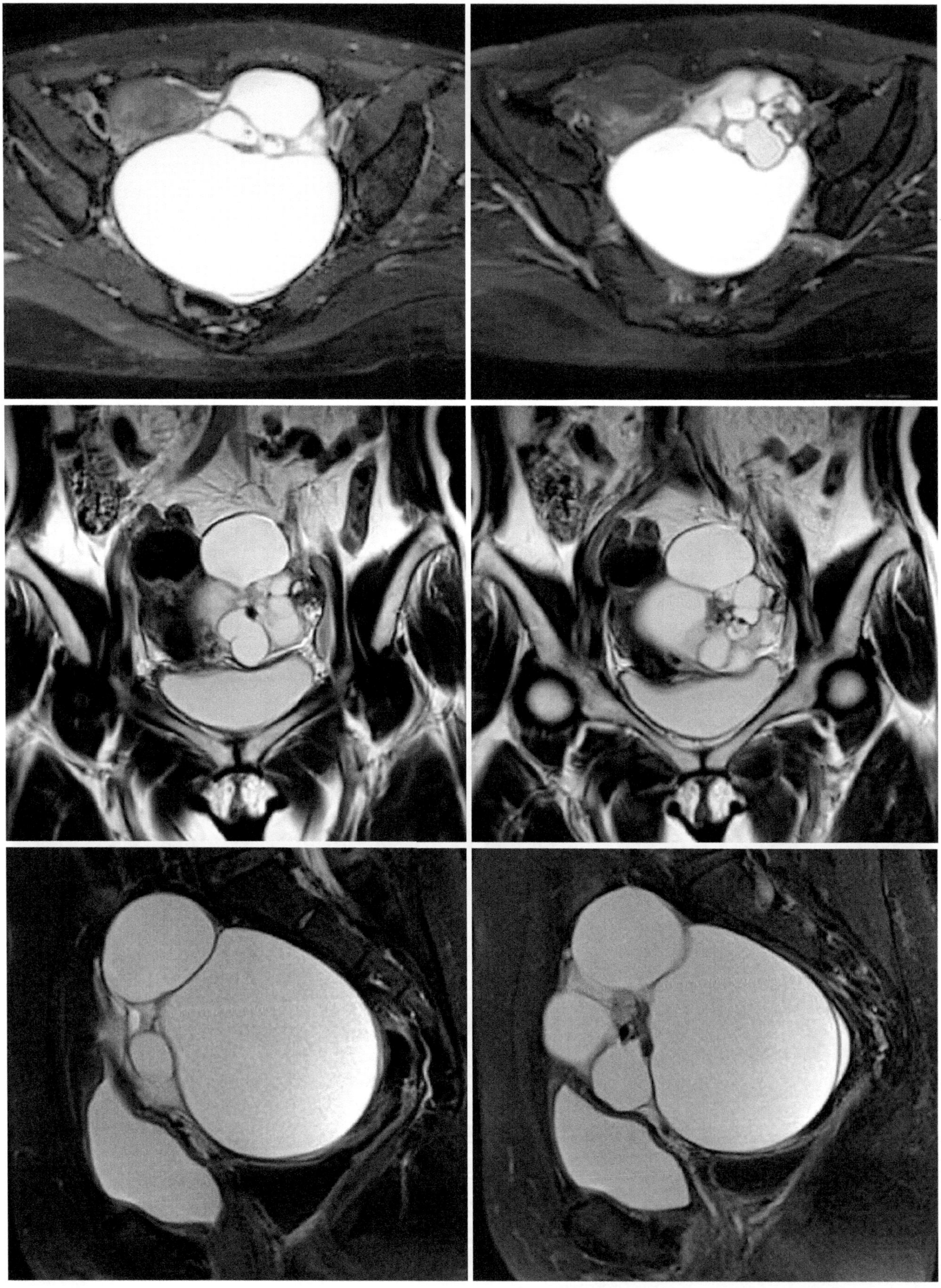

Figs. 16.3–16.8 Axial, coronal, and sagittal T2WI: the signal intensity is mainly hyperintensity and heterogeneous, and a small patchy of significant hypointensity was seen locally

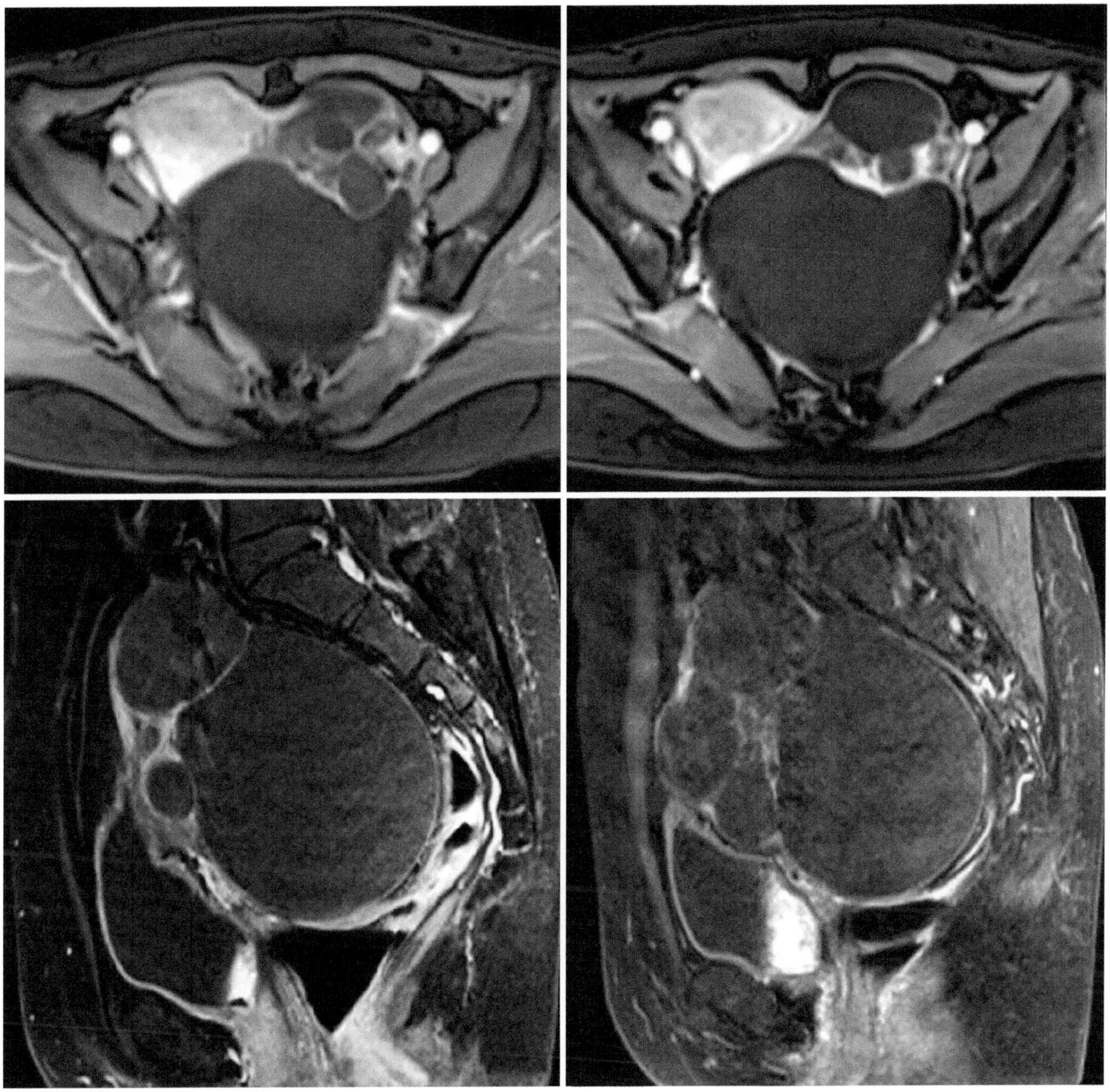

Figs. 16.9–16.12 Contrast-enhanced sagittal and axial T1WI images showed lesion septation and local part presented patchy and nodular enhancement

After admission, transabdominal total hysterectomy and bilateral salpingo-oophorectomy were performed. Intraoperative findings: the uterus was found in anterior position, 6 cm × 5 cm × 5 cm in size, with regular shape. The left ovary presented solid and cystic enlargement, measuring about 13 cm in diameter, smooth surface without laceration, and the posterior and inferior parts adhesion with pelvic peritoneum and was irregular in shape. No obvious abnormalities were observed in the appearance of the left fallopian tube. There was no abnormality in the right ovary and fallopian tube; no abnormality was observed in the bladder and rectouterine pouch.

Postoperative pathological result: cystic mature teratoma of the left ovary with abundant thyroid tissue.

16.2 Image Analysis

Struma ovarii is a special type of teratoma, which is named for containing different degrees of thyroid tissue [1]. Struma ovarii is the most common monodermal teratoma and is histologically characterized by thyroid tissue containing colloidal follicles. Thyroid tissue is usually less than 5–15% of teratoma tissue, but thyroid tissue accounts for more than

50% of teratoma tissue in struma ovarii [2]. Struma ovarii usually occurs in about 50 years old. Most patients have no specific symptoms. The most common symptoms are abdominal pain, abdominal distension, and occasionally vaginal discharge [3].

Struma ovarii is classified into simple struma ovarii and mixed struma ovarii (often associated with dermoid cyst) according to the content of thyroid tissue. The former showed a mixed solid and cystic mass on ultrasound examination, while the latter had a combined dermoid cyst presentation in about 63%, and the 37% showed pure thyroid tissue. The characteristic ultrasonography feature is the "thyroid pearl" sign in the solid area with smooth surface [4].

CT showed polycystic mass with solid area [5], and calcification was common in the solid area. Microscopically, the colloidal substance in the cyst contained birefringent calcium oxalate crystals, and the cystic area showed high density. Shen et al. [6] found that 68% of the patients presented with high density cysts (CT value 58–98 HU) and speculated that it was formed by X-ray attenuation of thyroglobulin and thyroid hormone in ovarian follicular thyroid tissue, which may be the characteristic CT manifestation of struma ovarii.

MRI is typically characterized by multiple intracystic solid areas, and the surface is formed by multiple small chambers. The signal intensity varies in the solid area, which can be presented as moderate or low signal on T2WI and moderate or low signal on T1WI [7], and pathological manifestations are colloidal substances. It may also be characterized by significant high signal on T2WI and moderate signal on T1WI [8]. The solid area showed obvious enhancement after contrast enhancement, which is corresponding to the thyroid tissue containing multiple small vessels on pathology. The cystic area showed various signal intensities on T1WI and T2WI due to the presence of pure fluid, hemorrhage, or mucous substances in the cystic cavity [7, 8]. Joja et al. [8] found that the difference of MR signal intensity in cystic area depended on the concentration of thyroglobulin and thyroid hormone and concluded that the variation of signal intensity in the cystic area was highly suggestive of struma ovarii. Occasionally, struma ovarii presents as a completely solid mass [9], or as a multilocular cystic mass, and rarely as a unilocular cystic mass [10].

16.3 Differential Diagnosis

Although struma ovarii has certain imaging characteristics, preoperative diagnosis is difficult. The differential diagnosis mainly includes cystic masses, such as ovarian mucinous cystadenoma, endometriosis cyst, tubal and ovarian abscess, and ovarian malignant cystic tumor. The typical manifestation of ovarian mucinous cystadenoma is multilocular cystic mass, presents as high signal intensity on T1WI, and high or moderate or slightly low signal intensity on T2WI because of mucus substances, and this manifestation is also seen in struma ovarii. However, the latter is more complex than the former and can contain plentiful solid tissue, while cystadenoma usually has no solid component. Endometriosis cysts can be distinguished by significantly low signal intensity on T2WI and high signal intensity on T1WI, and struma ovarii is usually moderate or slightly high signal intensity on T1WI. Tubal and ovarian abscess is often accompanied by typical clinical symptoms such as abdominal pain and fever and so on. The enhancement mode is significant ring enhancement of cyst wall. However, struma ovarii is usually asymptomatic, and lesion enhancement is moderate or significant enhancement of solid tissue. The most challenging is the differentiation with ovarian malignant cystic tumor, which can be manifested as a solid and cystic mass. When the cystic fluid contains hemorrhage or mucus substances, the imaging feature is similar to struma ovarii, and careful observation should be carried out. Whether there are other malignant signs such as ascites, enlarged lymph nodes and peritoneal implants can help to identify them.

References

1. Scully RE, Young RH, Clement PB. Tumors of the ovary, maldeveloped gonads, fallopian tubes and broad ligament. 3rd ed. Washington, DC: Armed Force Institute of Pathology; 1998. p. 239–312.
2. Yoo SC, Chang KH, Lyu MO, et al. Clinical characteristics of struma ovarii. J Gynecol Oncol. 2008;2:135–8.
3. Shanbhogue AK, Shanbhogue DKP, Prasad SR, et al. Clinical syndromes associated with ovarian neoplasms: a comprehensive review. Radiographics. 2010;30:903–19.
4. Zalel Y, Capsi B, Tepper R. Doppler flow characteristics of dermoid cysts: unique appearance of struma ovarii. J Ultrasound Med. 1997;16:355–8.
5. Van de Moortele K, et al. Struma ovarii: US and CT findings. JBR-BTR. 2003;86(4):209–10.
6. Shen J, Xia X, Lin Y, et al. Diagnosis of struma ovarii with medical imaging. Abdom Imaging. 2011;36:627–31.
7. Matsuki M, Kaji Y, Matsuo M, et al. Struma ovarii: MRI findings. Br J Radiol. 2000;73:87–90.
8. Joja I, Asakawa T, Mitsumori A, et al. Struma ovarii: appearance on MR images. Abdom Imaging. 1998;23:652–6.
9. Szyfelbein WM, Young RH, Scully RE. Struma ovarii simulating ovarian tumors of other types. A report of 30 cases. Am J Surg Pathol. 1995;19:21–9.
10. Okada S, Ohaki Y, Kawamura T, et al. Cystic struma ovarii: imaging findings. J Comput Assist Tomogr. 2000;24(3):413–5.

17 Ovarian Thecoma

Shuhui Zhao

17.1 Clinical History

Female patient, 87 years old, had been experiencing menopausal for 30 years and had no abnormal vaginal bleeding or discharge after menopause. The patient found a small amount of bright red blood on her underwear without obvious inducement, and she touched a mass at the vaginal orifice. Ultrasound examination showed that the endometrium was 15 mm, with obvious thickening and reticular pattern in the uterus and cervical canal and solid space-occupying lesion in the left adnexa area, 52 mm × 47 mm × 49 mm in size. Further examination was recommended. The outpatient clinic admitted her for "postmenopausal vaginal bleeding, endometrial thickening, anterior and posterior vaginal wall prolapse, and left adnexal mass." She underwent transabdominal total hysterectomy and bilateral salpingo-oophorectomy. Postoperative pathological result: endometrial atypical hyperplasia, left ovarian thecoma.

17.2 Imaging Analysis

Ovarian thecoma is a subtype of sex cord-stromal tumor [1]. Ovarian thecomas are composed of lipid-laden stromal cells that resemble theca cells, which usually encircle the ovarian follicles, and exhibit estrogenic activity in most cases. Ovarian thecomas account for 0.5–1% of all primary ovarian tumors. These tumors are more likely to occur in postmenopausal women and, with rare exceptions, are considered benign neoplasms. Affected women experience estrogen-related symptoms such as abnormal uterine bleeding, endometrial hyperplasia, and endometrial carcinoma; the latter has been reported to occur in 21% of cases [1]. Ovarian thecoma may be associated with ascites and pleural effusion, known as the Meigs syndrome. Typically, ascites and pleural effusion disappear with removal of tumor. Ovarian thecomas can mimic malignancy when present in Meigs syndrome. Generally, pure thecomas or thecomas with scanty fibrotic components do not have distinct US and CT appearances and mimic other solid ovarian tumors [1–3].

Most ovarian thecomas are homogeneous solid masses. On T1WI, they are isointense to hypointense compared with myometrium (Fig. 17.1). Fat elements can be identified on frequency selective fat-suppression or out-of-phase gradient echo sequences. When compared with predominant fibrous tumors, thecomas tend to exhibit greater hyperintensity on T2-weighted images (Figs. 17.2 and 17.3); more avid contrast enhancement may be observed (Figs. 17.4 and 17.5) [1, 4–7]. They are isointense to the myometrium on DWI (Fig. 17.6) and that the ADC values of thecomas did not significantly differ from those of other ovarian solid tumors and leiomyomas [3].

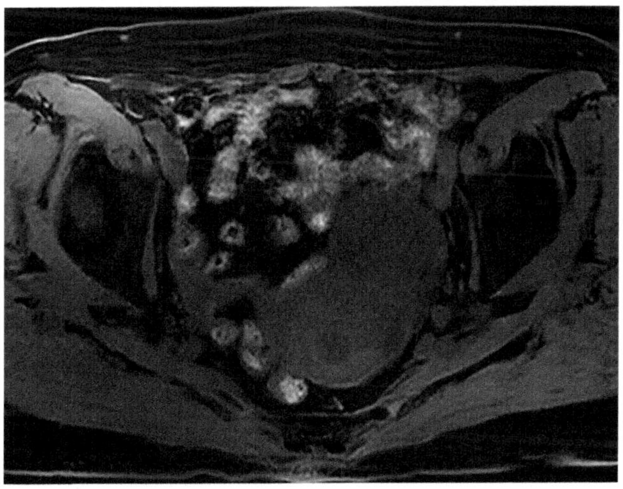

Fig. 17.1 Axial T1-weighted with fat suppression image showed an oval lesion of low signal intensity in the left adnexa area

S. Zhao (✉)
Department of Radiology, Xinhua Hospital, Medical College of Shanghai Jiao Tong University,
Shanghai, People's Republic of China

G. Zhang (ed.), *MRI of Gynaecological Diseases*, https://doi.org/10.1007/978-981-99-3644-1_17

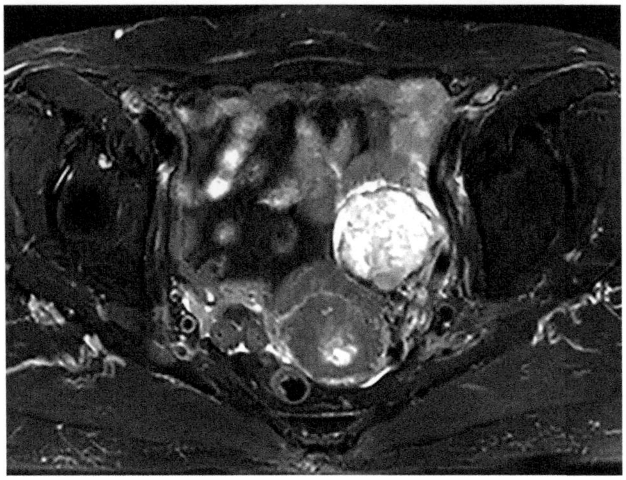

Fig. 17.2 T2-weighted with fat suppression image showed the mass had high signal intensity

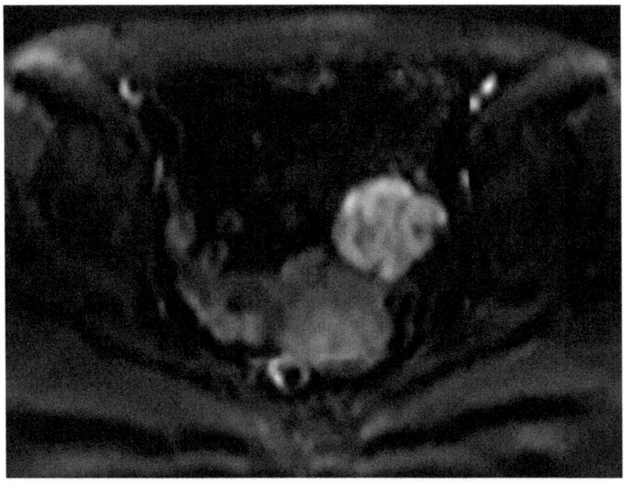

Fig. 17.3 Sagittal T2-weighted image showed the endometrial hyperplasia

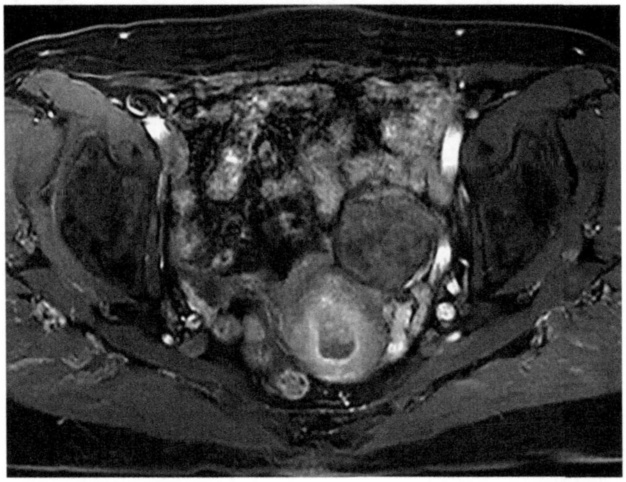

Fig. 17.4 T1-weighted contrast-enhanced image showed the mass enhanced less than myometrium

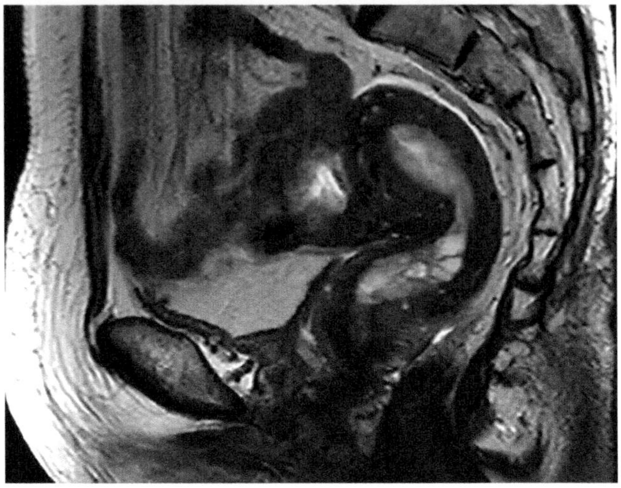

Fig. 17.5 Sagittal T1-weighted contrast-enhanced image showed the endometrial hyperplasia

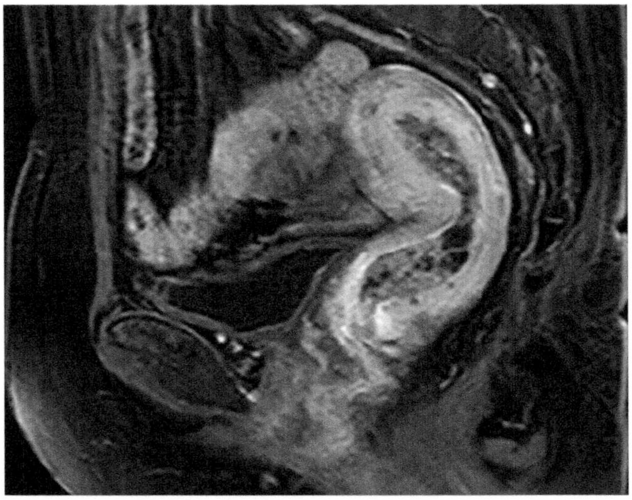

Fig. 17.6 The mass showed restricted diffusion on DWI

17.3 Differential Diagnosis

The main differential diagnosis includes a uterine pedunculated leiomyoma and ovarian cancer. Bridging vessel sign (vessels connect uterus and mass) helps establish uterine origin of a pelvic mass. A separate ovary will often be seen in subserosal leiomyoma cases [2]. It is difficult to distinguish thecoma from ovarian cancer on routine MRI [3]. On MR spectroscopy, the low choline-to-creatine ratio can help distinguish thecoma from ovarian cancer [8].

References

1. Horta M, Cunha TM. Sex cord-stromal tumors of the ovary: a comprehensive review and update for radiologists. Diagn Interv Radiol. 2015;21(4):277–86.
2. Shaaban AM. Diagnostic imaging: gynecology. Philadelphia, PA: Elsevier; 2015.
3. Zhang H, Zhang GF, Wang TP, Zhang H. Value of 3.0 T diffusion-weighted imaging in discriminating thecoma and fibrothecoma from other adnexal solid masses. J Ovarian Res. 2013;6(1):58.
4. Jung SE, Rha SE, Lee JM, Park SY, Oh SN, Cho KS, et al. CT and MRI findings of sex cord-stromal tumor of the ovary. Am J Roentgenol. 2005;185(1):207–15.
5. Shinagare AB, Meylaerts LJ, Laury AR, Mortele KJ. MRI features of ovarian fibroma and fibrothecoma with histopathologic correlation. Am J Roentgenol. 2012;198(3):W296–303.
6. Montoriol P-F, Mons A, Ines DD, Bourdel N, Tixier L, Garcier JM. Fibrous tumors of the ovary: aetiologies and MRI features. Clin Radiol. 2013;68(12):1276–83.
7. Chung BM, Park SB, Lee JB, Park HJ, Kim YS, Oh YJ. Magnetic resonance imaging features of ovarian fibroma, fibrothecoma, and thecoma. Abdom Imaging. 2015;40(5):1263–72.
8. Ma F, Qiang J, Cai S, Zhao S, Zhang G, Rao Y. MR spectroscopy for differentiating benign from malignant solid adnexal tumors. Am J Roentgenol. 2015;204(6):W724–30.

18 Ovarian Sclerosing Stromal Tumor

Shuhui Zhao

18.1 Clinical History

Female patient, 26 years old, came to our gynecology outpatient department due to menstrual irregularity. Ultrasound examination showed a solid space-occupying lesion in the right adnexa area. She underwent further MRI examination. MRI diagnosis: right adnexal mass, considered for broad ligament myoma with possible degeneration and necrosis; ovarian fibroma is not excluded. She underwent laparoscopic right oophorectomy. Postoperative pathological result: right ovarian sclerosing stromal tumor.

18.2 Imaging Analysis

Ovarian sclerosing stromal tumor is a benign neoplasm that accounts for less than 5% of ovarian sex cord-stromal tumors. Sclerosing stromal tumors are likely to occur in young women; approximately 80% of reported cases are under 30 years of age. Although sclerosing stromal tumors most commonly occur after menarche, a few cases have been reported in premenarchal girls. Typically, sclerosing stromal tumors manifest as unilateral masses [1, 2].

Pelvic pain and menstrual irregularities are frequent symptoms. A few hormonally active tumors that produce androgens and/or estrogens have been documented in the literature [3–5]. Ovarian sclerosing stromal tumors have also been associated with pregnancy. Although rare, ascites may be present [1–3]. Surgical removal of the tumor is curative, and there is no local or distant recurrence [3].

Sclerosing stromal tumors are mostly solid masses with yellowish foci, edema, and cystic areas [1]. Tumor size is variable and usually 3–5 cm [2]. The histopathology is characterized by the presence of an ill-defined pseudolobular pattern in the cellular areas, which are separated by edematous fibrous areas [1, 6]. These nodular portions contain collagen-producing spindle-shaped cells and vacuolated lipid-containing lutein cells. Prominent vascularization is seen within these areas [3–7] (Fig. 18.1).

Sclerosing stromal tumors demonstrate as a heterogeneous lesion on MRI. On T2-weighted image, the lesion has intermediate to high signal intensity (Figs. 18.2 and 18.3). The peripheral rim is hypointense on T2-weighted image. It may be the compressed ovarian cortex. Sclerosing stromal tumors display remarkable contrast enhancement with internal small cleft and cysts. On dynamic contrast-enhanced images (Figs. 18.4–18.6), the tumors demonstrate early peripheral enhancement with centripetal progression. Early marked enhancement represents the pseudolobular cellular areas rich in vascular networks. The area of delayed enhancement in the central portion of the lesion represents the collagenous hypocellular or acellular area [3–7].

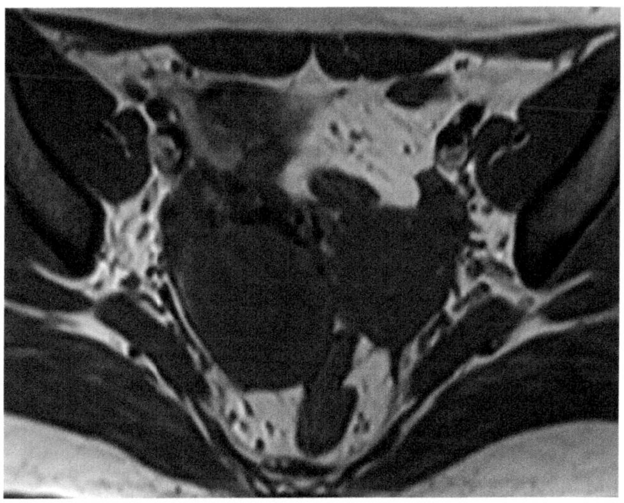

Fig. 18.1 Axial T1-weighted image showed an oval lesion of low signal intensity.

S. Zhao (✉)
Department of Radiology, Xinhua Hospital, Medical College of Shanghai Jiao Tong University,
Shanghai, People's Republic of China

G. Zhang (ed.), *MRI of Gynaecological Diseases*, https://doi.org/10.1007/978-981-99-3644-1_18

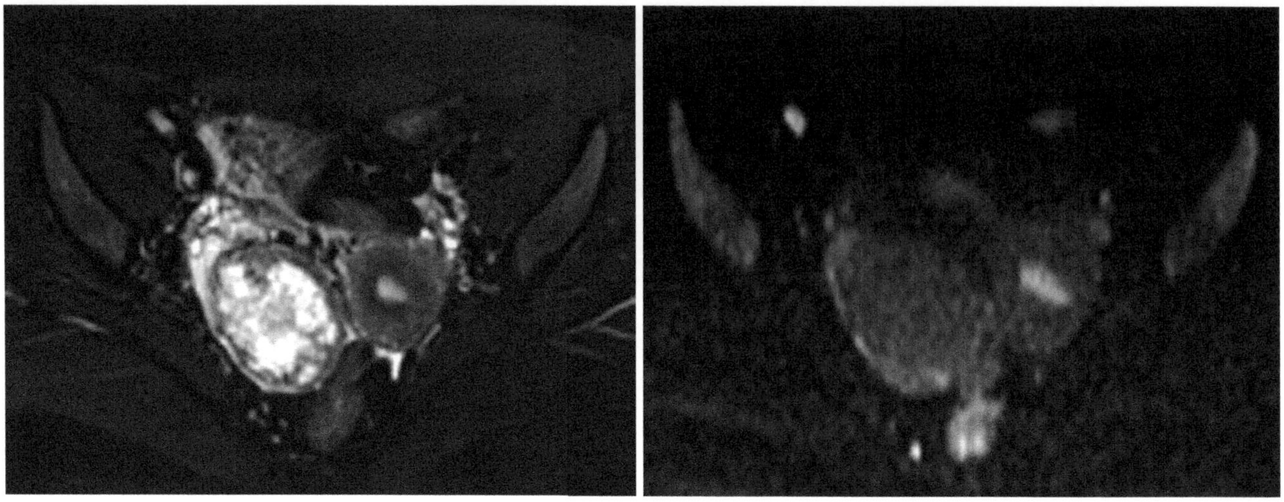

Figs. 18.2 and 18.3 T2-weighted with fat suppression image showed the mass had a rim of low signal intensity in the peripheral area and significant high signal intensity in the inner part. The mass showed low signal intensity on DWI

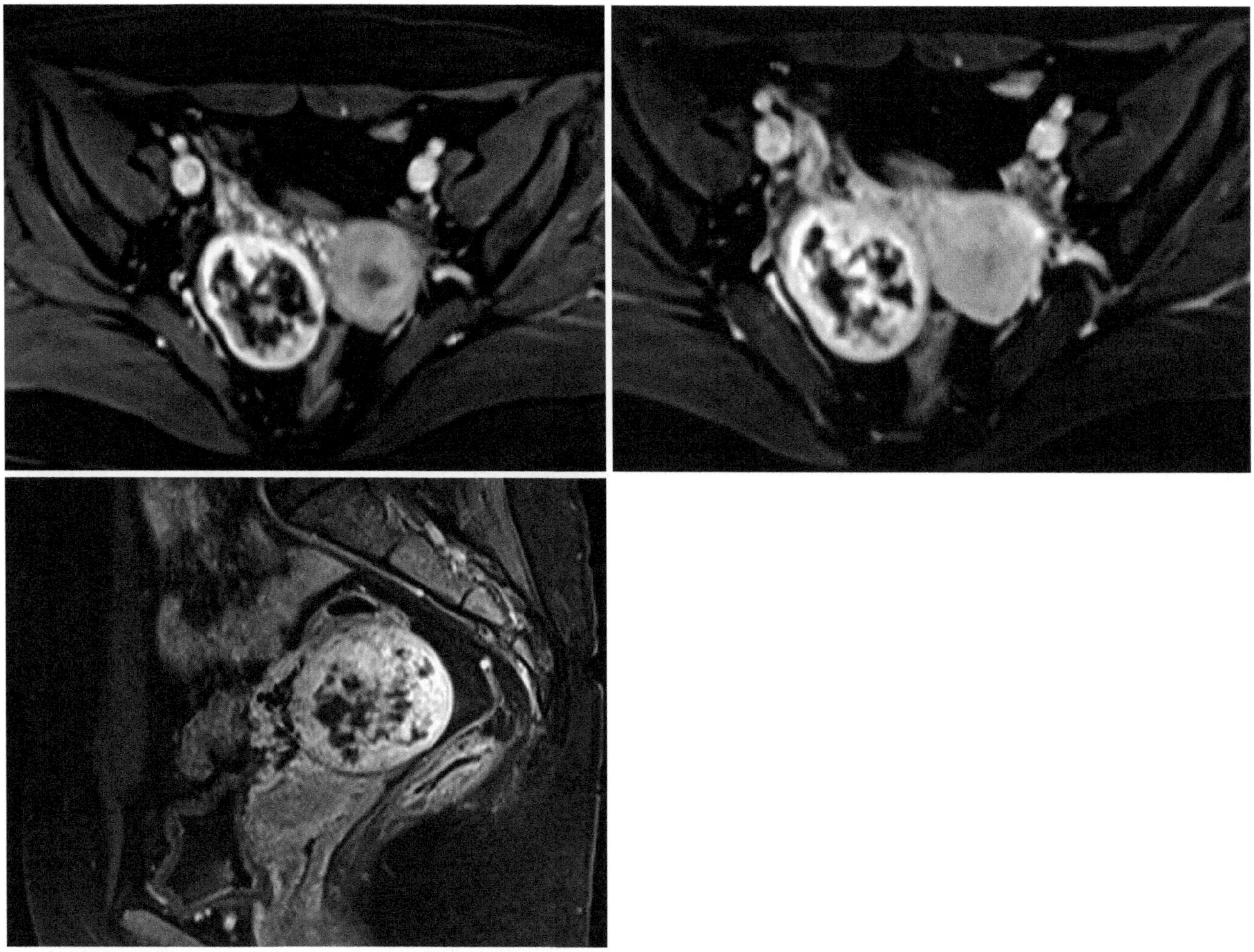

Figs. 18.4–18.6 Axial T1-weighted contrast-enhanced images and sagittal T1-weighted contrast-enhanced image showed the typical early avid enhancement of the outer part of the mass with centripetal progression

18.3 Differential Diagnosis

It is mainly differentiated from other ovarian tumors such as ovarian cancer and fibroma. The onset age of ovarian cancer is older than that of ovarian sclerosing stromal tumor, and the serum CA125 is elevated. The solid component of ovarian cancer is usually slightly high signal on T2WI, with internal hemorrhage and necrosis, and moderate enhancement after contrast enhancement. Pelvic implant metastasis and lymph node metastasis are found in advanced cancer. Ovarian fibromas are mostly solid, and a few can be edematous degeneration. On T2WI, low signal is shown in the non-edematous area, and high signal is shown in the edematous area. There is no or only slight enhancement after contrast enhancement. However, the low signal area of sclerosing stromal tumor on T2WI is vascularized, and the enhancement after contrast enhancement is very avid, which is different from fibroma. In addition, dynamic enhancement is helpful to differentiate ovarian sclerosing stromal tumor from fibroma. The former shows significant centripetal enhancement, and the latter shows slow and mild enhancement.

References

1. Horta M, Cunha TM. Sex cord-stromal tumors of the ovary: a comprehensive review and update for radiologists. Diagn Interv Radiol. 2015;21(4):277–86.
2. Shaaban AM. Diagnostic imaging: gynecology. Philadelphia, PA: Elsevier; 2015.
3. Jung SE, Rha SE, Lee JM, Park SY, Oh SN, Cho KS, et al. CT and MRI findings of sex cord-stromal tumor of the ovary. Am J Roentgenol. 2005;185(1):207–15.
4. Outwater EK, Marchetto B, Wagner BJ. Virilizing tumors of the ovary: imaging features. Ultrasound Obstet Gynecol. 2000;15(5):365–71.
5. Tanaka YO, Tsunoda H, Kitagawa Y, Ueno T, Yoshikawa H, Saida Y. Functioning ovarian tumors: direct and indirect findings at MR imaging. Radiographics. 2004;24(Suppl 1):147–66.
6. Ito K, Tanaka YO, Watanabe R, Tanaka H, Takazawa Y, Matsueda K. Variable distribution of pseudolobules in ovarian sclerosing stromal tumors: utility of diffusion-weighted imaging for differential diagnosis. Magn Reson Med Sci. 2018;17(2):107–8.
7. Zhao S, Li H, Qiang J, Wang D, Fan H. The value of MRI for differentiating benign from malignant sex cord-stromal tumors of the ovary: emphasis on diffusion-weighted MR imaging. J Ovarian Res. 2018;11(1):73.

19 Ovarian Endometrioid Cyst

Mengwei Zhang

19.1 Clinical History

Female patient, 24 years old, came to our hospital due to amenorrhea for 2 months and felt abdominal pain. Ultrasonography indicated bilateral ovarian cysts. Serum tumor markers: CA125: 1140 U/mL. She underwent laparoscopic bilateral ovarian cystectomy.

Postoperative pathological result: bilateral ovarian endometrioid cysts.

19.2 Imaging Analysis

Ovarian endometrioid cyst is defined as pseudocystic lesion formed by ectopic endometrial tissue growing on the ovarian cortex [1]. It is most common in premenopausal women, but also in postmenopausal women, with a reported incidence of 35% and 2%, respectively. Compared with ovarian malignant tumors, ovarian endometrioid cysts develop at a younger age and are more likely to be involved in the left ovary than the right. The most common clinical symptom is abdominal pain, especially in patients with abdominal lesions and deep infiltrative endometriosis (DIE) [2]. So far, the pathogenesis of endometrioid cyst is still uncertain. The main viewpoints generally include two kinds: one is the "cloning theory" proposed by McLeod et al. in 1946, which suggests that ovarian endometrioid cyst develops from functional cysts, and its ovarian cortex is invaded by endometrioid tissue; the second is the "implantation theory" proposed by Hughesdon. This viewpoint suggests that ectopic endometrioid tissue, which is repeatedly bleeding and surrounded by inflammatory tissue reaction, forms a pseudocyst that is chocolate cyst. There have been many reports of endometriosis associated with ovarian cancer. Therefore, MRI examination is very important for accurate preoperative assessment and identification of lesions.

On imaging, ovarian endometrioid cyst can be unilocular or multilocular. On T1WI (Fig. 19.1), >1 cm ovarian endometrioid cysts generally show homogeneous hyperintensity, namely the so-called "light bulb sign," whose signal is higher than the surrounding normal adipose tissue due to the accumulation of a large amount of paramagnetic hemoglobin in the cyst [3]. On T2WI (Fig. 19.2 and 19.3), the signal is iso- or hypointense. An important MRI sign of ovarian endometrioid cysts is the "shading effect"—loss of signal on T2WI, which is used to distinguish it from other functional ovarian cysts [4]. However, there are also some endometrioid cysts whose MR signals are not typical because they contain more water rather than hemoglobin degradation products. At this point, if there are multiple hyperintense cysts on T1WI, the diagnosis of endometrioid cysts is also suggested, because endometrioid cysts can

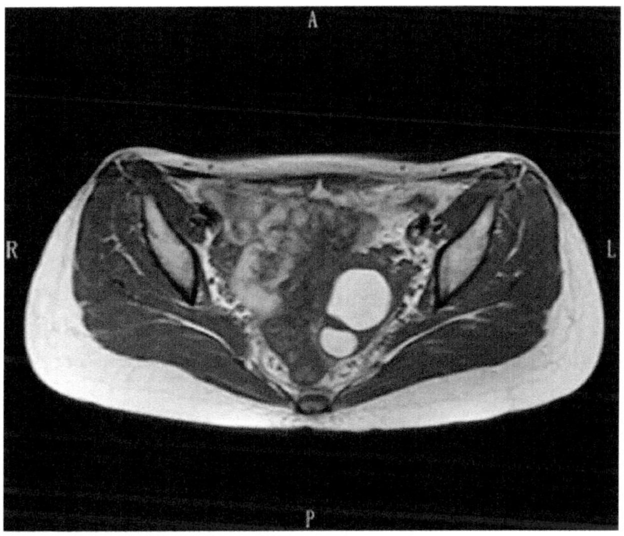

Fig. 19.1 The cystic mass in the left adnexa area showed homogeneous hyperintensity on T1WI with hypointense septation inside

M. Zhang (✉)
Department of Radiology, Obstetrics and Gynecology Hospital, Fudan University, Shanghai, People's Republic of China

G. Zhang (ed.), *MRI of Gynaecological Diseases*, https://doi.org/10.1007/978-981-99-3644-1_19

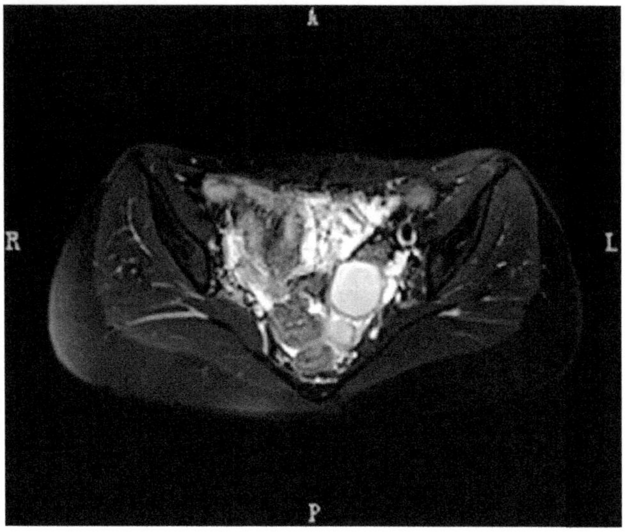

Fig. 19.2 High and low signals were shown on T2WI

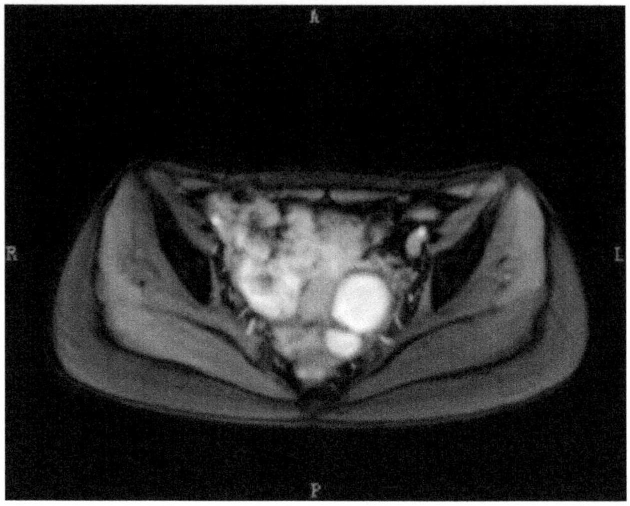

Fig. 19.4 After contrast enhancement, no significant enhancement was observed

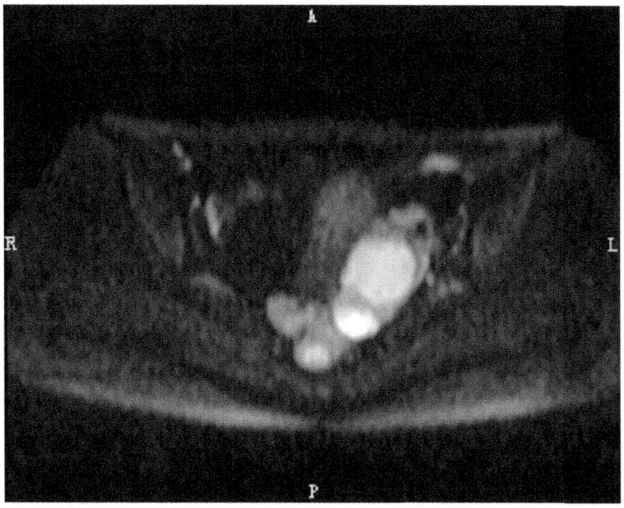

Fig. 19.3 High-bright signal was shown on DWI, and that is T2-shine through effect

often be repeatedly bleeding and cystic changes, resulting in multiple hyperintense cysts on T1WI. Ovarian endometrioid cysts can often be multiple, bilateral, and the formation of pelvic adhesions, which can form a typical "kissing sign"—two ovaries are joined together by adhesions caused by endometrioid cysts. After contrast enhancement (Fig. 19.4), the cystic wall formed by the fibrous component can be enhanced. The diagnosis of endometrioid cysts associated with ovarian cancer is similar to that of ovarian cancer, that is, solid nodules or masses with significant enhancement can be seen and usually do not have the typical T2 shading effect in the cystic fluid, because the hemorrhagic component in the cyst is basically replaced by the fluid secreted by the tumor tissue.

19.3 Differential Diagnosis

1. Ovarian dermoid cyst: The fat component within dermoid cysts is hypointense on fat suppression sequence. Therefore, it is easy to distinguish the two by adding fat suppression sequence.
2. Ovarian hemorrhagic cyst: Most of them are solitary, unilocular, and thin-walled and do not have the typical T2 shading effect of ovarian endometrioid cysts, because hemorrhagic cysts do not cause repeated intracystic hemorrhage. However, for endometrioid cysts without high signal on T1WI, it is difficult to distinguish them. Hemorrhagic cysts can be absorbed and decreased with the menstrual cycle, so timely ultrasound examination follow-up is necessary to confirm the diagnosis [5].
3. Ovarian cancer: Both epidemiological and retrospective studies have shown an increased incidence of secondary ovarian cancer in patients with endometriosis, particu-

larly the subtypes of endometrioid carcinoma (66.7%) and clear cell carcinoma (14.8%) [6]. Therefore, for patients with ovarian endometrioid cysts, the possibility of potential ovarian cancer must be excluded. The differential point is that for patients with tumors, irregular and hypervascularity mural nodules can be seen inside, which indicate ovarian cancer.

References

1. Cramer D, Missmer S. The epidemiology of endometriosis. Ann N Y Acad Sci. 2002;955:11–22.
2. Manganaro L, Fierro F, Tomei A, et al. Feasibility of 3.0T pelvic MR imaging in the evaluation of endometriosis. Eur J Radiol. 2012;81(6):1381–7.
3. Moteki T, Horikoshi H, Endo K. Relationship between apparent diffusion coefficient and signal intensity in endometrial and other pelvic cysts. Magn Reson Imaging. 2002;20(6):463–70.
4. Kinkel K, Frei K, Balleyguier C, et al. Diagnosis of endometriosis with imaging: a review. Eur Radiol. 2006;16(2):285–98.
5. Togashi K, Nishimura K, Kimura I, et al. Endometrial cysts: diagnosis with MR imaging. Radiology. 1991;180(1):73–8.
6. Tanaka YO, Okada S, Yagi T, et al. MRI of endometriotic cysts in association with ovarian carcinoma. Am J Roentgenol. 2010;194(2):355–61.

Part V

Malignant Tumors of the Ovary

20 Ovarian Serous Adenocarcinoma

Shulei Cai

20.1 Clinical History

A 52-year-old female patient had abdominal distension for 4 months and abdominal mass for 1 month. Physical examination showed tenderness in abdominal mass without other symptoms. Ultrasonography showed that there was a huge solid and cystic mass in the right adnexa area, about 13.5 cm × 10.2 cm in size, with a clear boundary and mixed echo. CT showed a huge multilocular solid and cystic mass in the pelvic cavity, about 15 cm × 8 cm × 12 cm in size, and the boundary between the lower edge of the lesion and the uterus was unclear. Serum CA125: 3638 U/mL, HE4: 535.8 pmol/L.

MRI examination showed that there was a huge lobulated solid and cystic mass in the pelvic cavity, with a clear boundary and size of 15 cm × 18 cm × 8.6 cm. On T1WI (Figs. 20.1–20.3), the solid component showed equal signal and the cystic part showed low signal; on T2WI (Figs. 20.4–20.9), the solid component showed slightly high signal, local strip-shaped low signal, and the cystic part high signal. The solid component and septation were significantly enhanced after contrast enhancement (Figs. 20.10–20.15). A small amount of effusion can be seen in the right paracolic gutter. No obvious enlarged lymph nodes were found in the pelvic cavity.

Hysterectomy, bilateral salpingo-oophorectomy, pelvic lymph node dissection, and greater omentum resection were performed. Ascites were light red, about 1000 mL. No abnormalities were found in the stomach, liver, and spleen. Scattered miliary nodules were touched in the diaphragm, with a maximum of about 1.5 cm. The uterus was in neutral position, about 5 cm × 4 cm × 4 cm in size and irregular in shape. Myoma-like protrusions with a diameter of 0.5–2 cm were scattered on the surface of the uterus. The left ovary was enlarged in cauliflower shape, about 5 cm × 4 cm × 4 cm in size. The left fallopian tube was stiff and adhered to the left ovary, wrapping part of the intestinal canal and the fundus of uterus. The rectouterine pouch and anterior wall of the rectum were scattered with miliary nodules.

Postoperative pathological results: (1) bilateral ovarian high-grade serous adenocarcinoma, involving uterine serosa (rectovaginal septum); (2) multiple uterine leiomyomas. Immunohistochemical results: CK7 (+), ER (80% +), PR (5% +), Ki-67 (50% +), p53 (+), WT1 (+), p16 (+), Pax-8 (+).

S. Cai (✉)
Department of Radiology, Obstetrics and Gynecology Hospital, Fudan University, Shanghai, People's Republic of China

G. Zhang (ed.), *MRI of Gynaecological Diseases*, https://doi.org/10.1007/978-981-99-3644-1_20

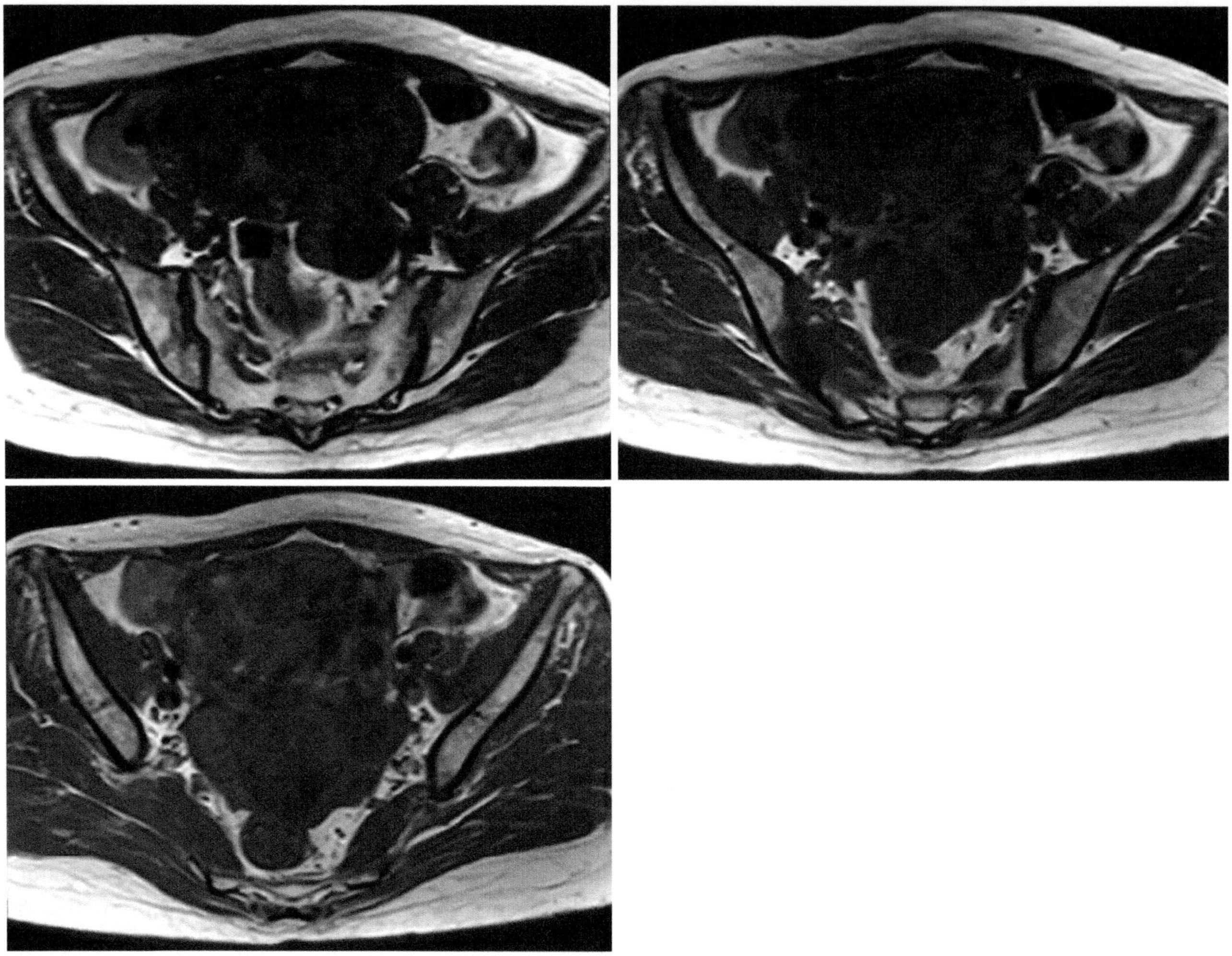

Figs. 20.1–20.3 Axial pre-contrast T1WI. The solid part showed equal signal, and the cystic part showed slightly low signal

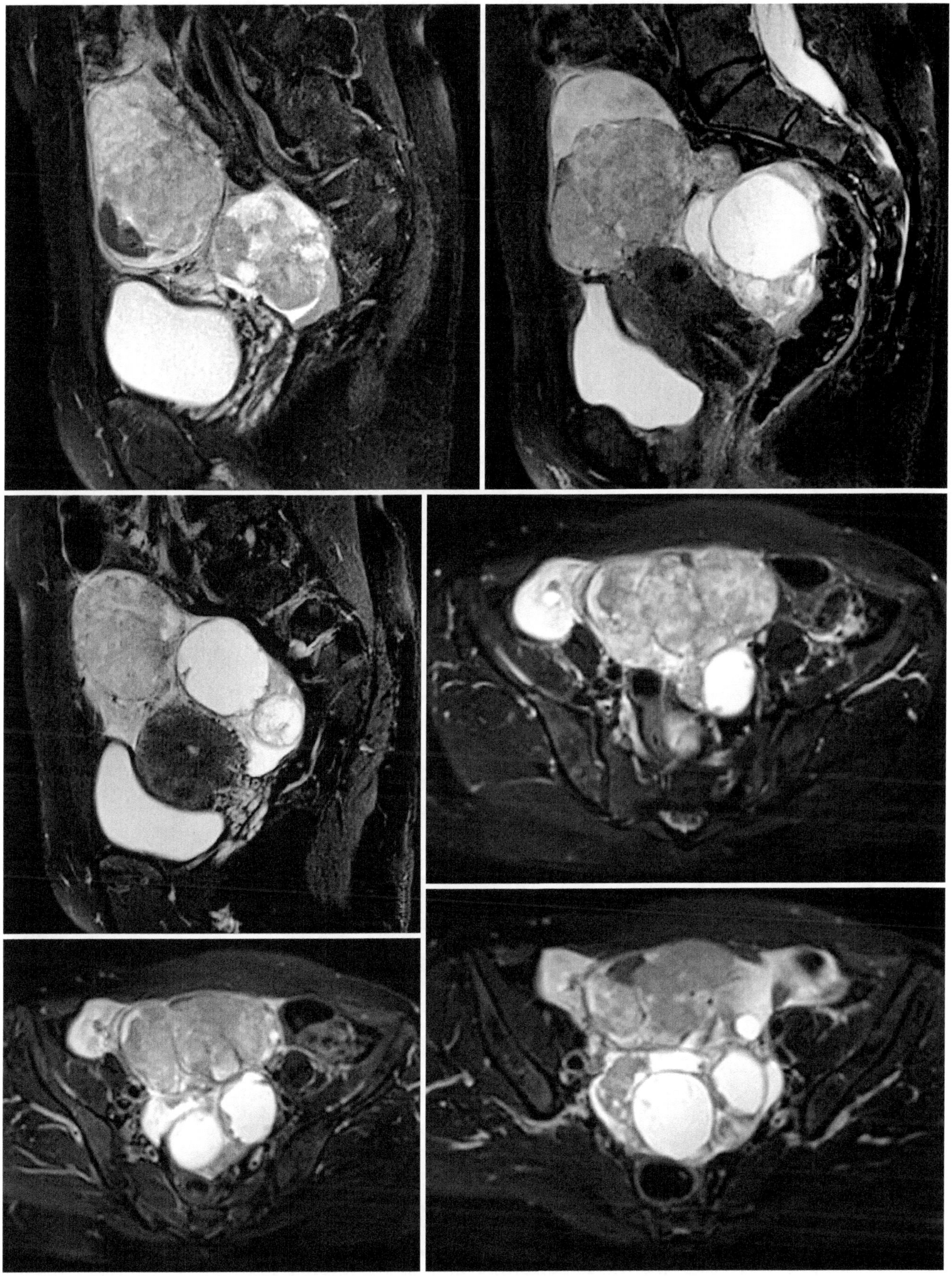

Figs. 20.4–20.9 Axial and sagittal fat suppression T2WI. A huge solid and cystic mass could be seen in the abdominal and pelvic cavity. The right lesion was mainly solid and the left was mainly cystic. The solid part showed uneven and slightly high signal, and strip-shaped low signal could be seen locally

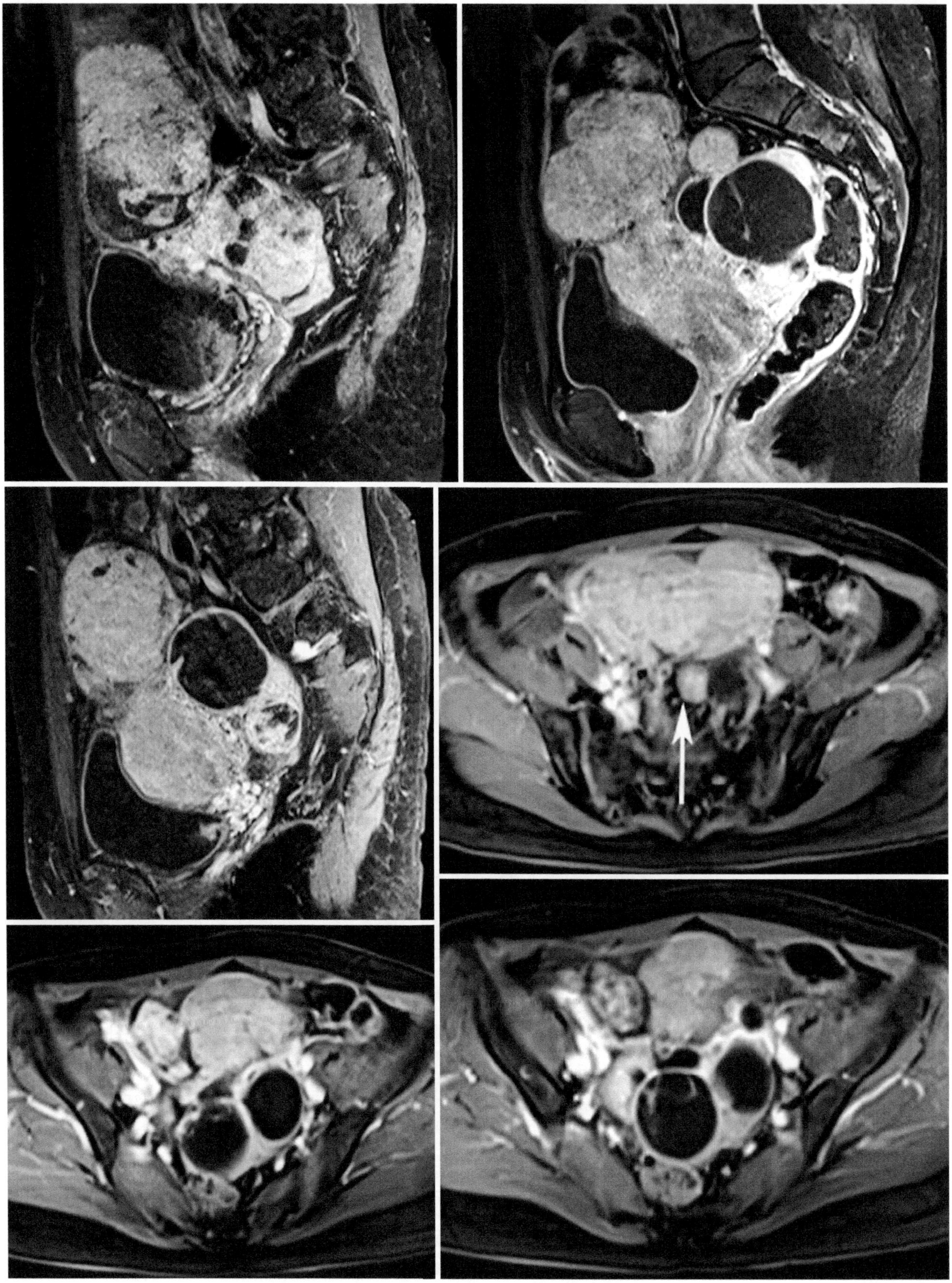

Figs. 20.10–20.15 On sagittal and axial fat suppression contrast-enhanced T1WI images, the solid part and septation were significantly enhanced, and small and significantly enhanced mural nodules could be seen in the cyst wall (arrow)

20.2 Imaging Analysis

Ovarian serous carcinoma (SC) is the most common ovarian malignancy, accounting for 17% of all ovarian tumors and about 70% of all epithelial ovarian malignancies [1]. It can occur from childhood to postmenopausal, mostly in postmenopausal middle-aged and elderly women. Ovarian epithelial cancer accounts for 90% of ovarian malignant tumors in women over 50 years old. Most patients have no special symptoms in the early stage. At the time of clinical diagnosis, 70% of patients are advanced ovarian cancer. Abdominal distension and pelvic and abdominal mass are the most common symptoms. When the tumor is huge, it can cause abdominal distension, abdominal pain, lower abdominal bulge, and compression symptoms, such as frequent urination, urgent urination, etc. A small number of cases develop acute abdominal symptoms, that is, abdominal pain, peritoneal irritation, and fever, as a result of tumor pedicle torsion or cyst infection. When the greater omentum metastasizes seriously and becomes a cake-like mass, the sensation of a floating ball or a large mass can be touched in the upper abdominal cavity. Ascites are a common sign of ovarian cancer. Many patients seek medical treatment because of a series of symptoms caused by ascites. When the amount of ascites is large, it can lead to severe abdominal distension, and sometimes accompanied by pleural effusion, with an incidence of about 10%. Patients with advanced ovarian cancer may have gastrointestinal symptoms such as low-grade fever, lack of appetite, and vomiting, and some may also have cachexia such as tabescence and weight loss.

At present, serous carcinoma is pathologically divided into high-grade serous carcinoma (HGSC) and low-grade serous carcinoma (LGSC) [2]. At the molecular level, LGSC and HGSC are two different diseases, not two types of the same disease. LGSC and serous borderline tumors are very similar and often exist together. The results of molecular pathology and immunohistochemistry showed that most of the primary lesions of HGSC came from the fimbria of the fallopian tube and had the trend of early intraperitoneal diffusion. The latest viewpoint is that HGSC from the fallopian tube or peritoneum was identified as the same disease as traditional ovarian HGSC in the past, and HGSC from the fallopian tube, peritoneum, or ovary should be collectively referred to as "pelvic HGSC" [3–5]. The gross pathology of HGSC can be divided into four types: (1) mainly cystic, the cystic fluid is serous, turbid and bloody fluid, unilocular or multilocular, fragile and soft, and papillary nodule protruding to the cystic cavity; (2) mixed solid and cystic; (3) completely solid, hemorrhage, and necrosis are common; (4) and completely exophytic (serous surface carcinoma), the ovary is normal or partially replaced by tumor tissue. The typical gross pathological manifestation is solid and cystic mass with hemorrhage and necrosis. The tumor tissue is soft and fragile, and bilateral and surface involvement is common. In most cases, the fimbria of the fallopian tube is involved at the same time, so it is impossible to distinguish between the fallopian tube and the ovarian mass. The greater omentum can be diffusely involved, with "omental cake" sign or diffuse nodules. At the same time, the peritoneum is often involved, with peritoneal implantation and metastasis.

The typical imaging features of ovarian serous tumors are bilateral, unilocular, or bilocular, mainly cystic tumors. The cystic fluid density shows watery density on CT, low signal on T1WI, and high signal on T2WI of MRI. The tumor can be evaluated in detail from the following signs: (1) bilaterality: about 58–67% of patients are bilateral ovarian masses [6]. Bilateral ovarian mass is an important sign of serous adenocarcinoma. (2) Size and morphology: the diameter of serous adenocarcinoma is usually less than 10 cm. The tumor size of HGSC is about 3–16 cm, with an average of about 8.8 cm. The tumor is usually irregular (81%). (3) Texture: according to the amount of solid components of the tumor, it can be divided into cystic (solid $\leq 1/3$), solid and cystic ($1/3 < \text{solid} < 2/3$), and solid (solid $>2/3$). (4) Mural nodules: mural nodules are typical imaging features of epithelial tumors. Mural nodules of HGSC can be endogenous or exogenous nodules growing outside the ovarian surface. The size of mural nodules is 0.2–4.5 cm, with an average of 1.2 cm [7]. Most of them are connected to the cyst wall with a wide base, and the surface is irregular. (5) Cyst wall and septation: it is generally believed that thin wall and fine septation (≤ 3 mm) are the characteristics of benign tumors, and the irregular thickening of cyst wall and septation (>3 mm) should consider the possibility of malignancy. (6) On contrast-enhanced images, the cystic dominant tumors are significantly enhanced by mural nodules, while the solid dominant tumors are homogeneously or unevenly enhanced of the solid part of the tumor. (7) Concomitant signs: ascites can occur in about 30% of cases, lymphadenopathy (30%), and peritoneal metastasis (20%). Peritoneal metastasis is typically manifested as a cake-like soft tissue mass between the transverse colon and the anterior abdominal wall or behind the anterior abdominal wall, which is corresponding to the greater omentum. (8) Others: intraperitoneal dissemination. In mild cases, the edge of the intestinal loop is blurred. In severe cases, irregular soft tissue masses or nodules can be seen in the abdominal cavity, which can be seen in various parts of the abdominal cavity, such as the rectouterine pouch, vesicouterine pouch, paracolic gutter, etc. Calcified metastasis: the upper abdomen is found on the edge of the liver and spleen, and the abdominal pelvic cavity is found at the peritoneum or greater omentum. The incidence of calcified metastasis is about 6%. Other metastases, such as bone metastasis, are generally osteolytic bone destruction.

20.3 Differential Diagnosis

The typical ovarian serous adenocarcinoma is characterized by irregular solid and cystic mass, which is not difficult to diagnose. When the tumor is multilocular cystic, it should be differentiated from benign serous and mucinous cystadenoma. The boundary of serous cystadenoma is generally round or oval, the cyst wall and septation are thin, and the enhancement is not significant after contrast enhancement, while serous adenocarcinoma generally has an uneven thickness of cyst wall and septation, which can be irregularly thickened locally, and the enhancement is significant after contrast enhancement and irregular shape in most cases. The vast majority of mucinous cystadenomas are thin-walled and multilocular, and the tumors are often huge. The cystic fluid density is higher and more uneven than that of serous tumors, and the grandson cysts within the daughter cysts can be seen. The latter is only found in mucinous cystadenomas, which is a characteristic manifestation. Endometriotic cysts are unilocular or multilocular. Multilocular cysts often show that the daughter chamber is located around the main chamber, the cyst wall is often blurred and thick, the cyst fluid density is often high, and sometimes higher density of fresh hemorrhage in the cyst fluid can be seen. MRI shows a high signal on T1WI and T2WI, and the cyst wall is usually not enhanced after contrast enhancement. When the tumor is bilateral, it needs to be differentiated from metastases. Bilaterality is also an important hint sign of metastases. The morphology of metastases at different primary tumor sites is changeable, and some imaging signs are helpful for diagnosis. For example, Krukenberg tumor is typically bilateral, solid masses with heterogeneous signals on T2WI. Metastatic tumors of colon cancer are usually bilateral cystic tumors with solid components of different sizes. Metastases from the appendix are often bilateral ovarian mucinous tumors with pseudomyxoma peritonei. Metastases of breast cancer usually are bilateral small solid lesions. Hematological diseases usually involve both ovaries and are characterized by homogeneous solid masses. Clinical and imaging features should be considered when distinguishing primary tumors from metastases.

References

1. Matulonis UA, Sood AK, Fallowfield L, Howitt BE, Sehouli J, Karlan BY. Ovarian cancer. Nat Rev Dis Primers. 2016;2:16061.
2. Kaldawy A, Segev Y, Lavie O, Auslender R, Sopik V, Narod SA. Low-grade serous ovarian cancer: a review. Gynecol Oncol. 2016;143(2):433–8.
3. Kim J, Park EY, Kim O, Schilder JM, Coffey DM, Cho CH, Bast RC Jr. Cell origins of high-grade serous ovarian cancer. Cancers (Basel). 2018;10(11):433.
4. Carlson JW, Miron A, Jarboe EA, et al. Serous tubal intraepithelial carcinoma: its potential role in primary peritoneal serous carcinoma and serous cancer prevention. J Clin Oncol. 2008;26(25):4160–5.
5. Salvador S, Gilks B, Köbel M, et al. The fallopian tube: primary site of most pelvic high-grade serous carcinomas. Int J Gynecol Cancer. 2009;19(1):58–64.
6. Amante S, Santos F, Cunha TM. Low-grade serous epithelial ovarian cancer: a comprehensive review and update for radiologists. Insights Imaging. 2021;12(1):60.
7. Sahin H, Akdogan AI, Smith J, Zawaideh JP, Addley H. Serous borderline ovarian tumours: an extensive review on MR imaging features. Br J Radiol. 2021;94(1125):20210116.

21 Ovarian Mucinous Adenocarcinoma

Shulei Cai

21.1 Clinical History

Female patient, 57 years old, had abdominal distention for 6 months and was found to have a pelvic mass for 1 week. CT showed a giant solid and cystic mass in the abdominal and pelvic cavity. CT diagnosis: ovarian cystadenocarcinoma is possible. Serum CA125: 176.8 U/mL, CA199: 1000 U/mL. Physical examination on admission: a giant mass was palpated in the middle of the pelvic cavity, which reached the anterior axillary line on both sides and the upper boundary reached three fingers above the navel. The mass was hard and had good mobility without tenderness.

MRI showed a giant oval multilocular cystic mass in the pelvic cavity, with clear boundary and a size of 20.5 cm × 10.8 cm × 20.6 cm. The mass demonstrated predominantly low signal on T1WI (Figs. 21.1–21.3) and high signal on T2WI (Figs. 21.4–21.9), although signal intensity varied on both sequences depending on the protein content of mucinous material. Solid components showed intermediate signal intensity. The thick septation and solid components showed significant enhancement after contrast enhancement (Figs. 21.10–21.12). There was no obvious effusion in the pelvic cavity and no obvious enlarged lymph nodes.

She underwent transabdominal hysterectomy, bilateral salpingo-oophorectomy, pelvic lymph node dissection, and greater omentum resection. Intraoperatively, the uterus was in neutral position, irregular in shape, with a size of 6 cm × 5 cm × 4 cm, and a nodule with a diameter of 2 cm was observed on the posterior wall of the uterus. The size of the left ovary was 2 cm × 1 cm × 1 cm, and no obvious abnormality was observed. A cystic mass with a diameter of 20 cm was found in the right ovary, with a small break on the surface. No obvious abnormality was found in the right fallopian tube.

Postoperative pathological result: (1) moderately differentiated mucinous adenocarcinoma of the right ovary; (2) uterine leiomyoma

S. Cai (✉)
Department of Radiology, Obstetrics and Gynecology Hospital, Fudan University, Shanghai, People's Republic of China

G. Zhang (ed.), *MRI of Gynaecological Diseases*, https://doi.org/10.1007/978-981-99-3644-1_21

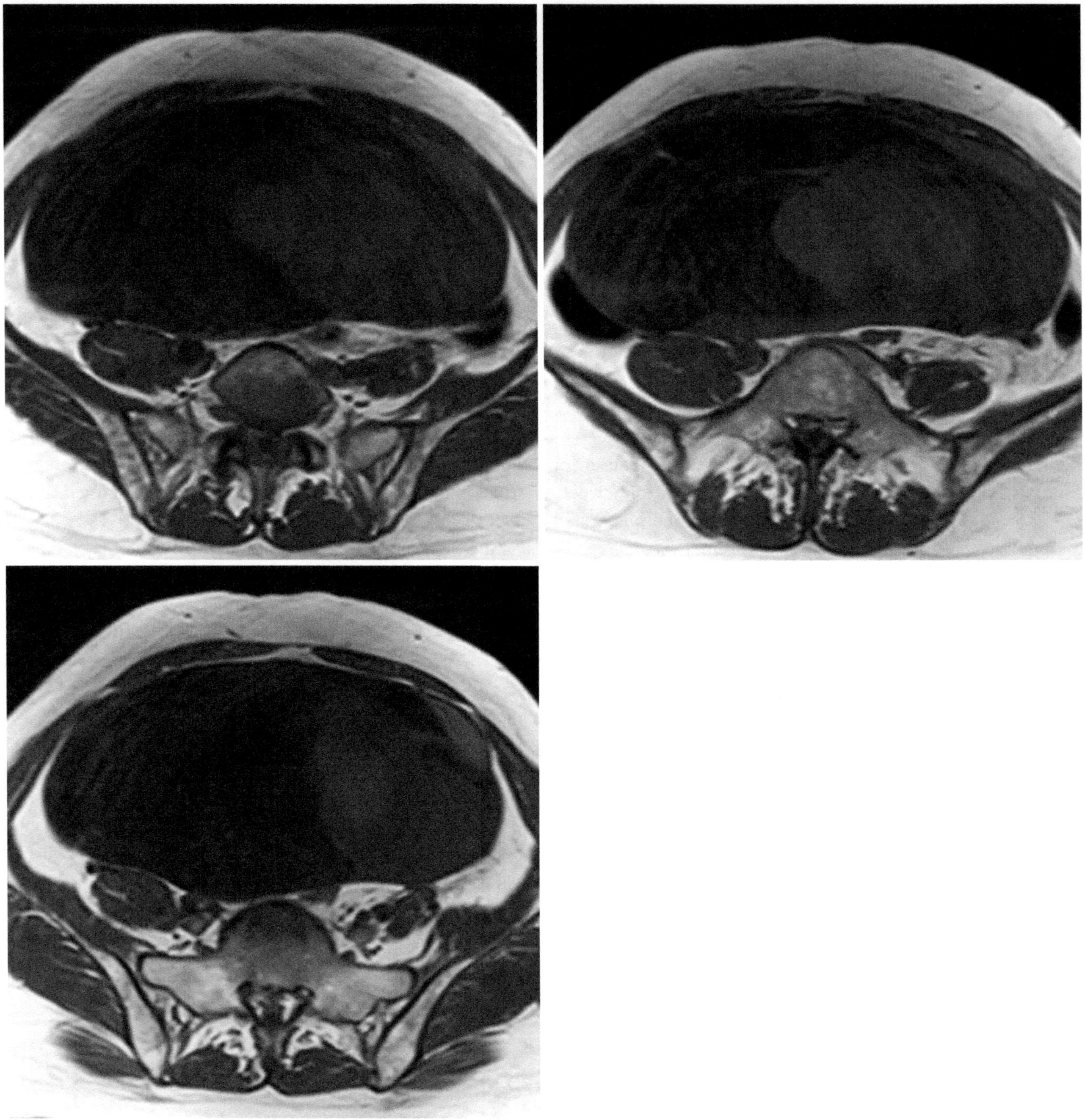

Figs. 21.1–21.3 Axial T1-weighted images showed that the cystic fluid was mainly low signal, and the local area was slightly high signal, and the signal was uniform

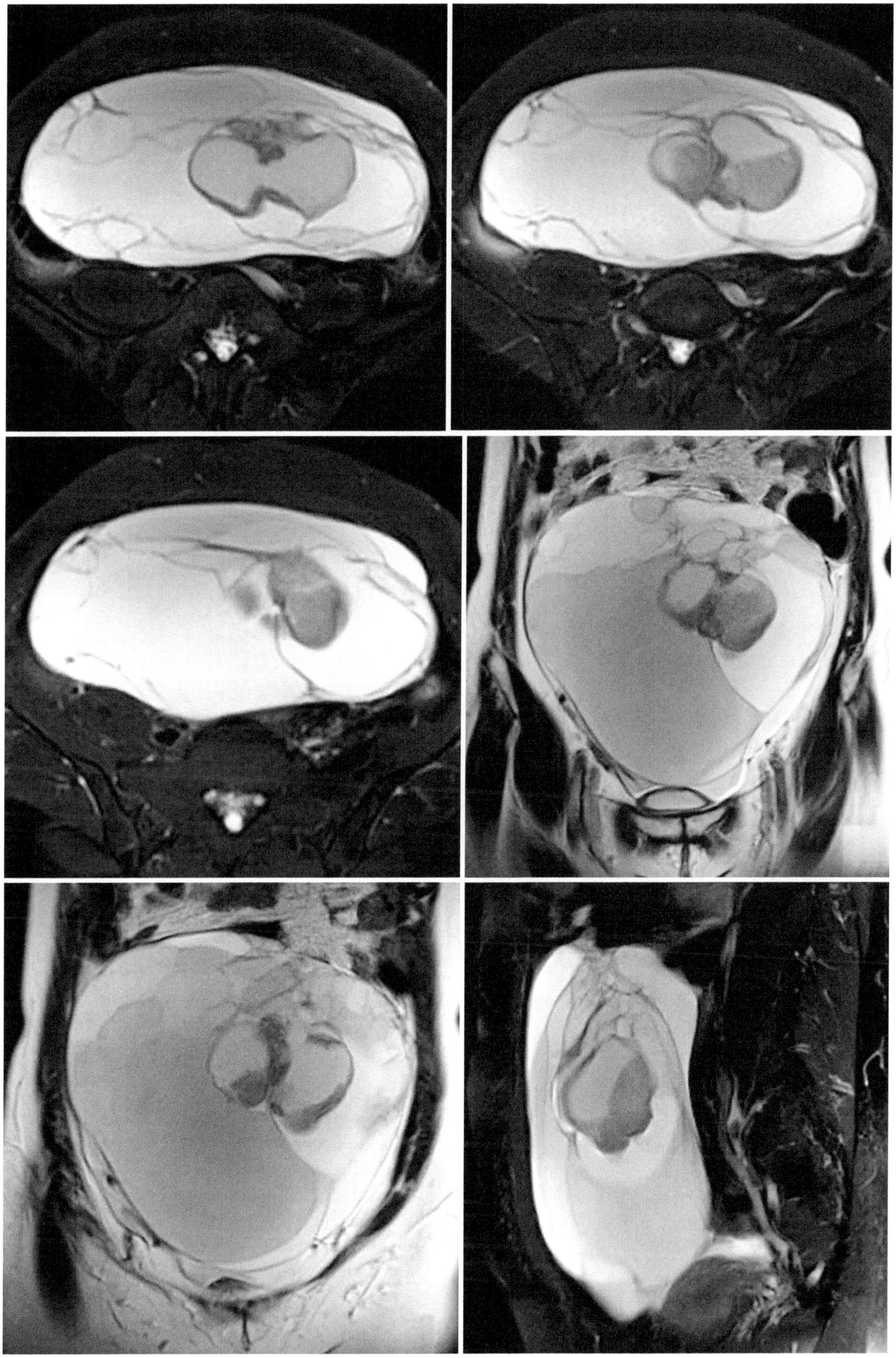

Figs. 21.4–21.9 Axial, coronal, and sagittal fat-suppressed T2-weighted images showed a giant multilocular cystic mass in the pelvic cavity, and the signal of adjacent chambers was different. The local cystic wall thickening showed isohypointensity

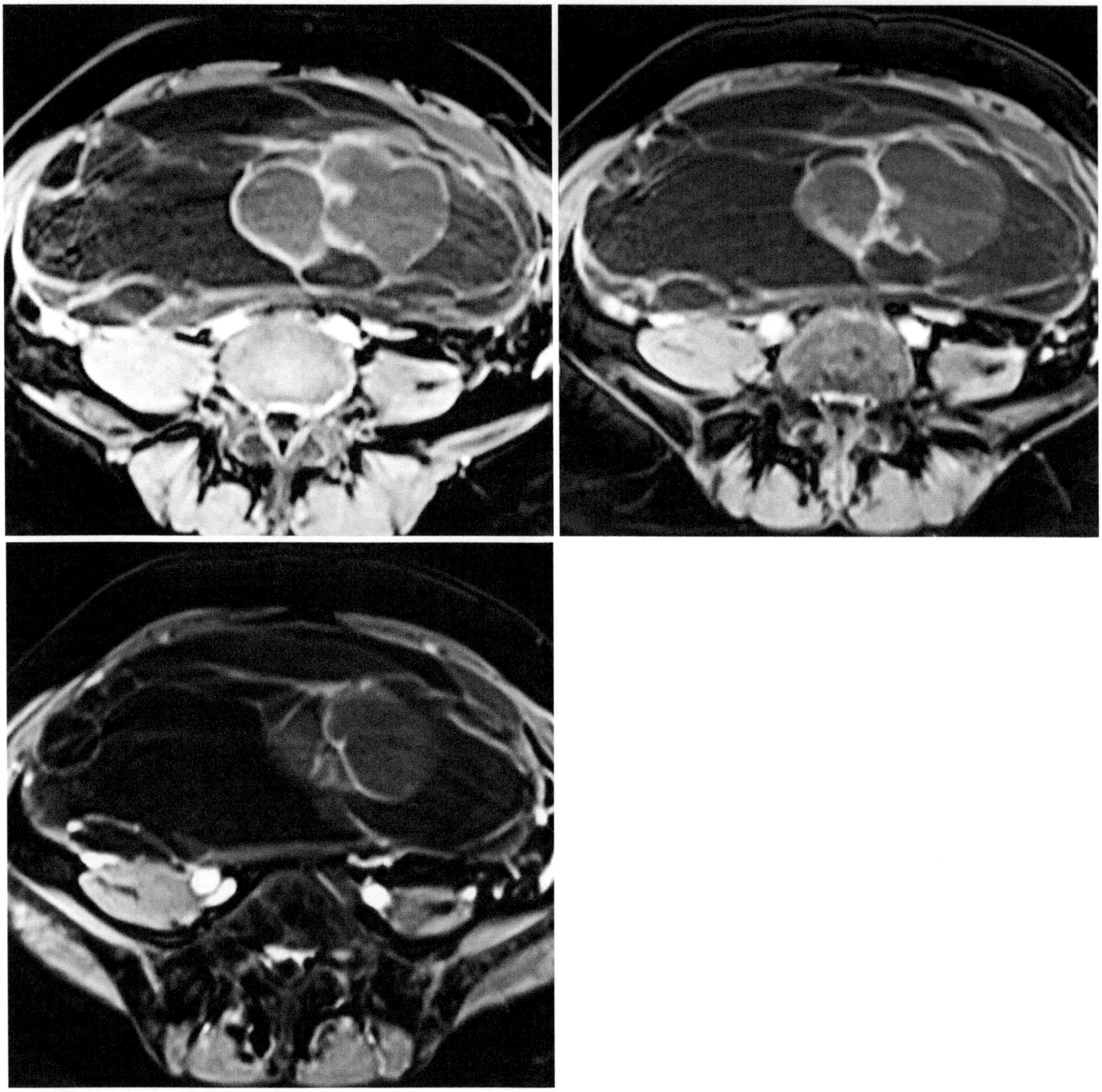

Figs. 21.10–21.12 The thick septation and solid components showed significant enhancement on contrast-enhanced fat-suppressed T1-weighted images

21.2 Imaging Analysis

Mucinous neoplasm is the second most common epithelial neoplasm of ovary, accounting for about 31%. According to histological features, they are classified as benign (23%), borderline (4%), and malignant (4%) [1, 2]. Compared with serous carcinoma, mucinous adenocarcinoma is more common in women before the age of 50 and occasionally in adolescents [3]. Compared with serous carcinoma, 55–63% of tumors belong to Stage I and have a better prognosis. If the tumors belong to Stage III or above, the prognosis is poor [1, 3]. The typical gross pathological manifestations are large multilocular cystic masses; solid areas and intracystic nodules are more common than cystadenomas and borderline tumors, and completely solid is rare [1, 2].

Compared with serous tumors, ovarian mucinous tumors are more common unilaterally, and typical MRI findings are multilocular cystic masses. The cystic fluid of each chamber shows different signal intensity on T2WI due to different mucus, hemorrhage, and protein content, that is, the so-called "stained glass" sign [3]. T1WI showed low, equal, and high mixed signals, and the cystic septation is irregularly thickened, with moderate to significant enhancement after contrast enhancement. This case was a multilocular cystic mass with a maximum diameter of 20.5 cm. The cystic fluid presented varying degrees of hyperintensity on T2WI, which is typical of mucinous tumors. The isohypointensity was dominant on T1WI, and slightly hyperintensity could be seen locally. However, multilocular cystic masses with irregular thickening of cyst wall and septation or presence of soft tissue components are highly suggestive of malignancy. Papillary mural nodules are typical of epithelial neoplasms. Mucinous neoplasms can also be seen, often in solid tissue, and rarely exist alone. A very few mucinous adenocarcinomas appear completely solid.

The rupture of cystic fluid can lead to pseudomyxoma peritonei [4], which is characterized by the presence of a large number of mucinous substances in the abdominal cavity. CT or MR images show irregularly localized or compartmented fluid in the abdominal cavity, with or without peritoneal or omental deposition. Ascites may give the liver a scalloping appearance. Pseudomyxoma peritonei was previously thought to be caused by mucinous adenocarcinoma of the ovary or rupture of the borderline tumor. In recent years, clinicopathological, immunohistochemical, and molecular studies have shown that pseudomyxoma peritonei is mostly derived from the appendix, while ovarian mucinous tumors are caused by peritoneal implantation secondary to the appendix tumor [5].

21.3 Differential Diagnosis

Benign ovarian mucinous cystadenoma is a multilocular cystic mass with thin cyst wall and septation, which is not difficult to distinguish from mucinous adenocarcinoma. Ovarian mucinous adenocarcinoma is mainly differentiated from metastatic mucinous adenocarcinoma. In clinical practice, metastatic tumors are more common than primary mucinous adenocarcinoma. Metastatic tumors are mostly from the gastrointestinal tract, appendix, and cervix, among which colon and rectum are the most common. The CT and MRI features of ovarian metastasis of colorectal cancer are very similar to those of ovarian mucinous adenocarcinoma, both of which are unilocular cystic or multilocular cystic masses with varying degrees of solid components [6]. Pathological comparison showed that cystic components were related to mucus secretion and necrosis. The differentiation of the two should be comprehensively judged in combination with clinical, immunohistochemical, and imaging.

References

1. Buy JN. Gynecological imaging. 2012. https://doi.org/10.1007/978-3-642-31012-6.394-397.
2. McCluggage WG. Morphological subtypes of ovarian carcinoma: a review with emphasis on new developments and pathogenesis. Pathology. 2011;43(5):420–32.
3. Schiavone MB, Herzog TJ, Lewin SN, et al. Natural history and outcome of mucinous carcinoma of the ovary. Am J Obstet Gynecol. 2011;205(480):e1–8.
4. Kim SH. Radiology illustrated gynecologic imaging. 2012
5. Jung ES, Bae JH, Lee A, Choi YJ, Park JS, Lee KY. Mucinous adenocarcinoma involving the ovary: comparative evaluation of the classification algorithms using tumor size and laterality. J Korean Med Sci. 2010;25(2):220–5.
6. Marko J, Marko KI, Pachigolla SL, Crothers BA, Mattu R, Wolfman DJ. Mucinous neoplasms of the ovary: radiologic-pathologic correlation. Radiographics. 2019;39(4):982–97.

22 Ovarian Endometrioid Adenocarcinoma

Fenghua Ma

22.1 Clinical History

Female patient, 32 years old, with abdominal distension for 2 days and pelvic mass found for 12 days. Abdominal distension was found in recent 2 months, occasionally bilateral pain in the lower abdomen, without abnormal vaginal discharge. Ultrasound examination in another hospital showed that cervical multilocular cyst; cystic mass in the left adnexa area, about 85 mm*55 mm in size; and ovarian cystadenoma were considered. She came to the outpatient clinic of our hospital, and the ultrasound re-examination showed a mixed mass in the left adnexa area, 91 mm × 89 mm × 76 mm in size, and ovarian cyst was considered. She was admitted to our hospital for treatment of ovarian tumor. Examination of serum tumor markers: CA125: 68.96 U/mL, CA199: 25.7 U/mL. Physical examination on admission: a 10 cm mass was palpable at the top of the vagina, with tough texture, moderate mobility, and no tenderness.

MRI examination: In the pelvic cavity, there was a rounded, unilocular cystic mass with regular boundary and 10 cm × 12 cm × 9 cm in size. Multiple mural nodules with different sizes were found. The larger mural nodules showed isointensity on T1WI (Figs. 22.1–22.3) and heterogeneous hyperintensity on T2WI (Figs. 22.4–22.8). The cystic part showed hyperintensity on both T1WI and T2WI. After contrast enhancement (Figs. 22.9–22.12), solid mural nodules were moderately homogeneously enhanced. There was no obvious effusion in the pelvic cavity and no obvious enlarged lymph nodes.

After admission, laparoscopic total hysterectomy, bilateral salpingo-oophorectomy, pelvic lymph node and para-aortic lymph node dissection, and greater omentum resection were performed. Intraoperative findings: the uterus was found in anterior position, 5 cm × 5 cm × 4 cm in size, with regular shape. The left ovary showed solid and cystic enlargement, about 9 cm × 9 cm × 8 cm in size, with smooth surface, dense adhesion to the lateral peritoneum and the posterior lobe of the left broad ligament, and normal morphology of the left fallopian tube. The right ovary was 3 cm × 2 cm × 2 cm in size, with normal morphology; corpus hemorrhagicum could be seen on the surface, and the right fallopian tube was with normal morphology. Scattered miliary lesions were seen in the peritoneum of the left vesicouterine pouch, and there were no abnormalities in the liver, spleen, stomach, and intestine. There was no obvious effusion in the pelvic cavity. Postoperative pathological result: (1) Endometrioid adenocarcinoma of the left ovary is grade II, originating from endometrioid cyst; (2) right periovaritis; (3) uterine localized adenomyosis. Immunohistochemical results: CK7(+), P63(+), VIH(+), PAX-8(+), ER(75%+), PR(85%+), Ki-67(5%+), P53(+), WT1(−).

F. Ma (✉)
Department of Radiology, Obstetrics and Gynecology Hospital, Fudan University, Shanghai, People's Republic of China

G. Zhang (ed.), *MRI of Gynaecological Diseases*, https://doi.org/10.1007/978-981-99-3644-1_22

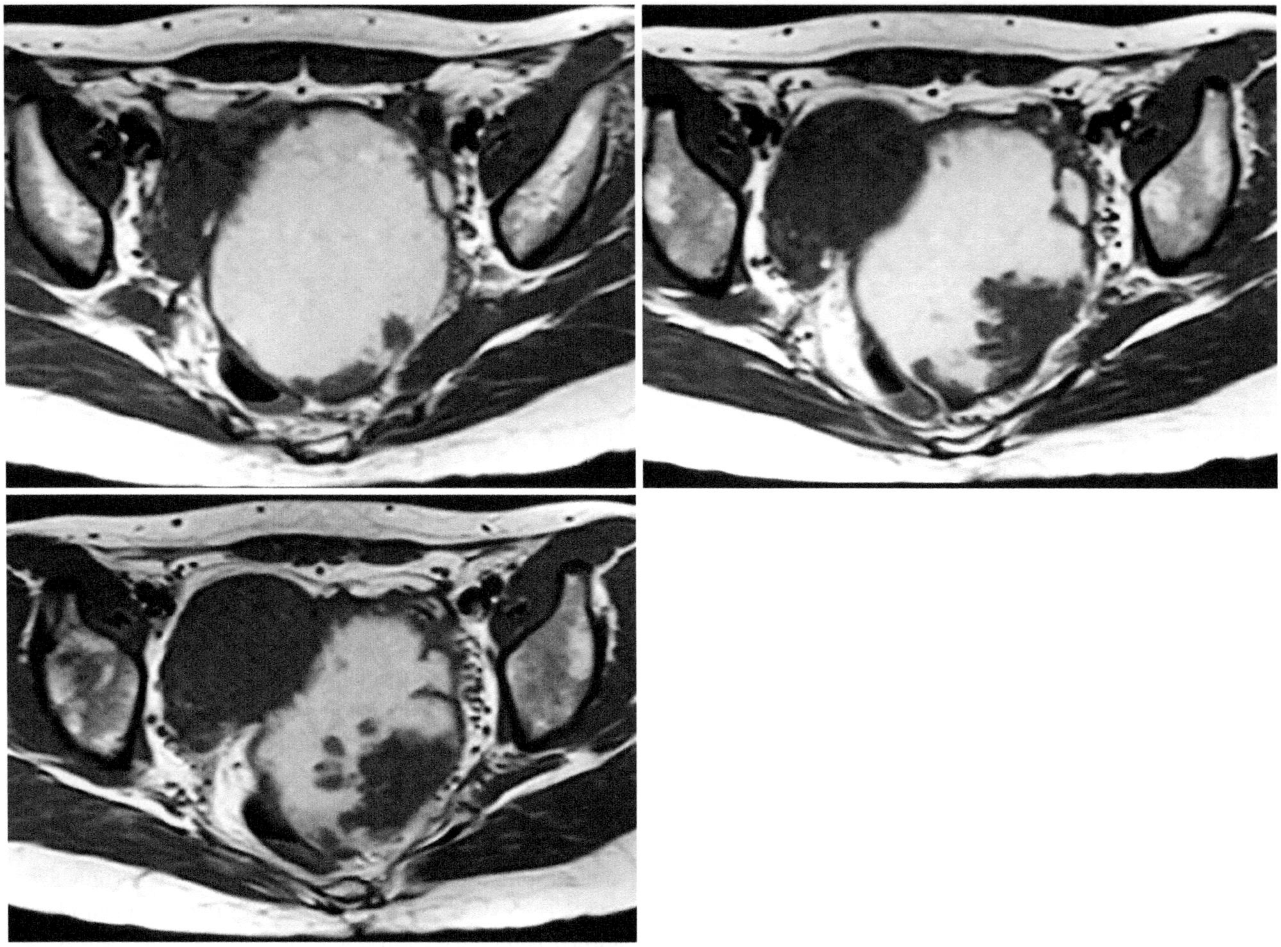

Figs. 22.1–22.3 Axial pre-contrast T1WI: There was a rounded cystic mass in the left adnexa area. Multiple mural nodules of different sizes were seen with iso-signal intensity, and the cystic fluid showed high signal intensity

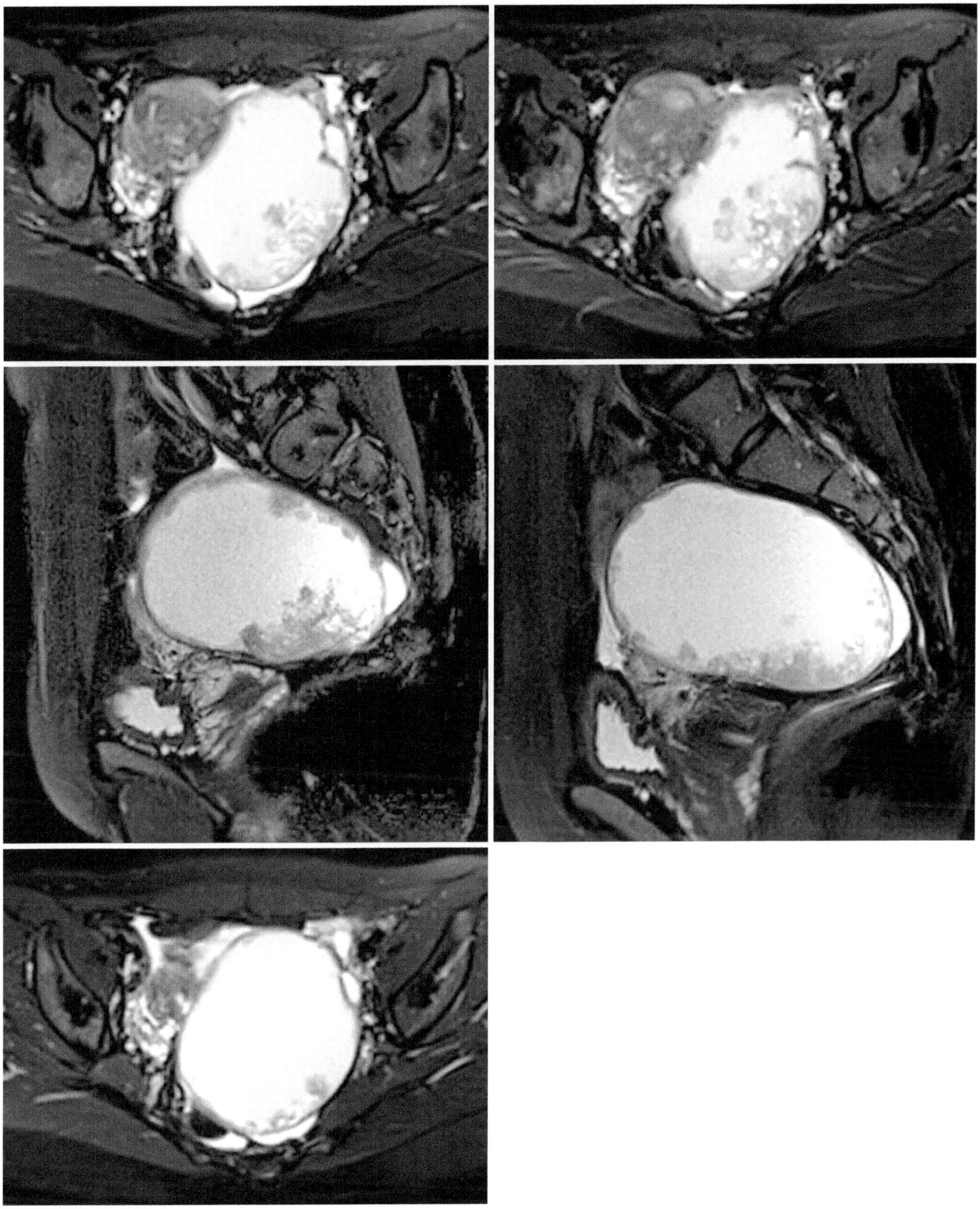

Figs. 22.4–22.8 Axial and sagittal T2WI: mural nodules showed heterogeneous hyperintensity, and the cystic fluid also showed hyperintensity

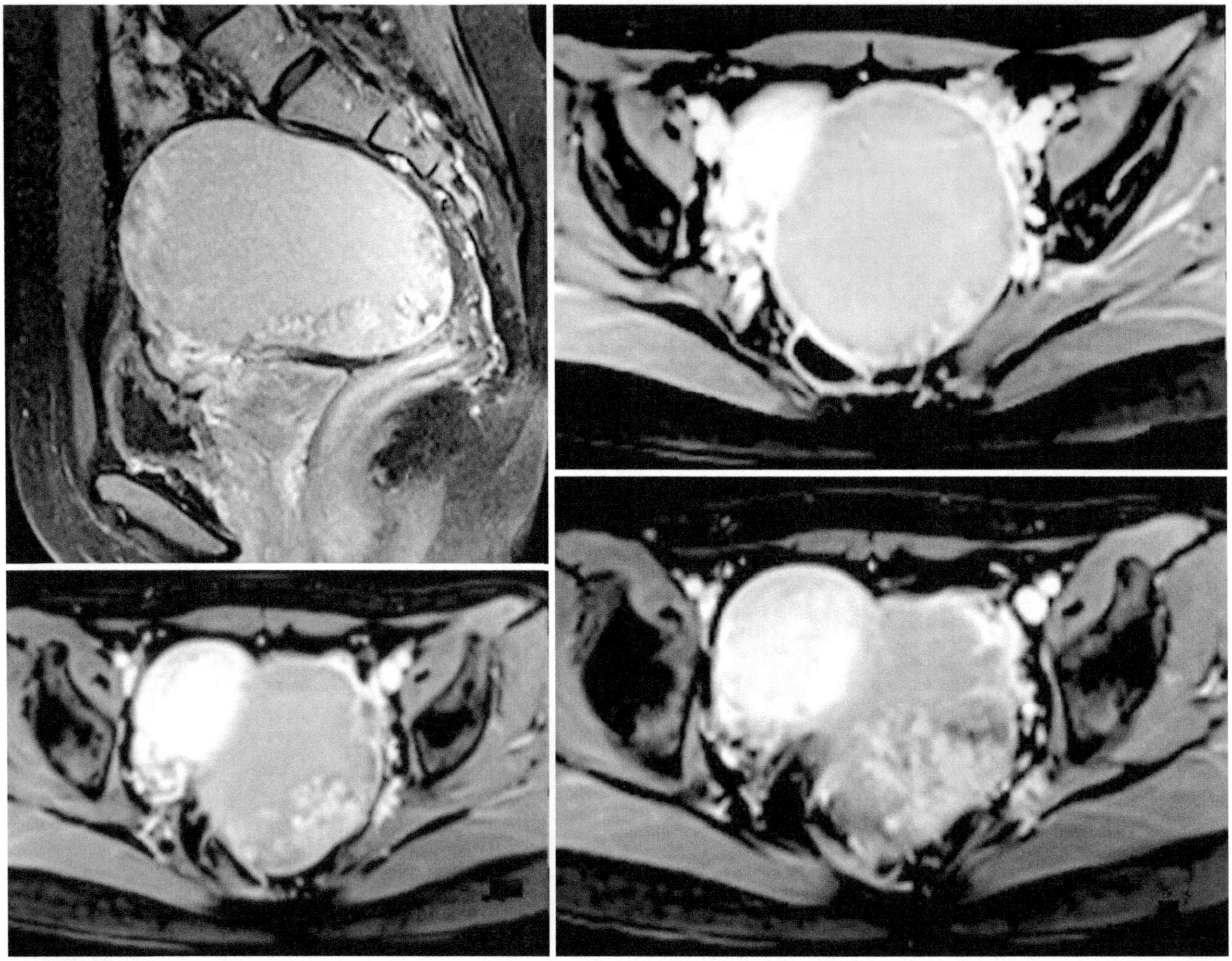

Figs. 22.9–22.12 Sagittal and axial T1WI contrast-enhanced images: mural nodules were significantly enhanced

22.2 Imaging Analysis

Ovarian endometrioid tumors are tumors that occur in the ovary, have epithelial cells, and their growth structures are similar to common and neoplastic hyperplasia of the endometrium. 75% of ovarian endometrioid tumors are malignant, and benign and borderline tumors are rare. Recent studies have shown that the incidence of ovarian endometrioid adenocarcinoma may have been overestimated, because tumor previously diagnosed as high-grade, advanced-stage ovarian endometrioid carcinoma is actually serous carcinoma. Nevertheless, ovarian endometrioid carcinoma is still the second most common ovarian malignant tumor after serous carcinoma, accounting for approximately 6% of all ovarian epithelial tumors [1]. About 15–20% cases are accompanied by low-grade endometrial carcinoma. Compared with serous carcinoma, endometrioid carcinoma is often detected earlier, with 36–67% of cases are stage I or II [2, 3].

The onset age of ovarian endometrioid carcinoma ranges from 8 to 86 years old, and it is most common in middle-aged and elderly women aged 50–60 years old. Carcinoma originating from endometriosis tends to occur in younger women, 5 to 10 years earlier than those not associated with endometriosis. Common clinical symptoms include abdominal distension, abdominal mass, menstrual disorders with abnormal vaginal bleeding, etc. The gross pathology presents a solid and cystic mass; the surface of most is smooth, round, or irregular shape and may have residual foci of endometriosis [4]. 60–90% of the cases are unilateral, solid, and cystic mass; the solid part of which is soft, brittle, and prone to hemorrhage, with papillary or nodular projections in the cystic cavity filled with thin or bloody fluid. When complicated with endometriosis, viscous chocolate-like liquid can be seen in the cystic cavity, and solid nodules on the local cyst wall reflect the malignant growth of the tumor. Sometimes the tumor is solid with much hemorrhage or necrosis. Microscopically, similar to endometrial carcinoma, there are many histologic types: (1) Well-differentiated type: irregular glands and dense glandular cavities are predominant, the adenoid structure is tubular or papillary, and the glands are round, oval, or irregular, the glandular epithelium is stratified, with a small amount of mitotic figures, and 30–50% were accompanied by squamous differentiation (2). Moderately differentiated type: the glands are irregular in shape, with non-squamous solid growth components ranging from 5% to 60% and increased mitotic figs [3]. Poorly differentiated type: glandular structure is rare; tumor cells proliferate in large numbers, forming diffuse lamellar mass and increased mitotic figures.

Compared with other ovarian malignant tumors, ovarian endometrioid carcinoma has no specific imaging features and consists mainly of two types: (1) mixed solid and cystic masses (solid predominant mass and cystic predominant mass with solid component or mural nodules) and (2) solid tumors with extensive hemorrhage or necrosis. Complicated with endometriosis is a good indication. In histopathology, ovarian endometrioid adenocarcinoma complicated with endometriosis is about 15–20%. Tanaka et al. [4] have shown that ovarian endometrioid carcinoma is the most common histological type of epithelial carcinoma originating from endometriotic cysts, and the patients complicated with endometriosis have a relatively older onset age, and the diameter of the cyst is usually >10 cm. Contrast-enhanced examination is helpful to distinguish clots and mural nodules in the cyst. Primary endometrial carcinoma is found in about 12% of patients with clinically diagnosed ovarian endometrioid carcinoma [5, 6]. Therefore, the identification of endometrial carcinoma complicated with ovarian endometrioid carcinoma with endometrial carcinoma metastasis to the ovary is often faced. The manifestations supporting primary endometrial carcinoma are as follows: (1) both sites show high-grade histological features; (2) bilateral ovarian tumors (only 13% of primary ovarian endometrioid carcinoma are bilateral masses); (3) the surface of the ovary, blood vessels, or the ovarian hilum is involved; (4) ovarian tumors show a multinodular growth pattern; and (5) absence of endometriosis. A summary analysis of 20 cases of ovarian endometrioid carcinoma by Li HM et al. [3] showed that 59% were ovoid masses, 68% were cystic with mural nodules, 33% were solid and cystic mixed masses, 9% were solid predominant masses, and about 50% were complicated with endometrial adenocarcinoma. For coexisting ovarian and uterine lesions, MRI plays an important role in displaying lesions and preoperative evaluation.

22.3 Differential Diagnosis

Because ovarian endometrioid carcinoma is mostly solid and cystic mass, it needs to be differentiated from clear cell carcinoma, metastatic colorectal cancer, granulosa cell tumor, and yolk sac tumor. Ovarian endometrioid carcinoma and clear cell carcinoma are the ovarian malignant tumors most closely related to endometriosis among epithelial cancers. Both of them can be presented as cystic tumors with mural nodules and accompanied by endometriosis. It is sometimes difficult to distinguish them. According to the literature, a unilocular cystic mass with single or multiple solid mural nodules of different sizes protruding into the cystic cavity is a typical sign of clear cell carcinoma [7, 8]. Manable et al. [8] compared the MR characteristics of ovarian endometrioid carcinoma and clear cell carcinoma and found that there were many imaging overlaps between them. After careful analysis, it was found that the growth mode of solid tissue of the former was centripetal pattern (multiple solid tissues grew along the cyst wall to the center of the cyst cavity), and the "an internal slit" sign appeared in the center of the cyst cavity during the growth process. However, the growth mode of the latter was mainly eccentric pattern (local solid tissue grew eccentrically to the cyst cavity), and solid nodules tend to be larger with internal cystic degeneration. Patients with ovarian metastasis from colorectal cancer often have clinical symptoms similar to those of primary ovarian tumors. In gross, it usually presents as bilateral ovarian cystic masses. Histologically, it closely resembles primary ovarian endometrioid carcinoma and mucinous adenocarcinoma [1, 9]. On both CT and MRI images, they are unilocular cystic or multilocular cystic masses, accompanied by varying degrees of solid components, and the solid components mainly show moderate enhancement (75%) [10]. Compared with pathology, cystic components are related to mucus secretion and necrosis. However, ovarian endometrioid carcinoma is mostly cystic tumor with multiple mural nodules, and the mural nodules show moderate or significant enhancement. Granulosa cell tumor and yolk sac tumor are both seen in adolescents and young women. Granulosa cell tumor causes clinical symptoms such as precocious puberty or abnormal menstruation due to the secretion of estrogen, and serum alpha-fetoprotein (AFP) does not increase. However, AFP is significantly increased in most patients with yolk sac tumor (AFP > 1000 mg/mL in young women, excluding liver lesions, which is suggestive).

References

1. Seidman JD, Horkayne-Szakaly I, Haiba M, et al. The histologic type and stage distribution of ovarian carcinomas of surface epithelial origin. Int J Gynecol Pathol. 2004;23:41–4.
2. Storey DJ, Rush R, Stewart M, et al. Endometrioid epithelial ovarian cancer: 20 years of prospectively collected data from a single center. Cancer. 2008;112:2211–20.
3. Li HM, Qiang JW, Xia GL, et al. Primary ovarian endometrioid adenocarcinoma: magnetic resonance imaging findings including a preliminary observation on diffusion-weighted imaging. J Comput Assist Tomogr. 2015;39:401–5.

4. Tanaka YO, Yoshizako T, Nishida M, et al. Ovarian carcinoma in patients with endometriosis: MR imaging findings. AJR Am J Roentgenol. 2000;175:1423–30.
5. Zaino R, Whitney C, Brady MF, et al. Simultaneously detected endometrial and ovarian carcinomas - a prospective clinicopathologic study of 74 cases: a gynecologic oncology group study. Gynecol Oncol. 2001;83:355–62.
6. Lim YK, Padma R, Foo L, et al. Survival outcome of women with synchronous cancers of endometrium and ovary: a 10 year retrospective cohort study. J Gynecol Oncol. 2011;22:239–43.
7. Matsuoka Y, Ohtomo K, Araki T, et al. MR imaging of clear cell carcinoma of the ovary. Eur Radiol. 2001;11:946–51.
8. Manable T, Hirose Y, Kiryun T, et al. Magnetic resonance imaging of endometrial cancer and clear cell cancer. J Comput Assist Tomogr. 2007;31:229–35.
9. Choi HJ, Lee JH, Lee JS, et al. CT findings of clear cell carcinoma of the ovary. J Comput Assist Tomogr. 2006;30:875–9.
10. Choi HJ, Lee JH, Seo SS, et al. Computed tomography findings of ovarian metastases from colon cancer: comparison with primary malignant ovarian tumors. J Comput Assist Tomogr. 2005;29(1):69–73.

23 Ovarian Clear Cell Carcinoma

Shulei Cai

23.1 Clinical History

Female patient, 60 years old, had been menopausal for 7 years, with a pelvic mass found on health checkup for 5 days. Serum CA125: 22.4 U/mL, CA199: 31.32 U/mL. Physical examination on admission showed that the hard mass in left adnexa area was about 4 months pregnant size. Ultrasound examination showed a giant solid and cystic mixed mass in abdominal and pelvic cavity, 15.3 cm × 13.7 cm × 11.1 cm in size, with dense punctate echoes inside. Irregular medium echo area with a size of 6.3 cm × 7.8 cm × 5.0 cm can be seen on the inner wall of the lesion, with abundant color blood flow, which was considered to be ovarian malignant tumor.

MRI showed the complex solid and cystic adnexal mass with thick walls, septation, and variable papillary projections (Figs. 23.1–23.3). The size of the lesion was 13 cm × 12 cm × 9 cm, with solid components showing low to intermediate signal (Figs. 23.4 and 23.5) and cystic components showing high signal on T2-weighted images (Figs. 23.6–23.8). On dynamic contrast-enhanced images (Figs. 23.9–23.12), the solid mural nodules were significantly enhanced. There was no obvious effusion in the pelvic cavity and no obvious enlarged lymph nodes.

She underwent transabdominal total hysterectomy, bilateral salpingo-oophorectomy, pelvic lymph node dissection, and greater omentum resection. The uterus was in anterior position, 4 cm × 4 cm × 3 cm in size, irregular in shape, and a protuberant nodule with a diameter of 1 cm could be seen on the posterior wall. Solid and cystic mass was seen in the left ovary, with a size of 20 cm × 19 cm × 15 cm. The appearance of left fallopian tube was normal. No abnormality was found in the right ovary and fallopian tube. No abnormality was found in the bladder and rectouterine pouch.

Postoperative pathological result: (1) Clear cell carcinoma of the left ovary, which originates from endometrioid cyst (2). Multiple intramural and subserosal leiomyomas.

S. Cai (✉)
Department of Radiology, Obstetrics and Gynecology Hospital, Fudan University, Shanghai, People's Republic of China
e-mail: gingerkite@126.co

G. Zhang (ed.), *MRI of Gynaecological Diseases*, https://doi.org/10.1007/978-981-99-3644-1_23

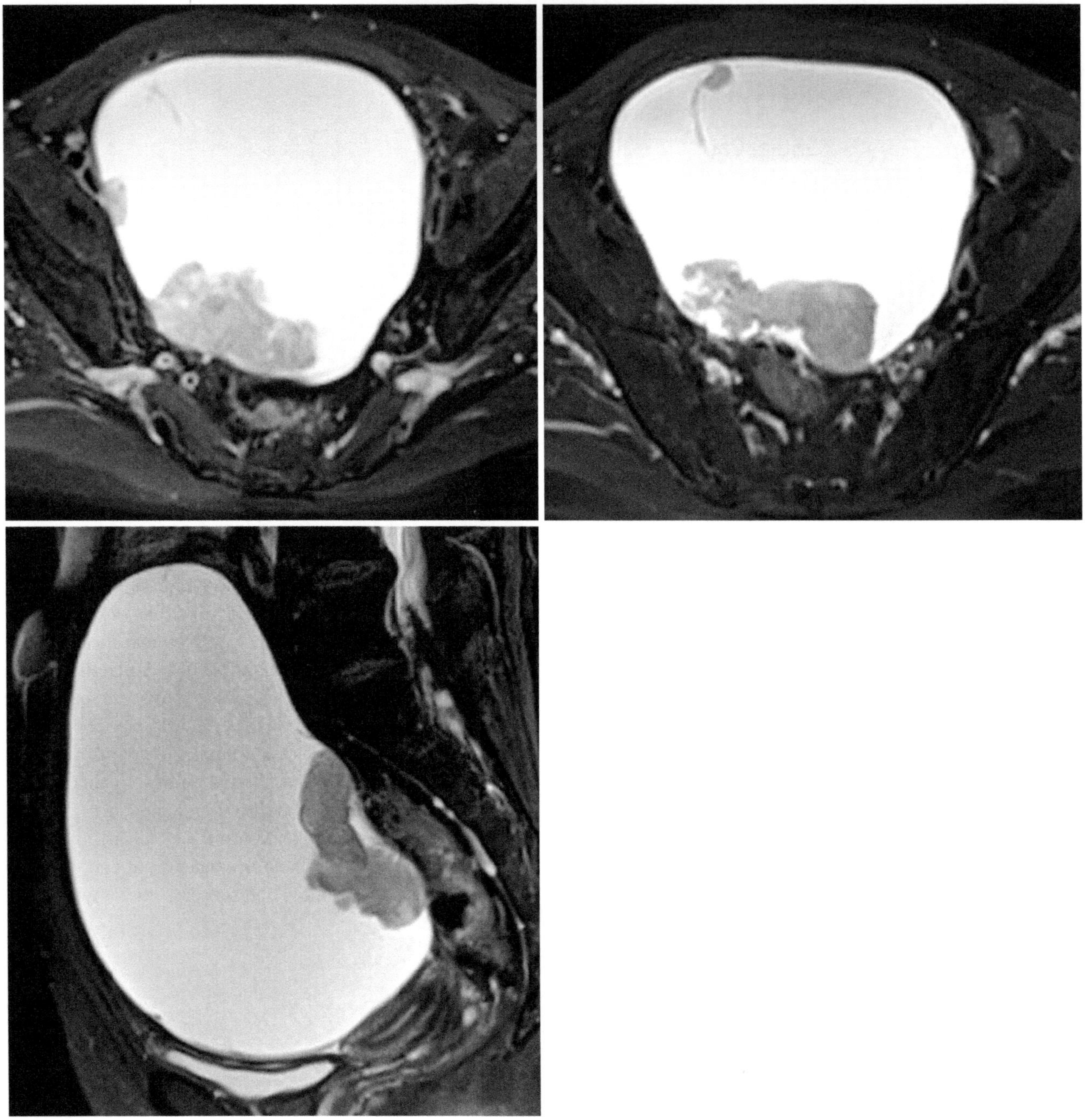

Figs. 23.1–23.3 Axial fat-suppressed T2WI; sagittal fat-suppressed T2WI. An oval unilocular cystic mass in the left adnexa area, with multiple mural nodules of varying sizes. The cystic fluid showed high signal intensity on T2WI and low signal intensity on T1WI. Mural nodules showed uniform and slightly high signal on T2WI, equal signal on T1WI, and punctate slightly high signal could be seen locally

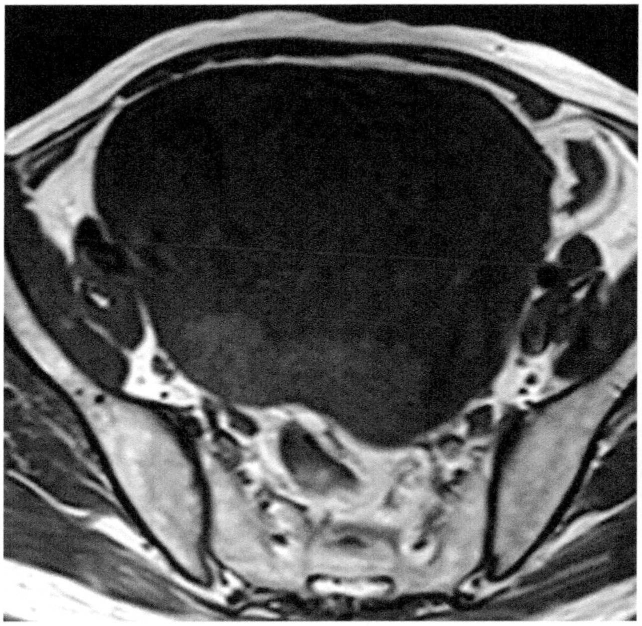

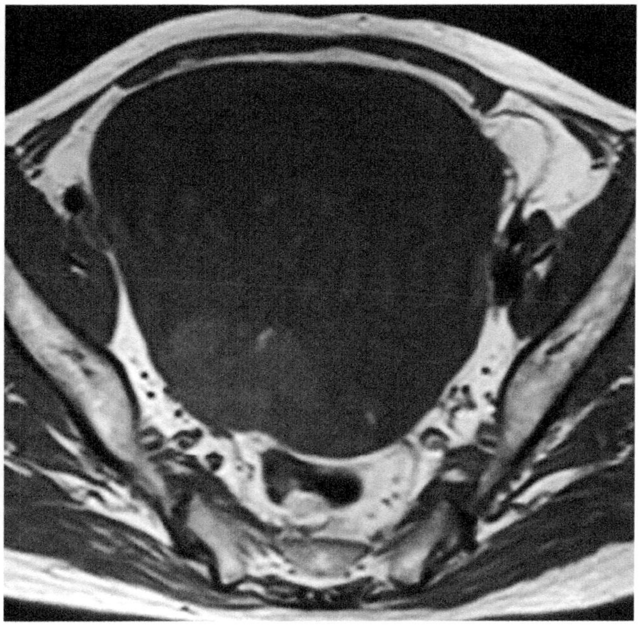

Figs. 23.4 and 23.5 Axial T1WI

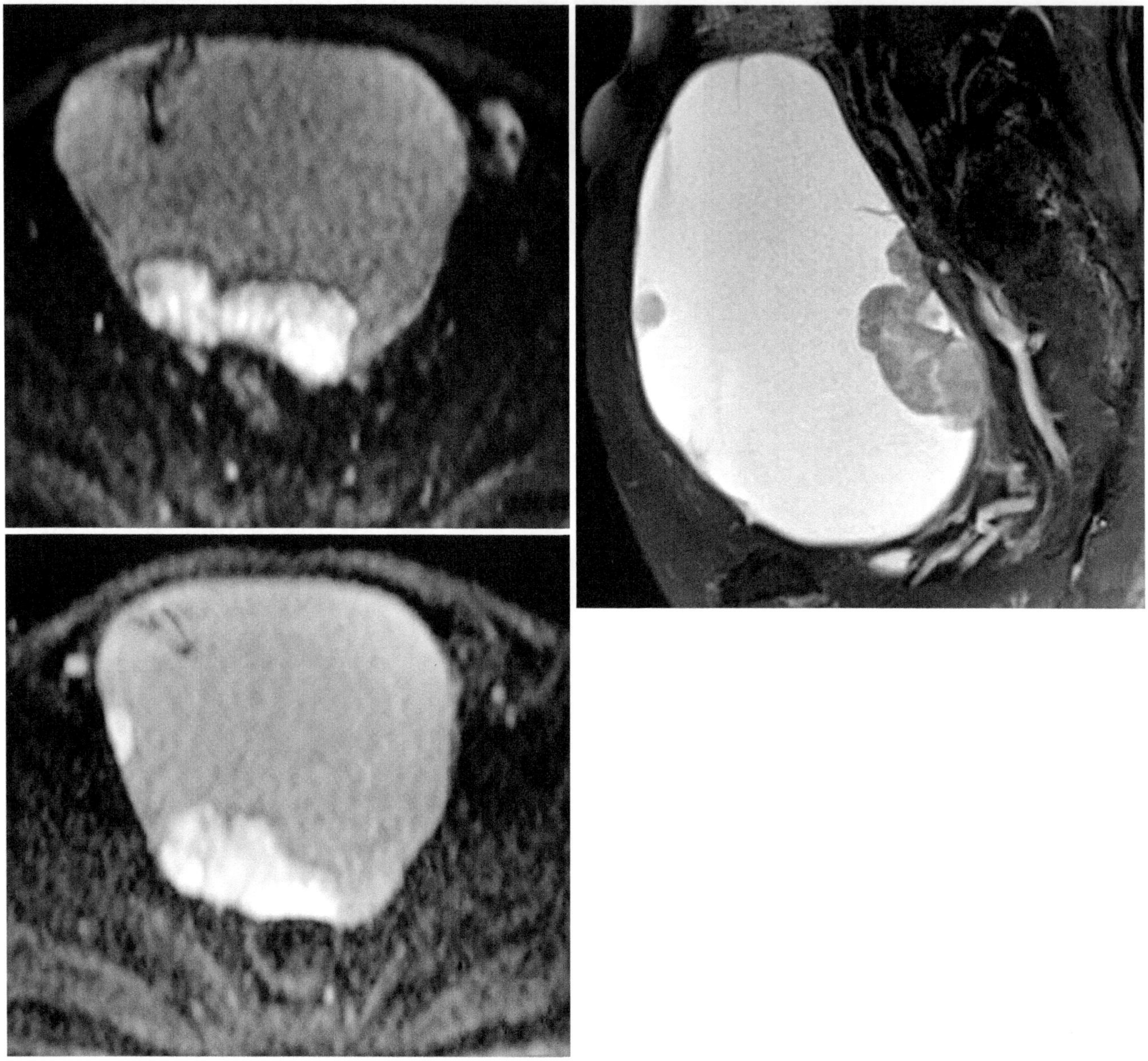

Figs. 23.6–23.8 Sagittal fat-suppressed T2WI. An oval unilocular cystic mass in the left adnexa area, with multiple mural nodules of varying sizes. The cystic fluid showed high signal intensity on T2WI and low signal intensity on T1WI. Mural nodules showed uniform and slightly high signal on T2WI, equal signal on T1WI, and punctate slightly high signal could be seen locally. On DWI, mural nodules showed high signal intensity

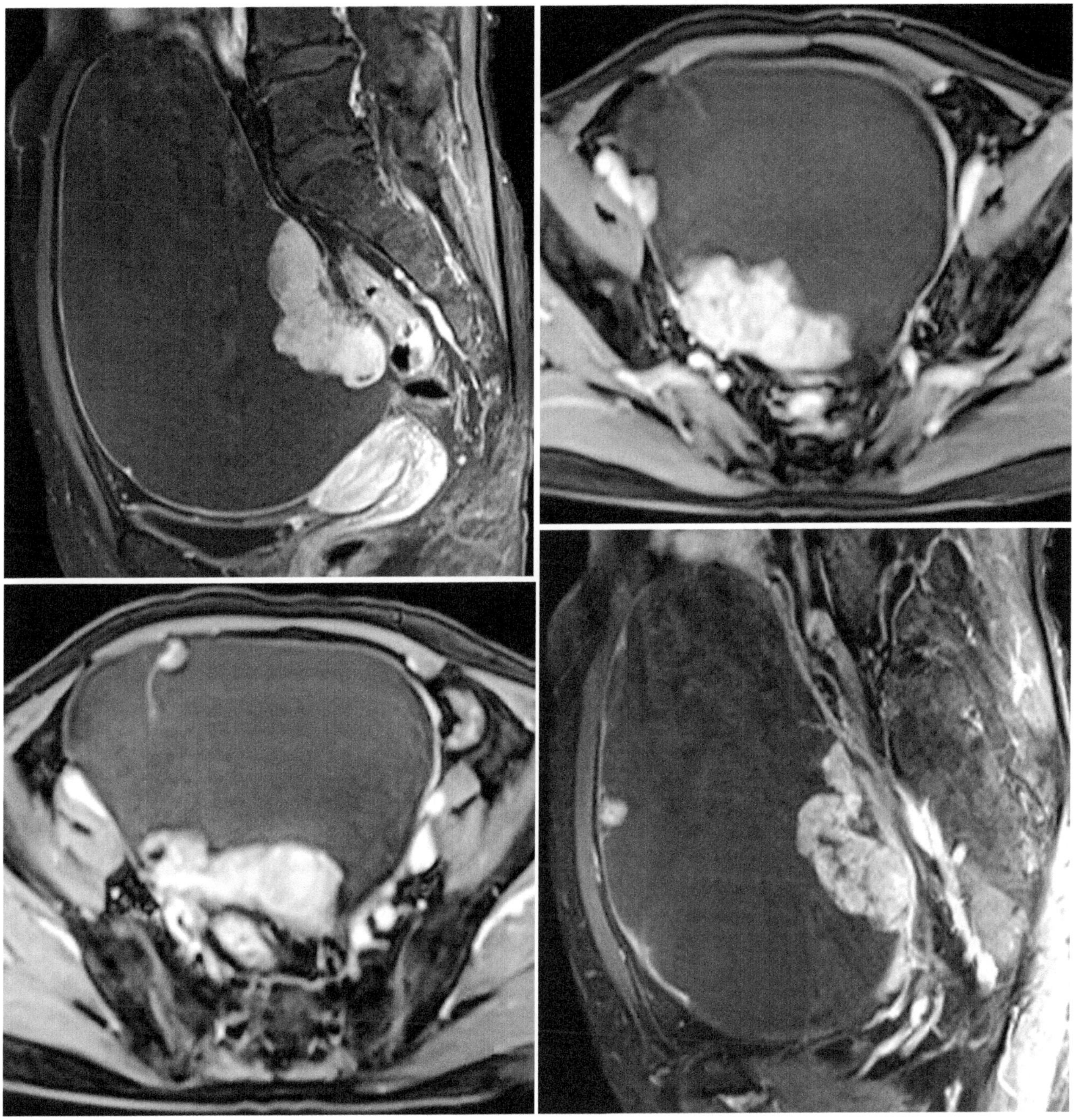

Figs. 23.9–23.12 Sagittal and axial T1WI fat-suppressed dynamic enhancement showed significant enhancement of mural nodules, and small patchy low enhancement areas were seen in larger mural nodules

23.2 Imaging Analysis

Clear cell carcinoma (CCC) is a special histological type of epithelial ovarian cancer, accounting for 5–25% of all epithelial ovarian tumors [1, 2], mainly composed of glycogen-rich clear cells and shoe nail-like cells. Most of the lesions are limited to ovary at the time of CCC diagnosis, and the FIGO stage mostly belongs to stage I–II [3, 4]. Clear cell carcinoma is similar to ovarian endometrioid carcinoma, often accompanied by endometriosis [3, 5, 6]. It has been reported to be associated with endometriosis up to 50–70%, and it is the tumor most closely related to endometriosis among ovarian epithelial tumors.

CCC is more common in perimenopausal or postmenopausal women, with the onset age ranging from 50 to 70 years, with an average age of 57 years. Clinical symptoms are nonspecific, often manifested as abdominal distension, abdominal pain, abdominal mass, or frequent urination.

Some patients have abnormal vaginal bleeding or discharge, and ascites are often complicated in the late stage. In gross pathology, the tumor diameter ranges from 4 cm to 25 cm, with an average diameter of 15 cm. The appearance is lobulated or round-like, solid, solid and cystic, or cystic. The solid part is fish flesh-like, brittle, or tough, often accompanied by hemorrhage or necrosis. The cystic part is unilocular or multilocular, with prominent stained yellow nodules in the capsule, and cyst cavity contains watery or myxoid and turbid bloody colloidal substances. The tumor with endometriosis contains chocolate-like brown fluid in cyst cavity.

Tumor morphology is an important sign for differentiating benign and malignant tumors. Benign tumors such as thecomas and fibromas are usually round-like or oval in shape, while most ovarian cancers are irregular in shape. Some researchers summarized and analyzed a group of CCC [5, 6]. The majority of CCC was oval (74%), and 81% was unilocular cystic, with single or multiple large solid mural nodules, and the maximum diameter of mural nodules was 5.06 ± 0.4 cm. 50–70% of CCC are complicated with pelvic or ovarian endometriosis. Therefore, CCC cystic fluid shows high density on CT and high signal on MRI T1WI due to periodic bleeding. The T1WI high signal of CCC cystic fluid accounts for about 50%. Matsuoka et al. [7] reported that 40% of CCC cystic fluid showed high signal on T1WI. Choi et al. [8] reported that the cystic fluid density of CCC was 13–34 HU, with an average of 24 HU, and considered that it was the result of tumor hemorrhage or necrosis, which may be the distinguishing point from other epithelial tumors such as serous adenocarcinoma, whose density is close to that of water. In terms of enhancement degree, CCC was mainly significantly enhanced (82%). Peritoneal implantation and massive ascites are rare in CCC. We speculate that the possible reason is that most of the lesions are limited to ovary at the time of CCC diagnosis, and FIGO stage mostly belongs to stage I–II, whereas peritoneal implantation and massive ascites are common signs of advanced ovarian cancer.

23.3 Differential Diagnosis

CCC is mostly cystic, so it is mainly differentiated from ovarian cystic tumors. On imaging, it should also be differentiated from non-epithelial tumors or tumor-like lesions: (1) Metastatic tumor: it often originates from gastrointestinal tract, breast, etc. Metastases from different primary sites have their own imaging characteristics [9, 10]. For example, Krukenberg tumor is typically characterized by bilateral, solid, and heterogeneous signals on T2WI. Metastases of colon cancer are usually bilateral cystic tumors with solid components of different sizes. Metastases from the appendix are usually bilateral ovarian mucinous tumors with pseudomyxoma peritonei. Metastases from breast cancer are usually bilateral small solid lesions. (2) Primordial germ cell tumors, such as yolk sac tumor and dysgerminoma, both of which have a relatively young age of onset and tend to occur in young women. The former is mostly single, large solid and cystic, or solid mass with hemorrhage and necrosis, with abundant blood supply. The "bright dot sign" is seen on contrast-enhanced CT, that is, the significantly enhanced small dot or tubular shadow inside the tumor, representing increased dilated blood vessels inside the tumor [11]. Simple dysgerminoma is mainly composed of solid components. On pre-contrast CT, it is an irregular lobulated slightly low-density soft tissue mass, while on contrast-enhanced image, the internal fibrovascular septation is significantly enhanced [12]. (3) Endometriosis cyst: unilocular or multilocular. Multilocular often shows that the daughter chamber is located around the main chamber, the cyst wall is often blurred and thick, the cyst fluid density is often high, and sometimes a higher density of fresh bleeding in the cyst fluid can be seen. MRI shows high signal intensity on T1WI and T2WI without obvious solid components, which is different from the significant enhancement of solid components in CCC.

References

1. Mccluggage WG. Morphological subtypes of ovarian carcinoma: a review with emphasis on new developments and pathogenesis. Pathology. 2011;43:420–32.
2. Mabuchi S, Sugiyama T, Kimura T. Clear cell carcinoma of the ovary: molecular insights and future therapeutic perspectives. J Gynecol Oncol. 2016;27(3):e31.
3. Rauh-Hain AJ, Winograd D, Growdon WB, et al. Prognostic determinants in patients with uterine and ovarian clear cell carcinoma. Gynecol Oncol. 2012;125:376–80.
4. del Carmen MG, Birrer M, Schorge JO. Clear cell carcinoma of the ovary: a review of the literature. Gynecol Oncol. 2012;126:481–90.
5. Okamoto A, Glasspool RM, Mabuchi S, Matsumura N, Nomura H, Itamochi H, Takano M, Takano T, Susumu N, Aoki D, Konishi I, Covens A, Ledermann J, Mezzanzanica D, Steer C, Millan D, McNeish IA, Pfisterer J, Kang S, Gladieff L, Bryce J, Oza A. Gynecologic cancer InterGroup (GCIG) consensus review for clear cell carcinoma of the ovary. Int J Gynecol Cancer. 2014;24(9 Suppl 3):S20–5.
6. Bulun SE, Wan Y, Matei D. Epithelial mutations in endometriosis: link to ovarian cancer. Endocrinology. 2019;160(3):626–38.
7. Matsuoka Y, Ohtomo K, Araki T, et al. MR imaging of clear cell carcinoma of the ovary. Eur Radiol. 2001;11:946–51.
8. Choi HJ, Lee JH, Lee JS, et al. CT findings of clear cell carcinoma of the ovary. J Comput Assist Tomogr. 2006;30:875–9.
9. Willmott F, Allouni KA, Rockall A. Radiological manifestations of metastasis to the ovary. J Clin Pathol. 2012;65:585–90.
10. Choi HJ, Lee JH, Kang S, et al. Contrast-enhanced CT for differentiation of ovarian metastasis from gastrointestinal tract cancer: stomach cancer versus colon cancer. Am J Roentgenol. 2006;187:741–5.
11. Kim SH. Radiology illustrated: Gynecologic imaging. (eBook). https://doi.org/10.1007/978-3-642-05325-2.
12. Guerriero S, Testa AC, Timmerman D, et al. Imaing of gynecological disease (6): clinical and ultrasound characteristics of ovarian dysgerimnoma. Ultrasound Obstet Gynecol. 2011;37:596–602.

24 Ovarian Dysgerminoma

Mengwei Zhang

24.1 Clinical History

Female patient, 29 years old, presented with a self-palpable lower abdominal mass for 4 months. CA125: 22.4 U/mL, CA199: 31.32 U/mL. Ultrasonography showed a huge solid and cystic mixed mass in the abdominal and pelvic cavity, 153 mm × 137 mm × 111 mm in size, with dense punctate echoes, irregular medium echoes of 63 mm × 78 mm × 50 mm on the inner wall, and abundant color blood flow, considering malignant tumor of ovarian origin.

She underwent transabdominal hysterectomy, bilateral salpingo-oophorectomy, pelvic lymph node dissection, and greater omentum resection. Intraoperative findings: the uterus was in anterior position, 4 cm × 4 cm × 3 cm in size, and irregular shape. The left ovary was with enlarged, 20 cm × 19 cm × 15 cm in size, solid and cystic, smooth surface, and the appearance of left fallopian tube is normal. No abnormality was found in the right ovary and fallopian tube. No abnormality was found in the bladder and rectouterine pouch.

Postoperative pathological result: left ovarian dysgerminoma.

MRI examination: an irregular lobulated solid mass was shown in the left adnexa area, 16 cm* 14 cm × 12 cm in size. It showed equal signal on T1WI (Figs. 24.1 and 24.2), slightly high signal on T2WI (Figs. 24.3–24.5), significantly high signal on DWI (Fig. 24.6), significantly reduced ADC value (Fig. 24.7), and mild uneven enhancement after contrast enhancement (Figs. 24.8 and 24.9).

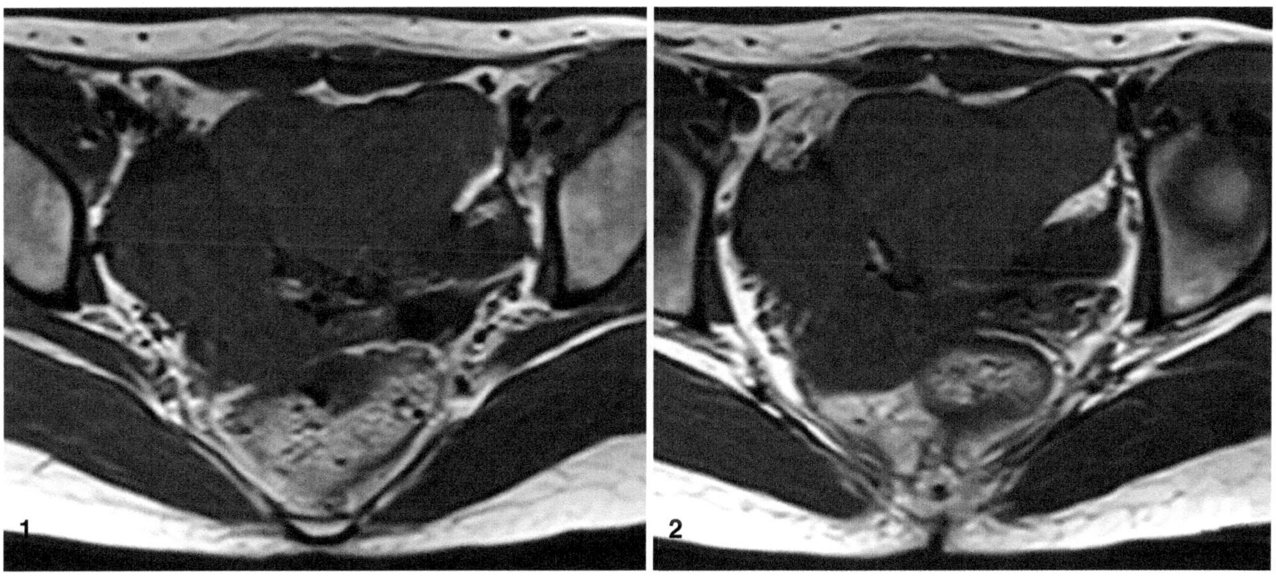

Figs. 24.1 and 24.2 Axial T1WI: An irregular solid mass was shown in the left adnexa area, with homogeneous and isointense signal

M. Zhang (✉)
Department of Radiology, Obstetrics and Gynecology Hospital, Fudan University, Shanghai, People's Republic of China

G. Zhang (ed.), *MRI of Gynaecological Diseases*, https://doi.org/10.1007/978-981-99-3644-1_24

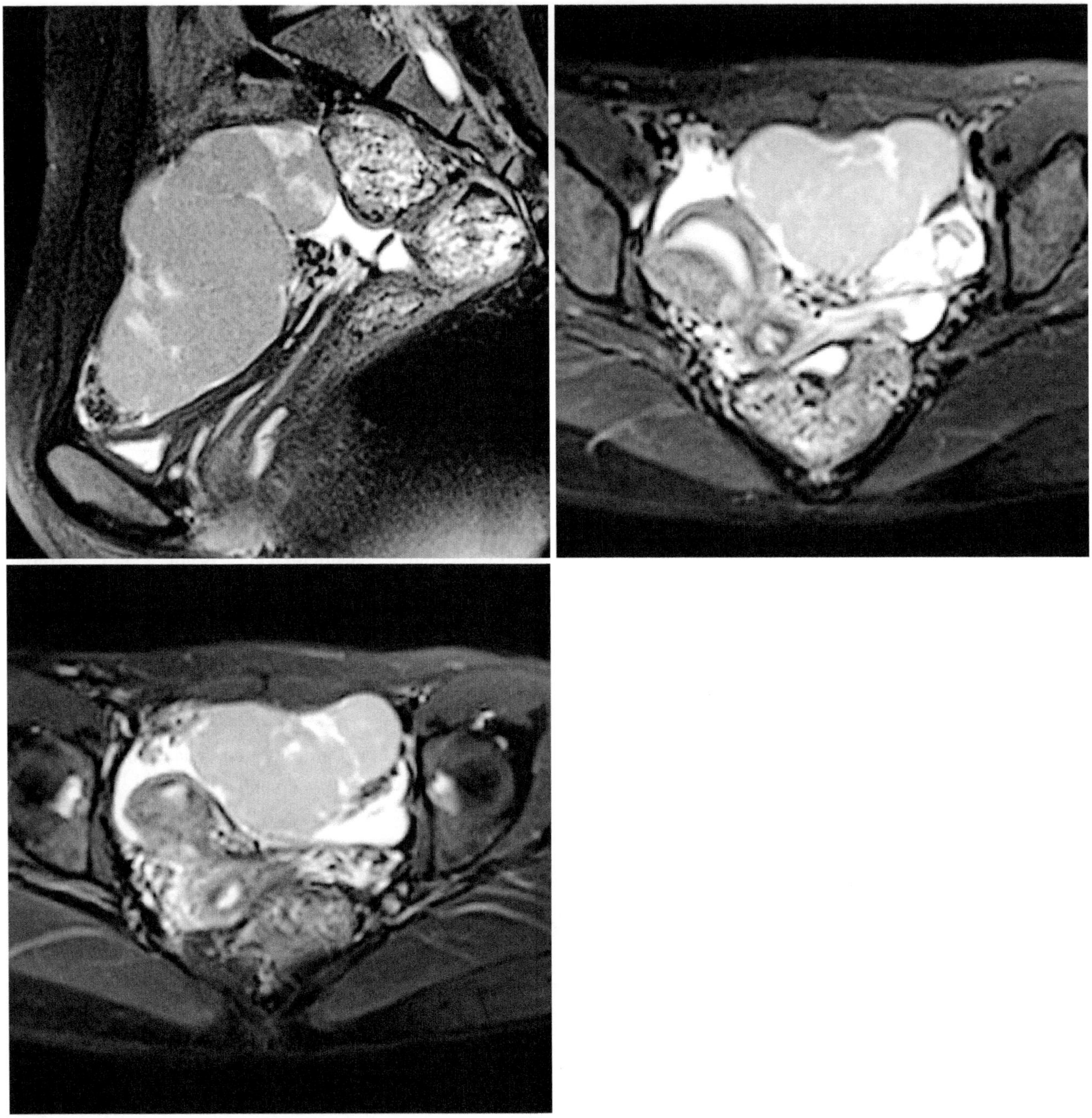

Figs. 24.3–24.5 Axial and sagittal T2WI: the mass was slightly high signal, the signal is homogeneous, with a slight patchy hyperintensity locally

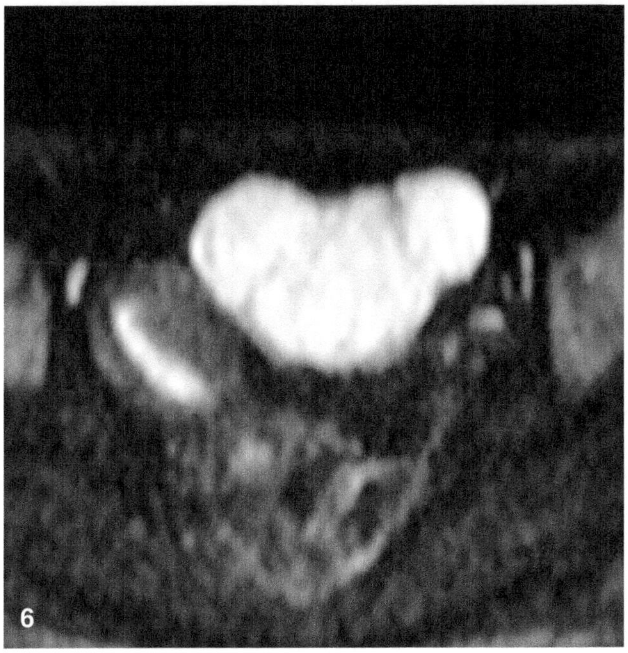

Fig. 24.6 DWI: The tumor showed significant high signal

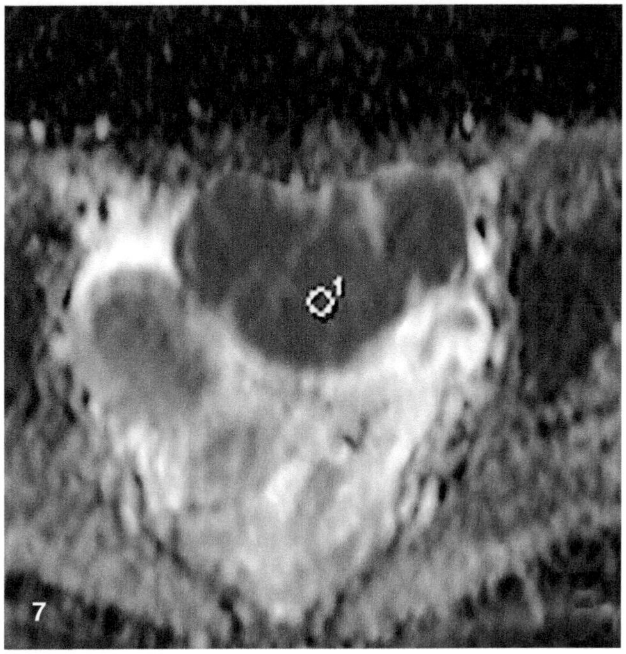

Fig. 24.7 ADC map: ADC map showed low signal, ADC value of the lesion = 0.770×10^{-3} mm^2/s

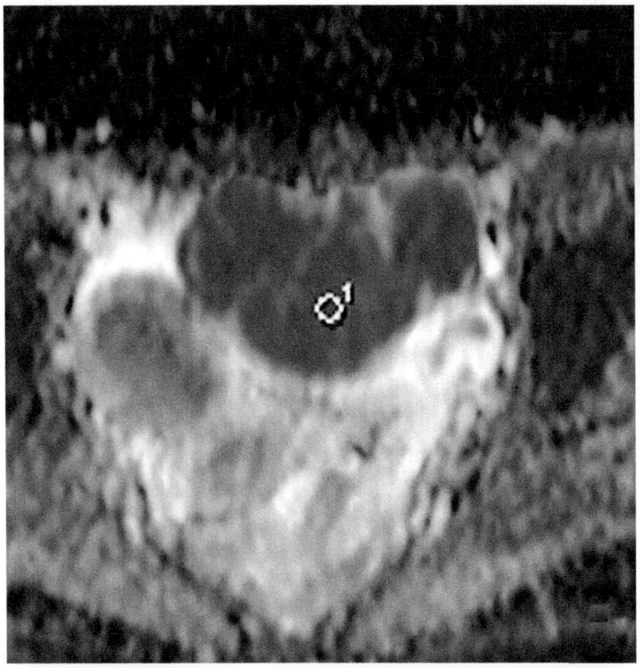

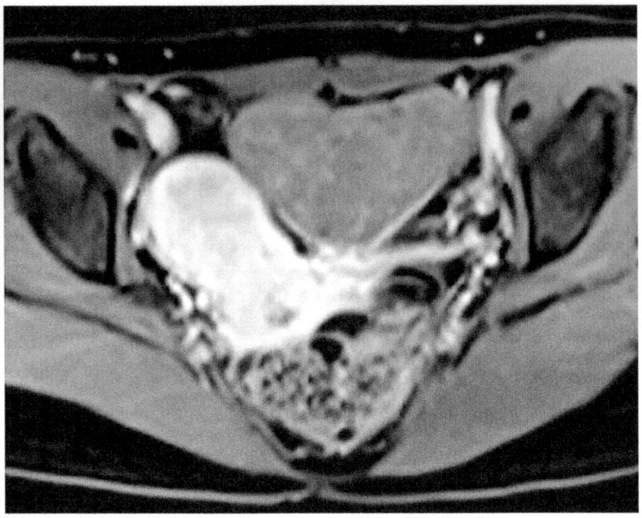

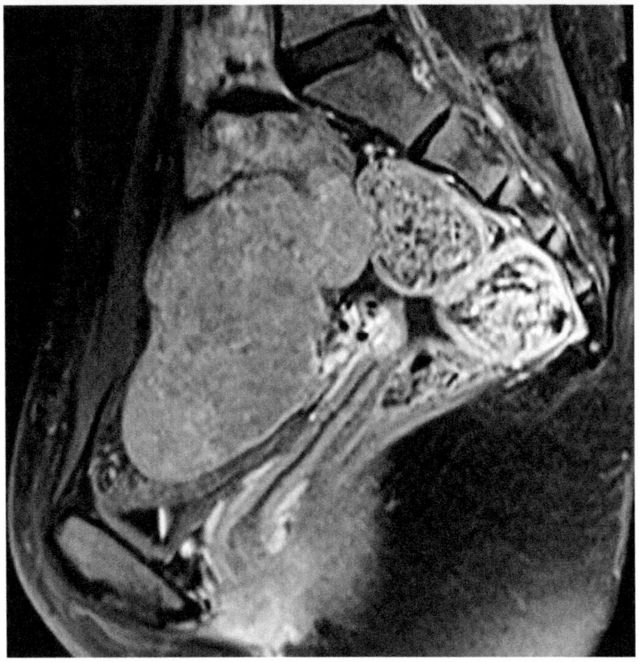

Figs. 24.8 and 24.9 Axial and sagittal contrast-enhanced T1WI, the lesion was mildly and uniformly enhanced

24.2 Imaging Analysis

Ovarian dysgerminoma is a neoplasm formed by abnormal hyperplasia of primordial germ cells, which corresponds to spermatogonia tumor of male [1]. The etiology is not clear, and it has been suggested by some researchers to be related to reproductive system malformations, which may be accompanied by bisexual reproductive system malformation [2]. It occurs in women of adolescence and childbearing age, and young women of 20–30 years old are the most common, accounting for about 75% [1].

Most patients have no obvious gynecological symptoms, and the most common clinical manifestation is abdominal mass, which can be accompanied by weight loss and occasionally with menstrual and endocrine abnormalities. Some patients are referred for primary amenorrhea. 95% of patients have elevated lactate dehydrogenase (LDH), alkaline phosphatase, alpha-fetoprotein (AFP), or β-hCG [3], and some patients have elevated CA125. Pathologically, it is divided into simple type and mixed type. The latter is often associated with endodermal sinus tumor or choriocarcinoma, which is mainly composed of round or polygonal tumor cells. The tumor cells are nest-like, strip-like, or diffuse growth, and large and uniform in size, abundant in cytoplasm, transparent, and nuclear mitotic figures are common, nucleolus can be seen, and vascular fibrous tissue hyperplasia and lymphocyte infiltration can be seen in the interstitium of tumor cells.

Ovarian dysgerminoma is usually unilateral; 5–10% is bilateral. The tumor is usually large in size, and the maximum diameter is often greater than 10 cm. Simple dysgerminoma is mainly composed of solid components and may be accompanied by varying degrees of cystic degeneration and necrosis. Ultrasonography shows mainly solid, lobulated, with multiple septation mass [4]. Pre-contrast CT shows irregular lobulated slightly low-density soft tissue mass, the solid area is slightly to moderately enhanced on contrast enhancement, and the internal fibrovascular septation is significantly enhanced. The increase of CT value is up to 14–40 HU, and some are combined with scattered spotted calcification. Typically, the mass is iso-low signal on T1WI, moderate, or high signal on T2WI. The fibrovascular septation is typically low signal on T1WI and T2WI, with significant enhancement after contrast enhancement, while enhancement of the tumor itself is weaker than that of the fibrovascular septation. Mixed type ovarian dysgerminoma mostly presents as solid and cystic mass, cystic necrosis is common, cystic wall and intracystic septation are with uneven thickness and unclear boundaries, ascites and lymph node metastasis are common, and cystic wall and intracystic septation show mild enhancement after contrast enhancement. The tumor is highly malignant and easy to relapse after surgery [5].

24.3 Differential Diagnosis

Ovarian dysgerminoma should be differentiated from the following solid predominant tumors: (1) Ovarian sex cord-stromal tumors: these are more common in perimenopausal women over 50 years old and are often associated with elevated estrogen and endometrial hyperplasia and may present as solid or solid and cystic masses characterized by a mild or moderate progressive enhancement of the solid part, but the boundary is more well-defined, and the T2WI low signal is characteristic. However, ovarian dysgerminoma is mostly lobulated solid mass, with significantly enhanced fibrovascular septation after contrast enhancement (2). Broad ligament or subserous leiomyoma: It can be seen in women of any age, with clear and well-defined boundary, iso-signal on T1WI, iso-hyposignal on T2WI, and significant homogeneous enhancement after contrast enhancement. Careful observation of the relationship between the mass and the uterus is generally not difficult to distinguish (3). Malignant epithelial tumors, such as ovarian serous adenocarcinoma, are usually associated with significantly elevated CA125, iso-signal on T1WI, slightly high signal on T2WI, irregular boundary, uneven signal, and obvious heterogeneous enhancement after contrast enhancement, and ancillary signs such as ascites, peritoneal lesions, enlarged lymph nodes, and so on are helpful for the diagnosis of ovarian cancer [6]. (4) Metastatic tumors, such as Krukenberg tumor, are usually solid, typically bilateral, lobulated, solid tumors that are low or high signal on T2WI due to edema, collagen reaction and mucus secretion, and heterogeneous enhancement after contrast enhancement [7].

References

1. Scully RE, Young RH, Clement PB. Tumors of the ovary, maldeveloped gonads, fallopian tubes and broad ligament, vol. 18. 3rd ed. Washington, DC: Armed Force Institute of Pathology; 1998. p. 239–312.
2. Buy JN, Ghossain M. Gynecological Imaging [OL]. 2013.
3. Pressley RH, Muntz HG, Falkenberry S, et al. Serum lactic dehydrogenase as a tumor marker in dysgerminoma. Gynecol Oncol. 1992;44:281–3.
4. Guerriero S, Testa AC, Timmerman D, et al. Imaging of gynecological disease (6): clinical and ultrasound characteristics of ovarian dysgerimnoma. Ultrasound Obstet Gynecol. 2011;37(5):596–602.
5. Alvarado CI, Valencia CR, Mohs AM, et al. Ovarian dysgerminoma associated with fifibrosarcoma: a case report. Int J Gynecol Pathol. 2011;30(5):466–9.
6. Carter JS, Koopmeiners JS, Kuehn-Hajder JE, et al. Quantitative multiparametric MRI of ovarian cancer. J Magn Reson Imaging. 2013;38:1501–9.
7. Jung ES, Bae JH, Lee A, et al. Mucinous adenocarcinoma involving the ovary: comparative evaluation of the classifification algorithms using tumor size and laterality. J Korean Med Sci. 2010;25(2):220–5.

25 Ovarian Granulosa Cell Tumors

Mengwei Zhang

25.1 Clinical History

Female patient, 32 years old, self-conscious abdominal bulge, and palpation of an abdominal mass for 2 weeks. She had lower abdominal pain, lumbar discomfort, which was aggravated by prolonged sitting or fatigue and relieved after rest. Ultrasonography revealed: an irregular space-occupying lesion with mixed echo was shown in the left posterior area of uterus, with a size of 150 mm × 98 mm × 69 mm and possible origin of ovary; the parenchymal structure of vesicouterine pouch was 28 mm × 21 mm × 21 mm, and enlarged ovary was possible; the deepest ascites was 67 mm. CA125: 479.6 U/mL, CA199: 8.55 U/mL.

She underwent laparotomy of total hysterectomy, bilateral salpingo-oophorectomy, pelvic lymph node dissection, greater omentum resection, partial sigmoid colon resection, middle and upper rectum resection, and low anastomosis.

Postoperative pathological results: (1) Malignant juvenile granulosa cell tumor of the right ovary with extensive dissemination of surrounding tissues (2). Malignant juvenile granulosa cell tumor was found on the serosal surface of part of the sigmoid colon and the middle and upper part of rectum.

MRI examination: A huge solid and cystic mixed mass was seen above the uterus in the pelvic cavity, which was mainly solid, with irregular shape and unclear boundary, and 16.1 cm × 10.6 cm × 9.6 cm in size. The solid part was isointense on T1WI (Figs. 25.1–25.3) and slightly hyperintense on T2WI (Figs. 25.4–25.9). After contrast enhancement, it was significantly heterogeneous enhanced and showed honeycomb-like change (Figs. 25.10–25.15). The cystic part showed hypointense on T1WI and hyperintense on T2WI. There was a moderate amount of effusion in the pelvic and abdominal cavity, and no obvious enlarged lymph nodes were noted. Part of the peritoneal thickening showed nodular and cake-like changes, which were significantly enhanced after contrast enhancement.

M. Zhang (✉)
Department of Radiology, Obstetrics and Gynecology Hospital, Fudan University, Shanghai, People's Republic of China

G. Zhang (ed.), *MRI of Gynaecological Diseases*, https://doi.org/10.1007/978-981-99-3644-1_25

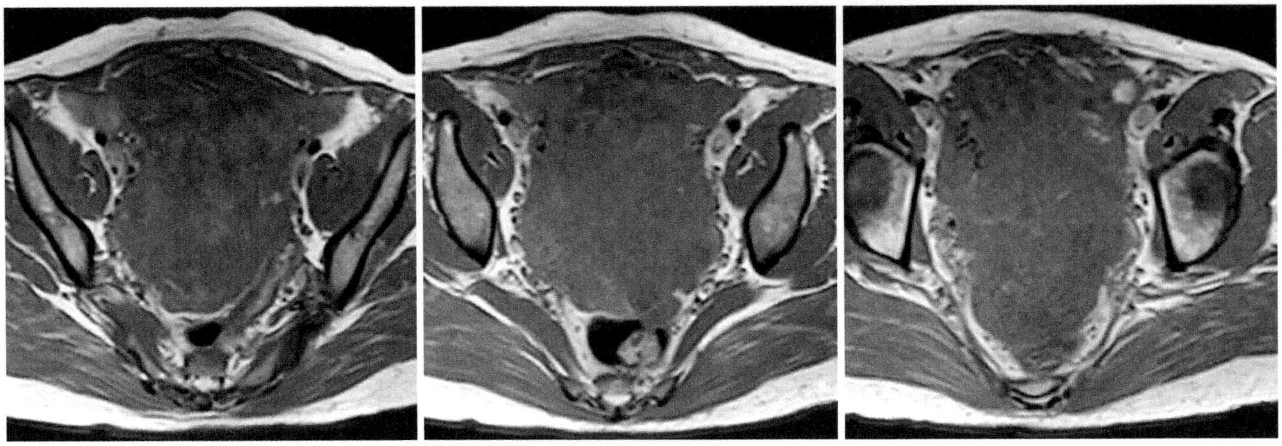

Figs. 25.1–25.3 Axial T1WI: A huge solid and cystic mixed mass was seen in the pelvic and abdominal cavity, which was mainly solid, showed isointense signal, and the signal intensity is homogeneous

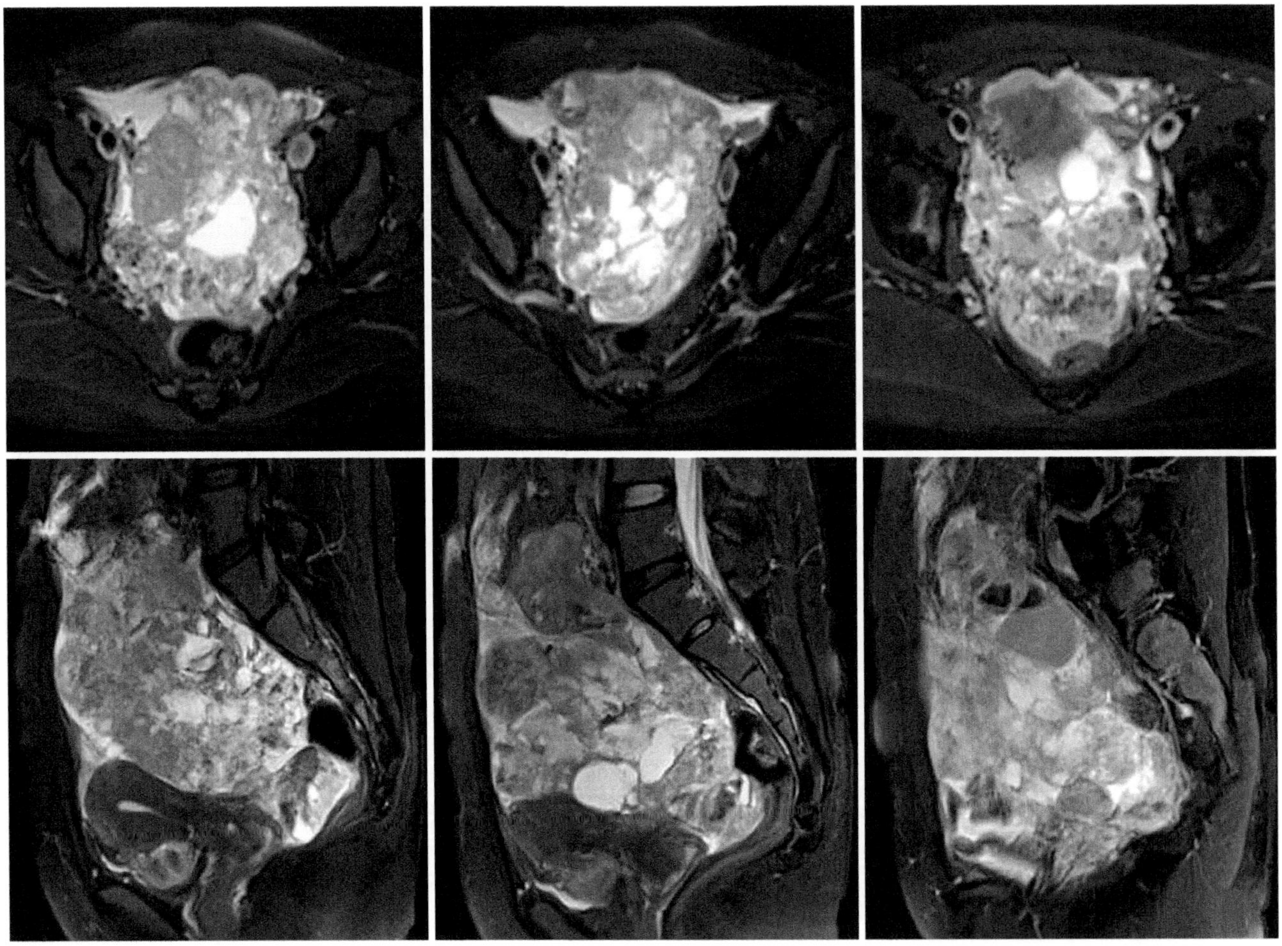

Figs. 25.4–25.9 Axial and sagittal fat-suppressed T2WI: Mainly with slightly high signal, and the signal is heterogeneous. Multiple patchy high signal cystic areas and multiple small patchy, punctate iso- and hypointense foci can be seen locally

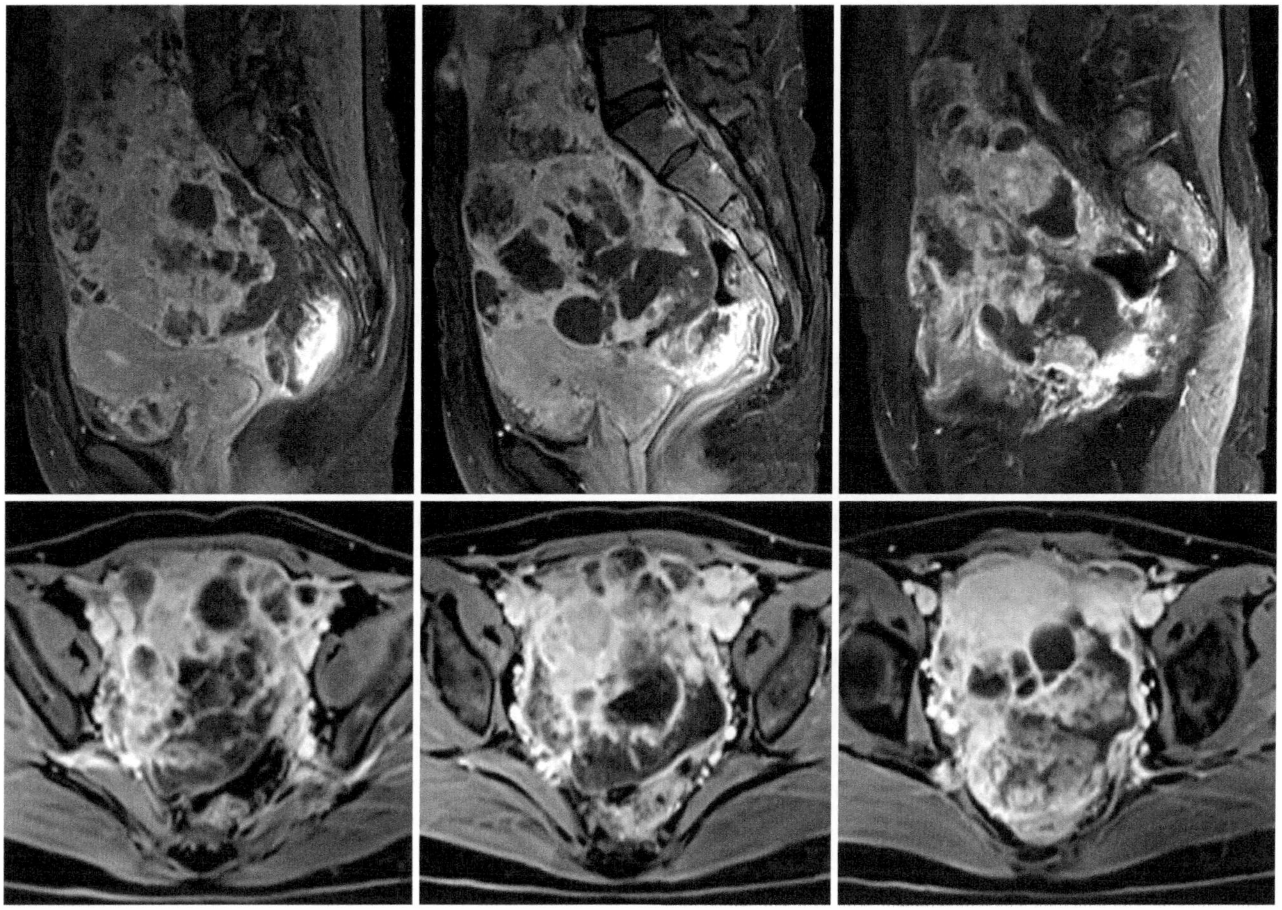

Figs. 25.10–25.15 Contrast-enhanced sagittal and axial fat-suppressed T1WI: The lesion was significantly heterogeneously enhanced, with local honeycomb-like enhancement

25.2 Imaging Analysis

Ovarian granulosa cell tumors (GCTs) are the second most common sex cord-stromal tumors, accounting for about 12% of all sex cord-stromal tumors and 2–5% of all ovarian malignancies [1]. However, they are the most common sex cord-stromal tumors apart from fibroma and thecoma. According to clinical and pathological features, GCTs are divided into two types: adult GCTs (95%) and juvenile GCTs (5%) [2]. Adult GCTs are more common in perimenopausal or postmenopausal women, with an average age of 55 years, and can also be seen in any age group after puberty. GCTs are the most common estrogen-secreting ovarian tumors, followed by thecoma [3]. The clinical manifestations include postmenopausal uterine bleeding, abnormal vaginal discharge, and amenorrhea in women of childbearing age. The typical manifestation of endometrium is cystic hyperplasia, which can be manifested as precancerous atypia in severe cases [4]. In addition to endocrine symptoms, other symptoms are associated with the tumor itself, such as abdominal pain and distention. Juvenile GCTs are more common in children and young women before the age of 30 and 80% in prepubertal children, leading to precocious puberty characterized by the development of secondary sexual characteristics without ovulation.

GCTs usually occur in unilateral ovary, and about 9% occur in bilateral ovaries. Approximately 93% of the tumors are stage I. According to the pathological diagnostic criteria, granulosa cells account for at least 10% of GCT tumors [5], and the stromal composition varies widely, with either stromal or fibrous predominance, or more typically contains components similar to theca or luteal cells. Thus, the gross appearance varies greatly, mainly depending on the percentage of theca cells or luteinized cells and the presence or absence of necrosis. Tumors are usually solid or solid and cystic, and tumors rich in theca cells or luteinized cells are usually yellowish and hard. Microscopically, the nuclei of granulosa cell tumors are very homogeneous, with minimal chromatin complexity, and varying degrees of nuclear grooves or nuclear folds, which is an important feature of granulosa cell tumors. The cells of diffuse granulosa cell tumors are nestlike, and reticular staining can clearly outline the cell nest. Granulosa cell and theca cell components can coexist in the same tumor, and if either component accounts for more than 10%, it is called theca-granulosa cell tumor. Juvenile GCT differs histologically from adult GCT in the following ways: (1) The nuclei are larger, slightly richer in chromatin, often no obvious nuclear groove, and the cytoplasm is more eosinophilic or sometimes vacuolar (2). The cells are nodular, with variable cytoplasmic content, and are solid sheets containing follicles of varying sizes (3). The cells may be distinctly heteromorphic, with exotic nuclei.

GCT is divided into the following three types: (1) solid and cystic, (2) solid, and (3) cystic.

1. Solid and cystic mass: 1. Multilocular cystic with local tissue thickening or irregular thickening of the septation, MR cystic fluid with hemorrhage shows high signal on T1WI, fat suppression T1WI and T2WI, slightly high density on CT, and medium high signal on T2WI. After contrast enhancement, the lesion shows significant enhancement in the early stage and still enhanced in the late and delayed stages. 2. Locally or as a whole, the tumor presents as multilocular small cystic areas, typically with spongy changes on T2WI [6, 7].
2. Solid mass: The tumor is either completely solid or predominantly solid, with iso-low density on pre-contrast CT, iso-low signal intensity on MR T1WI, and slightly high signal intensity on T2WI. After contrast enhancement, the lesion shows significant enhancement and irregular blood vessels on arterial phase, and the degree of enhancement is higher than that of the myometrium. The lesion is still enhanced in the late and delayed phases.
3. Cystic mass: Sometimes the tumor is multilocular cystic, and imaging findings are similar to mucinous cystadenoma. Others such as endometrial hyperplasia or thickening with the formation of small sacs are occasionally accompanied by a large or small amount of ascites.

25.3 Differential Diagnosis

When the tumor is solid and cystic mass, it is mainly differentiated from yolk sac tumor and solid- cystic serous adenocarcinoma. Granulosa cell tumor and yolk sac tumor are both found in adolescents and young women. Granulosa cell tumor causes clinical symptoms such as precocious puberty or menstrual abnormalities due to the secretion of estrogen, and serum alpha-fetoprotein (AFP) does not increase. However, most patients with yolk sac tumor have significantly increased AFP (>1000 mg/mL in young women, excluding liver lesions, which is suggestive). Serous adenocarcinoma is the most common ovarian malignant tumor in postmenopausal middle-aged and elderly women. Serum CA125 can be significantly increased because it does not have endocrine functions such as estrogen secretion and does not have signs such as endometrial hyperplasia and is usually irregular in boundary. It is often accompanied by massive ascites, peritoneal and omental implantation metastasis, and peri-iliac vascular lymphadenopathy. It is not difficult to distinguish the two. When the tumor is multilocular solid and cystic or multilocular cystic mass, it is mainly differentiated from mucinous tumors.

The typical MRI manifestations of mucinous tumors are multilocular cystic masses. The cystic fluid in each chamber presents different signal intensity on T2WI due to different mucus, hemorrhage, and protein content, which is the so-called "stained glass" sign [8]. It presents low, equal, and high mixed signals on T1WI, and the septa between the chambers were irregularly thickened. After contrast enhancement, it is moderately or significantly enhanced. However, multilocular cystic masses with irregular thickening of cystic wall and septa or presence of soft tissue components are highly suggestive of malignancy. When the tumor is solid mass, it is mainly differentiated from solid fibroma, thecoma, and solid serous adenocarcinoma. Fibroma and thecoma show characteristic isointensity or hypointensity on T2WI, and delayed enhancement after contrast enhancement is helpful to distinguish them. Solid serous adenocarcinoma is usually irregular in shape and is often accompanied by malignant signs such as massive ascites, implantation metastasis of peritoneum and greater omentum, and peri-iliac vascular lymphadenopathy. It is not difficult to distinguish the two.

References

1. Louis DN, Ohgaki H, Wiestler OD, et al. The 2007 WHO classification of tumours of the central nervous system. Acta Neuropathol. 2007;114(2):97–109.
2. Zhang D, Henning TD, Zou LG, et al. Intracranial ganglioglioma: clinicopathological and MRI findings in 16 patients. Clin Radiol. 2008;63(1):80–91.
3. Luyken C, Blümcke I, Fimmers R, et al. Supratentorial gangliogliomas: histopathologic grading and tumor recurrence in 184 patients with a median follow-up of 8 years. Cancer. 2004;101(1):146–55.
4. Koeller KK, Sandberg GD. Armed forces Institute of Pathology. From the archives of the AFIP. Cerebral intraventricular neoplasms: radiologic-pathologic correlation. Radiographics. 2002;22(6):1473–505.
5. Oliva E, Young RH. Endocrine pathology of the ovary. Endocr Pathol. 2014;25(1):102–19.
6. Kim SH. Kim SH (2002) granulosa cell tumor of the ovary: common findings and unusual appearances on CT and MR. J Comput Assist Tomogr. 2002;26(5):756–61.
7. Sugimura K. MRI diagnosis of the ovary (Japanese). In: Sugimura K, editor. MRI diagnosis of pelvis. Tokyo: Igaku-Shoin; 1993. p. 88–132.
8. Schiavone MB, Herzog TJ, Lewin SN, et al. Natural history and outcome of mucinous carcinoma of the ovary. Am J Obstet Gynecol. 2011;205(480):e1–8.

Recurrent Ovarian Granulosa Cell Tumor

26

Shuhui Zhao

26.1 Clinical History

Female patient, 58 years old, was admitted to the hospital with a pelvic mass found for 7 days, 4 years after chemotherapy after ovarian granulosa cell tumor cytoreductive surgery. Postoperative pathology after cytoreductive surgery 4 years ago: left ovarian adult granulosa cell tumor, involving the uterine seromuscular layer and serous layer of the left fallopian tube. No tumor metastasis was found in the pelvic lymph nodes and greater omentum. Ultrasonography examination showed that the whole uterus and bilateral adnexa had been removed. Pelvic effusion: anechoic area above the vagina, 72 mm × 62 mm × 17 mm in size. A mixed echo area of 93 mm × 65 mm × 58 mm was found on the right side of pelvic cavity, with abundant color blood flow; a moderate hypoechoic area was found on the posterior wall of the bladder protruding to pelvic cavity: 25 mm × 26 mm × 16 mm, with punctate color blood flow. Weak echo area was seen on the left side of pelvic cavity: 23 mm × 21 mm × 23 mm, with colored blood flow in the margin. PET-CT: ovarian postoperative change; solid and cystic mass and multiple nodules on the right side of pelvic cavity, with partially increased FDG uptake; and metastasis were considered. Postoperative pathological result: the stump of greater omentum, bladder apex mass, the mass of the anterior wall of sigmoid colon, and the mass of rectouterine pouch, consistent with recurrence of ovarian granulosa cell tumor in correlation with medical history.

26.2 Imaging Analysis

Granulosa cell tumors are the most common malignant ovarian sex cord-stromal tumors. They account for less than 5% of all malignant ovarian tumors [1, 2]. Granulosa cell tumors are low malignant. Histologically, they have two subtypes of adult and juvenile. 95% of ovarian granulosa cell tumors are adult granulosa cell tumors [1–4]. Adult granulosa cell tumors often affect early postmenopausal women. Juvenile granulosa cell tumors often affect children and women younger than 30 years old [1–4]. Granulosa cell tumors can produce estrogen. Patients often present with abnormal vaginal bleeding. High level of estrogen can lead to endometrial hyperplasia, polyps, and even carcinoma. Clinically, ovarian granulosa cell tumors can behave like a malignant lesion. Prognosis depends on stage and age at the time of the diagnosis. Prognosis is excellent in most patients. 10-year survival rate is higher than 90%. However, adult granulosa cell tumors can relapse even in 10–20 years after diagnosis [4–7].

Granulosa cell tumors are typically unilateral masses (average size, 12 cm) [1]. They have various imaging manifestations. They can have the appearance of multilocular cystic lesions with solid components, solid masses, solid with a sponge-like appearance resembling Swiss cheese, and completely cystic tumors with thick rind of soft tissue. A solid tumor can become heterogeneous if there are intratumoral hemorrhage, infarct, fibrous degeneration, and irregularly arranged tumor cells. On T2WI images, the solid component shows isointense signal intensity (Figs. 26.1, 26.2). Thickened septations may show hypointense signal intensity on T2WI images [1, 2, 4, 5, 7]. Fluid-fluid levels may present in the cystic portion of the tumor. Areas of intracystic hemorrhage show hyperintense signal intensity on T1WI images (Fig. 26.3). After contrast enhancement (Fig. 26.4), solid components demonstrate enhancement [1, 2, 4, 5, 7].

Recurrent ovarian granulosa cell tumors display as discrete peritoneal or retroperitoneal masses. There is no ascites or a small amount of ascites. Like primary ovarian granulosa cell tumors, recurrent tumors have various imaging findings. They can be solid masses, solid masses with cystic portions, or completely cystic lesions. In patients with history of ovarian granulosa cell tumor,

S. Zhao (✉)
Department of Radiology, Xinhua Hospital, Medical College of Shanghai Jiao Tong University, Shanghai, People's Republic of China

G. Zhang (ed.), *MRI of Gynaecological Diseases*, https://doi.org/10.1007/978-981-99-3644-1_26

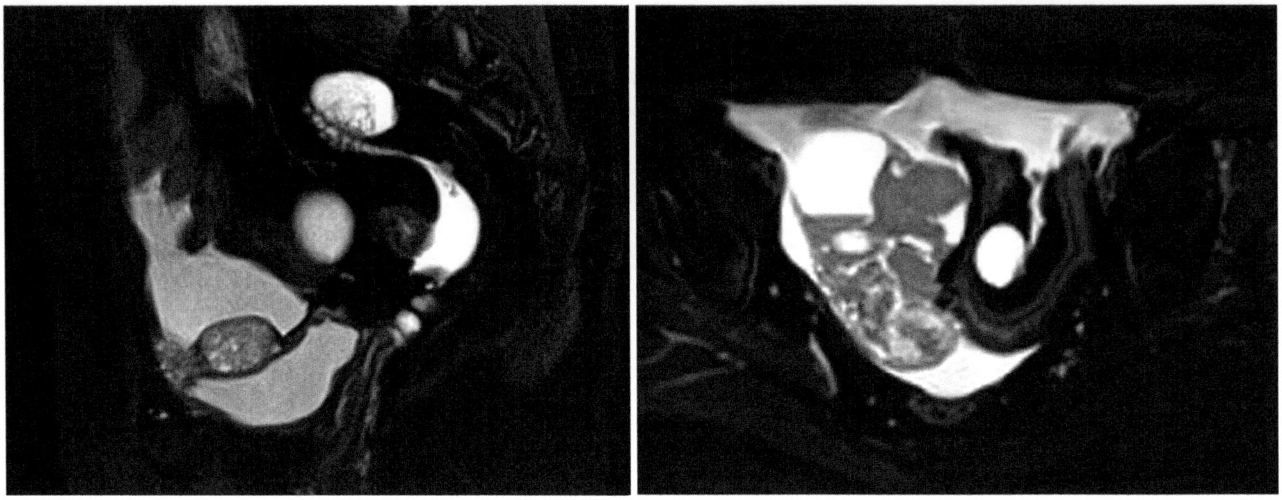

Figs. 26.1 and 26.2 Sagittal and axial T2-weighted with fat suppression images showed multiple variable-sized nodular recurrent masses with heterogeneous signal intensity in the pelvic cavity. Ascites was seen

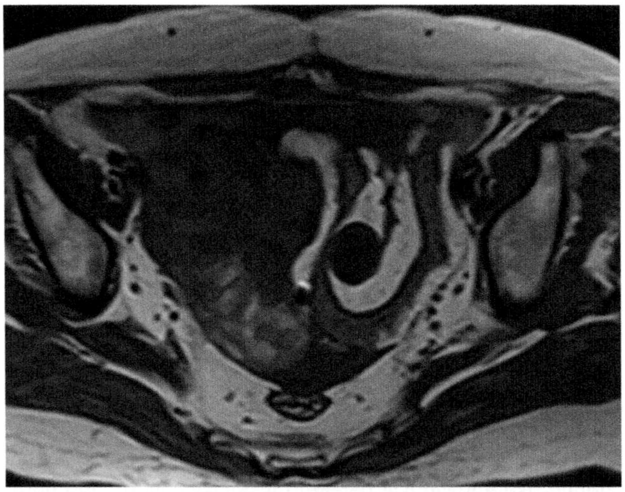

Fig. 26.3 Axial T1-weighted image showed heterogeneous signal intensity caused by intratumoral hemorrhage

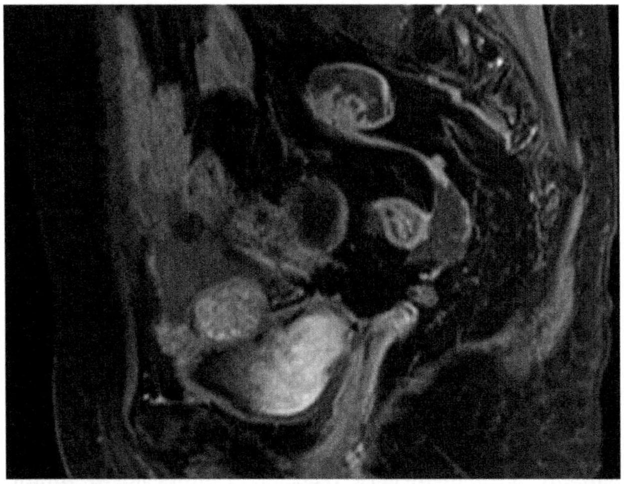

Fig. 26.4 T1-weighted contrast-enhanced image showed the recurrent masses had heterogeneous enhancement

recurrence should be considered if new peritoneal or retroperitoneal masses are present, even if the time is long after initial diagnosis [7].

26.3 Differential Diagnosis

It is mainly differentiated from gastrointestinal stromal tumor (GIST) and primary or metastatic ovarian cancer. GIST can occur in any part of the digestive tract from esophagus to rectum, mostly in stomach and small intestine, as well as in colon, esophagus, omentum, and mesentery inside the peritoneal cavity. Pathologically, it is mainly composed of spindle cells. Necrosis, cystic degeneration, and myxoid degeneration may also occur and are sometimes difficult to identify. Careful identification of the relationship between base of the tumor and the small intestine and ovary is crucial for the origin of the tumor. However, clinical history of ovarian granulosa cell tumor is crucial for the diagnosis of recurrence. Primary or metastatic ovarian cancer, which often involves both ovaries, may also be solid, cystic, or solid and cystic. Therefore, it is difficult to distinguish on imaging and needs to be combined with clinical history. Likewise, clinical history of ovarian granulosa cell tumor is crucial for the diagnosis of recurrence.

References

1. Horta M, Cunha TM. Sex cord-stromal tumors of the ovary: a comprehensive review and update for radiologists. Diagn Interv Radiol. 2015;21(4):277–86.
2. Shaaban AM. Diagnostic imaging: Gynecology. 2015
3. Matsuki M, Numoto I, Suzuki A, Hamakawa T, Matsukubo Y, Tsurusaki M, et al. Magnetic resonance imaging of recurrent adult

granulosa cell tumor of the ovary: a retrospective analysis of 11 cases. J Comput Assist Tomogr. 2020;44(6):887–92.
4. Jung SE, Rha SE, Lee JM, Park SY, Oh SN, Cho KS, et al. CT and MRI findings of sex cord-stromal tumor of the ovary. Am J Roentgenol. 2005;185(1):207–15.
5. Tanaka YO, Tsunoda H, Kitagawa Y, Ueno T, Yoshikawa H, Saida Y. Functioning ovarian tumors: direct and indirect findings at MR imaging. Radiographics. 2004;24(Suppl 1):147–66.
6. Rha SE, Oh SN, Jung SE, Lee YJ, Lee AW, Byun JY. Recurrent ovarian granulosa cell tumors: clinical and imaging features. Abdom Imaging. 2008;33(1):119–25.
7. Zhao S, Li H, Qiang J, Wang D, Fan H. The value of MRI for differentiating benign from malignant sex cord-stromal tumors of the ovary: emphasis on diffusion-weighted MR imaging. J Ovarian Res. 2018;11(1):73.

27 Ovarian Sertoli-Leydig Cell Tumor

Shuhui Zhao

27.1 Clinical History

Female patient, 56 years old, had been experiencing menopausal for 2 years, and uterine myomas were found progressively larger for more than 10 years. The patient was followed up regularly. In recent 3 months, there was frequent urination, without urgency and pain of urination, without hematuria, no postmenopausal abnormal vaginal bleeding and discharge, no abdominal pain, and no leucorrhea abnormalities. MRI examination showed that there was a huge soft tissue tumor in the front of the uterus. MRI diagnosis: (1) Malignant tumor from the adnexa was considered possible, malignant transformation of subserosal myoma to be excluded (2). Multiple uterine myomas. She underwent laparoscopic total hysterectomy and bilateral salpingo-oophorectomy. Postoperative pathological result: poorly differentiated Sertoli-Leydig cell tumor of right ovary.

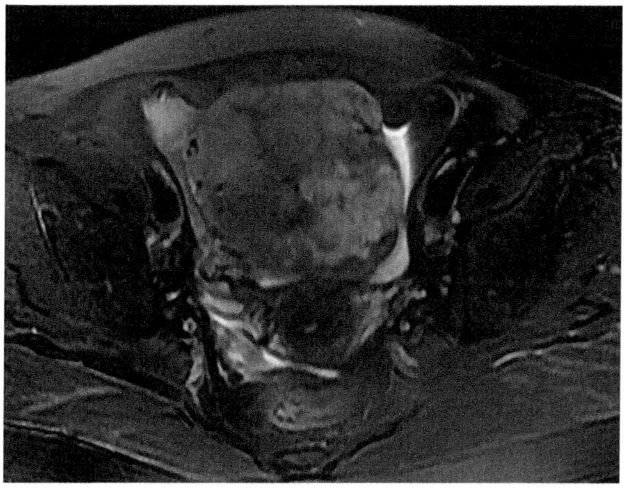

Fig. 27.1 T2-weighted with fat suppression image showed the mass had heterogeneous high signal intensity

27.2 Imaging Analysis

Ovarian Sertoli-Leydig cell tumor is a rare malignant sex cord-stromal tumor. It accounts for approximately 0.5% of all ovarian neoplasms. It is the most common virilizing ovarian tumor. Approximately, 30%–50% of ovarian Sertoli-Leydig cell tumor can produce androgens. Clinical symptoms of virilization are present in more than one-third of cases with abnormal androgen level [1–5]. In patients with non-functioning tumors, abdominal pain and swelling are frequent clinical symptoms. They often have a benign clinical behavior [1–3]. Unlike granulosa cell tumors, they may have early recurrence after initial diagnosis. Ovarian Sertoli-Leydig cell tumors are usually unilateral lesions. They appear as solid, solid and cystic, or even cystic mass [1–3]. Pathologically, ovarian Sertoli-Leydig cell tumors could be well-differentiated, moderately differentiated or poorly differentiated. Ovarian Sertoli-Leydig cell tumors are often combined with heterologous elements such as carcinoid, mesenchymal, and mucinous epithelial tissues [2, 6]. Mucinous epithelial tissues are the most common heterologous elements.

Ovarian Sertoli-Leydig cell tumor has a nonspecific appearance. Tumor size varies and can reach up to 15 cm [3]. On CT images; ovarian Sertoli-Leydig cell tumors display as a multilocular cystic mass or a soft-tissue attenuating adnexal mass with intratumoral cysts. The solid component has marked enhancement [1, 2]. MR signals of the solid portion are correlated with the fibrous and fatty content. Fibrous stroma has low signal on T2WI images (Figs. 27.1 and 27.2) [1, 2]. On DWI images (Fig. 27.3), ovarian Sertoli-Leydig cell tumors have diffusion restriction in solid area [7]. Cystic areas show low signal on T1WI images (Fig. 27.4) and high signal on T2WI images. On T1WI images, cystic component may also show slightly high signal [1]. Solid areas have avid contrast enhancement. Enhancement can be homogeneous or heterogeneous (Figs. 27.5 and 27.6) [1–3].

S. Zhao (✉)
Department of Radiology, Xinhua Hospital, Medical College of Shanghai Jiao Tong University,
Shanghai, People's Republic of China

G. Zhang (ed.), *MRI of Gynaecological Diseases*, https://doi.org/10.1007/978-981-99-3644-1_27

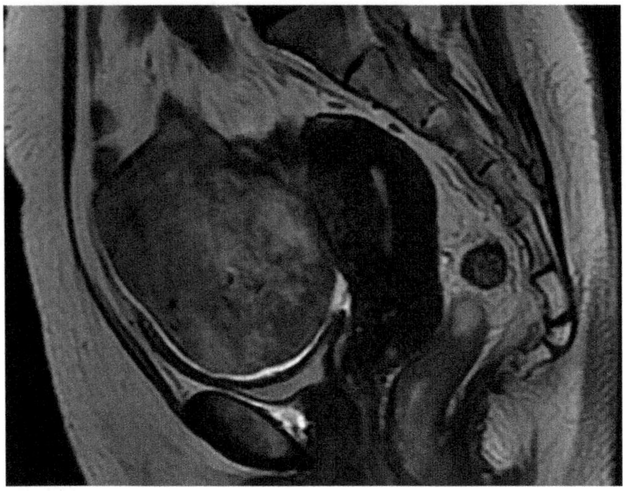

Fig. 27.2 Sagittal T2-weighted image showed the mass was heterogeneous. It had marked enhancement equal to myometrium after contrast enhancement

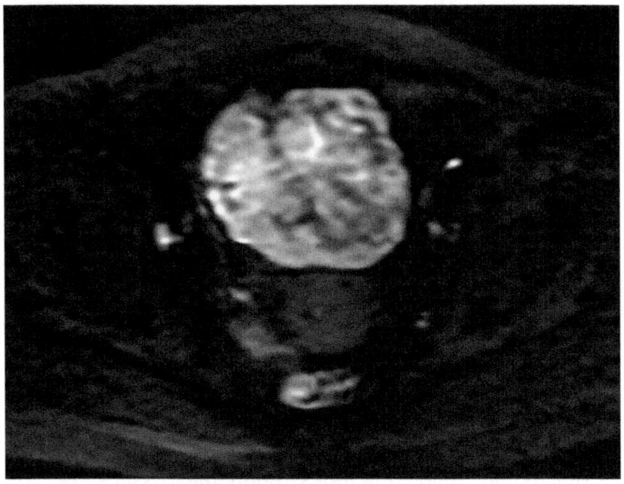

Fig. 27.3 The mass showed restricted diffusion on DWI

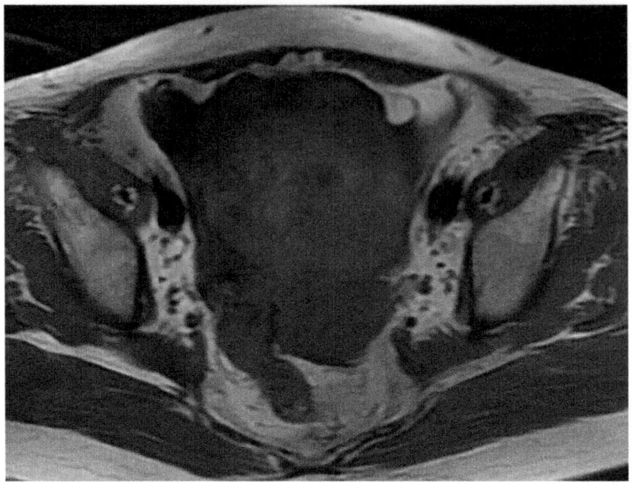

Fig. 27.4 Axial T1-weighted image showed an oval lesion of slightly high signal intensity

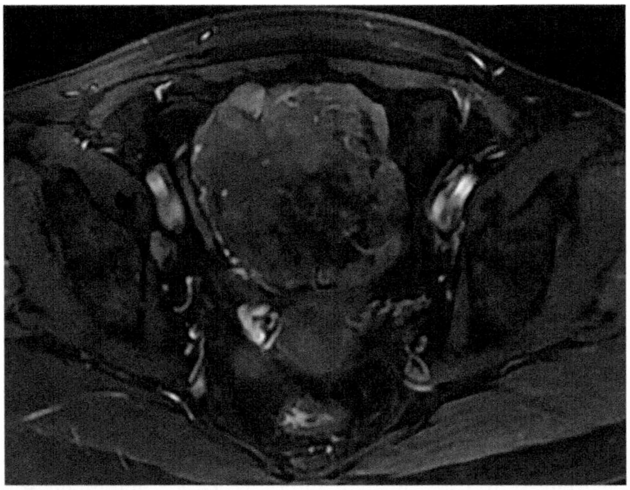

Fig. 27.5 T1-weighted contrast-enhanced image showed the mass had heterogeneous enhancement

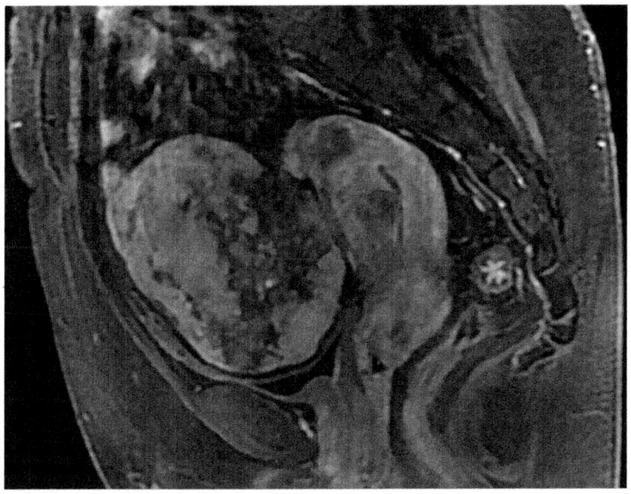

Fig. 27.6 Sagittal T1-weighted contrast-enhanced image showed the mass was heterogeneous. It had marked enhancement equal to myometrium after contrast enhancement

27.3 Differential Diagnosis

The main differential diagnosis includes granulosa cell tumors and sclerosing stromal tumor of the ovary. Ovarian granulosa cell tumors most commonly present with estrogenic manifestations. They can have various appearances including solid, mixed solid and cystic, or completely cystic tumors [3]. Ovarian sclerosing stromal tumors demonstrate as masses with cystic and heterogeneous solid components. They demonstrate early peripheral enhancement with centripetal progression [3].

References

1. Jung SE, Rha SE, Lee JM, Park SY, Oh SN, Cho KS, et al. CT and MRI findings of sex cord-stromal tumor of the ovary. Am J Roentgenol. 2005;185(1):207–15.
2. Horta M, Cunha TM. Sex cord-stromal tumors of the ovary: a comprehensive review and update for radiologists. Diagn Interv Radiol. 2015;21(4):277–86.
3. Shaaban AM. Diagnostic imaging: Gynecology. 2015
4. Outwater EK, Marchetto B, Wagner BJ. Virilizing tumors of the ovary: imaging features. Ultrasound Obstet Gynecol. 2000;15(5):365–71.
5. Tanaka YO, Tsunoda H, Kitagawa Y, Ueno T, Yoshikawa H, Saida Y. Functioning ovarian tumors: direct and indirect findings at MR imaging. Radiographics. 2004;24(Suppl 1):147–66.
6. Cai S, Zhao S, Qiang J, Zhang G, Wang L. Ovarian sertoli–leydig cell tumors: MRI findings and pathological correlation. J Ovarian Res. 2013;6(1):73.
7. Zhao S, Li H, Qiang J, Wang D, Fan H. The value of MRI for differentiating benign from malignant sex cord-stromal tumors of the ovary: emphasis on diffusion-weighted MR imaging. J Ovarian Res. 2018;11(1):73.

28 Ovarian Yolk Sac Tumor

Mengwei Zhang

28.1 Clinical History

Female patient, 19 years old, presented with right lower abdominal pain for 11 days. She developed severe right lower abdominal pain without obvious cause, accompanied by vomiting and no diarrhea. Ultrasonography revealed a multilocular cystic mass above the uterus, 190 mm × 160 mm × 115 mm in size, and multiple septation was seen inside. The boundary of the mass was clear, the shape was regular, and ovaries were not detected. Diagnosis of ultrasound examination: the mass was originated from the ovary possible. AFP > 3000 ng/mL.

She underwent transabdominal right salpingo-oophorectomy, left ovarian biopsy, pelvic lymph node dissection, and greater omentum resection. Intraoperative findings: small amount of ascites, clear color, and no obvious abnormalities in liver, spleen, or stomach. The uterus was in anterior position, 5 cm × 4 cm × 3 cm in size, and with normal shape. The size of left ovary was 3.5 cm × 3 cm × 3 cm, and there was no obvious abnormality in appearance; the size of the right ovary was 30 cm × 20 cm × 20 cm, which was solid and cystic and adherent to the anterior abdominal peritoneum. There was no abnormality in the right fallopian tube and no abnormality in bladder and rectouterine pouch.

Postoperative pathological result: right ovarian yolk sac tumor.

28.2 Imaging Analysis

Ovarian yolk sac tumor, as also known as endodermal sinus tumor (EST), is a primordial malignant germ cell tumor, which is considered to result from differentiation of primordial germ cells along the yolk sac or yolk direction. It is the second most common malignant germ cell tumor of the ovary after dysgerminoma. It most commonly occurs in 11–30 years old, followed by 1–10 and 31–40 years old. It is rarely seen in middle-aged or elderly women, and the degree of malignancy is high, accounting for approximately 1% of all ovarian malignancies. The most common clinical symptoms are abdominal pain and distention, and a few present with abdominal or pelvic masses. Most patients show a significant increase in alpha-fetoprotein (AFP, >1000 ng/mL in young women, excluding liver lesions, which has a suggestive role), and CA125 is elevated in some patients [1]. At diagnosis, approximately 50% of patients have lesions limited to the ovary (Stage I). Ovarian yolk sac tumor is highly malignant, and the tumors often spread through ovary to surrounding tissues and organs, including peripheral peritoneum and greater omentum, and 10% of patients were confined to the pelvic cavity (Stage II), metastases to para-aortic and common iliac lymph nodes through lymphatic system first, distant metastases to mediastinal and supraclavicular lymph nodes, and blood metastases to liver and lungs (Stage III and IV, 40%) [2]. Ovarian yolk sac tumor is not sensitive to radiotherapy and has a poor prognosis, with a 3-year survival rate of only 13% [3]. In recent years, with the development of combination chemotherapy, the survival rate of stage I has increased to 80%, and late stages have also reached 50% [4]. Serum AFP level can be used to monitor therapeutic effect and recurrence.

Pathologically, ovarian yolk sac tumor is the second most common primordial germ cell tumor, but clinical studies have shown that it is the third most common malignant germ cell tumor after malignant teratoma and dysgerminoma [2, 5]. The typical gross pathological manifestation is a large mass with smooth appearance, with an average diameter of 15 cm. The sectional surface is solid and cystic, brown, white, or gray. Multiple cyst cavities of different sizes are common in solid areas, with hemorrhage and necrosis inside. Honeycomb-like lobulation and complete cystic are rare manifestations [6].

Most ovarian yolk sac tumor is unilateral, and about 1% is bilateral, 7–28 cm in diameter, with an average of 15 cm. On

M. Zhang (✉)
Department of Radiology, Obstetrics and Gynecology Hospital, Fudan University, Shanghai, People's Republic of China

G. Zhang (ed.), *MRI of Gynaecological Diseases*, https://doi.org/10.1007/978-981-99-3644-1_28

imaging, typical manifestation of ovarian yolk sac tumor is predominantly solid, with multiple cyst cavities of different sizes. The diameters of cyst cavities range from several millimeters to 2 cm, which could be diffusely distributed in the solid area, so that the tumor presents a honeycomb-like change [3]. Different degrees of hemorrhage are seen within the tumor, which show high signal intensity on T1WI (Figs. 28.1 and 28.2), while the entire tumor shows different degrees of high signal intensity on T2WI (Figs. 28.3–28.6). Another characteristic feature of ovarian yolk sac tumor is significant enhancement of the tumor and multiple signal loss structures (Figs. 28.7–28.10), corresponding to the "bright dot sign" seen on CT. The so-called "bright dots" are small dots or tubular shadows significantly enhanced inside the tumor, representing increased blood vessels within the tumor [7].

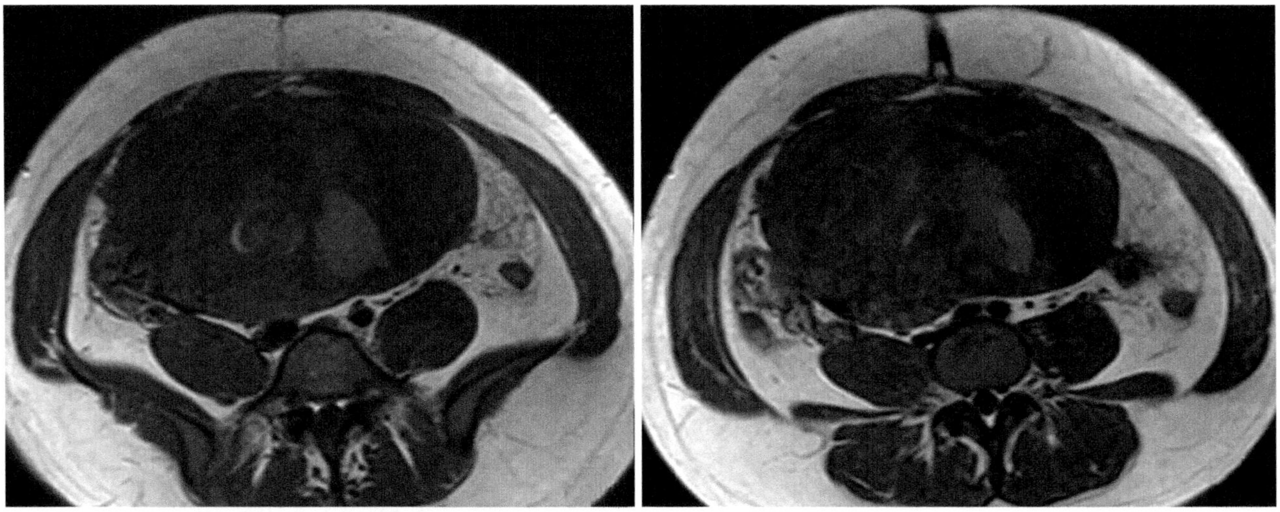

Figs. 28.1 and 28.2 Axial pre-contrast T1WI: an oval multilocular cystic mass was seen in the pelvic and abdominal cavity, with iso- and hypointense predominance, and small patches of slightly hyperintense signal can be seen locally

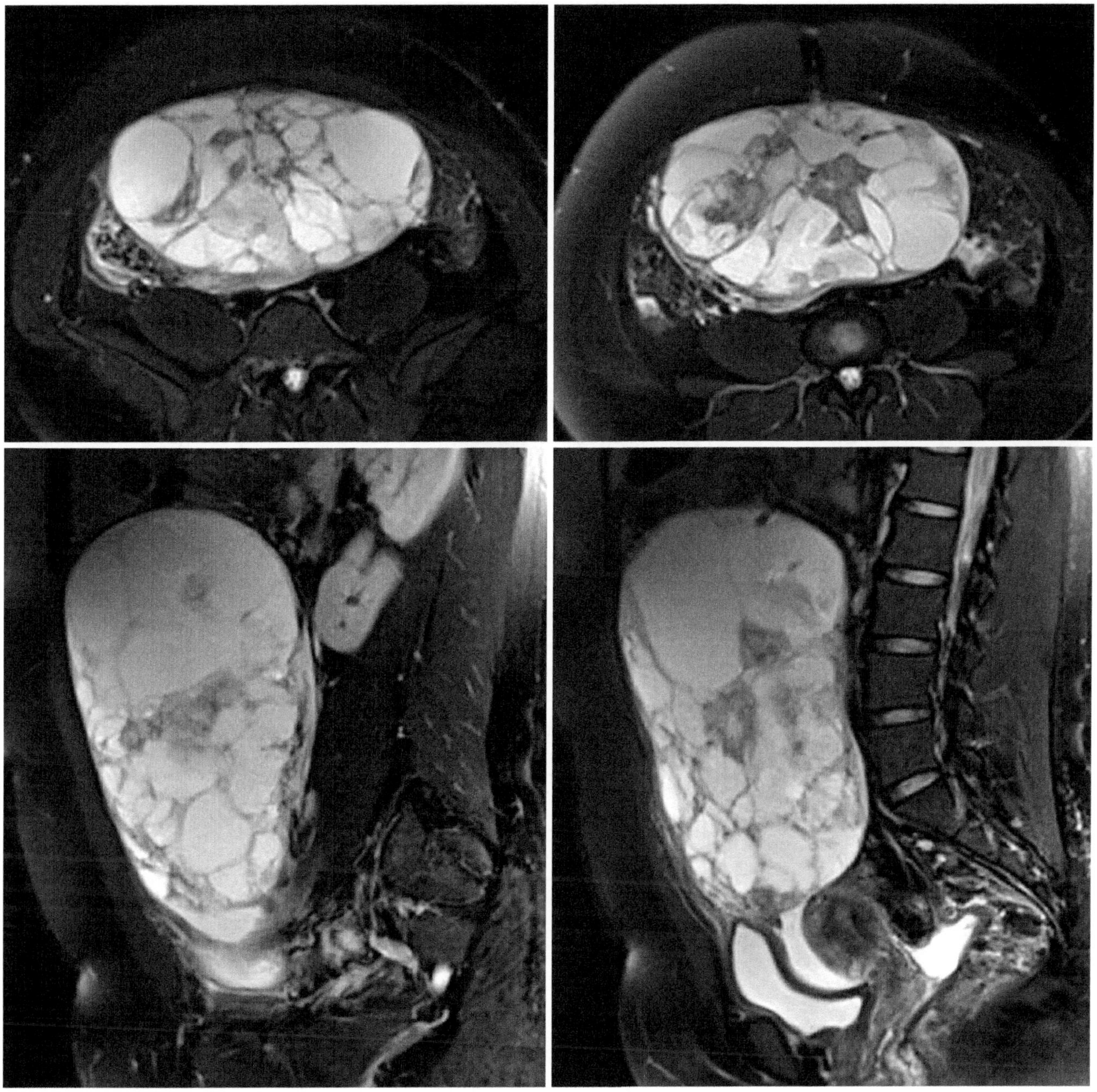

Figs. 28.3–28.6 Axial and sagittal pre-contrast T2WI: the mass is predominantly high signal intensity; small patches of slightly low signal can be seen locally, with multiple low signal septation

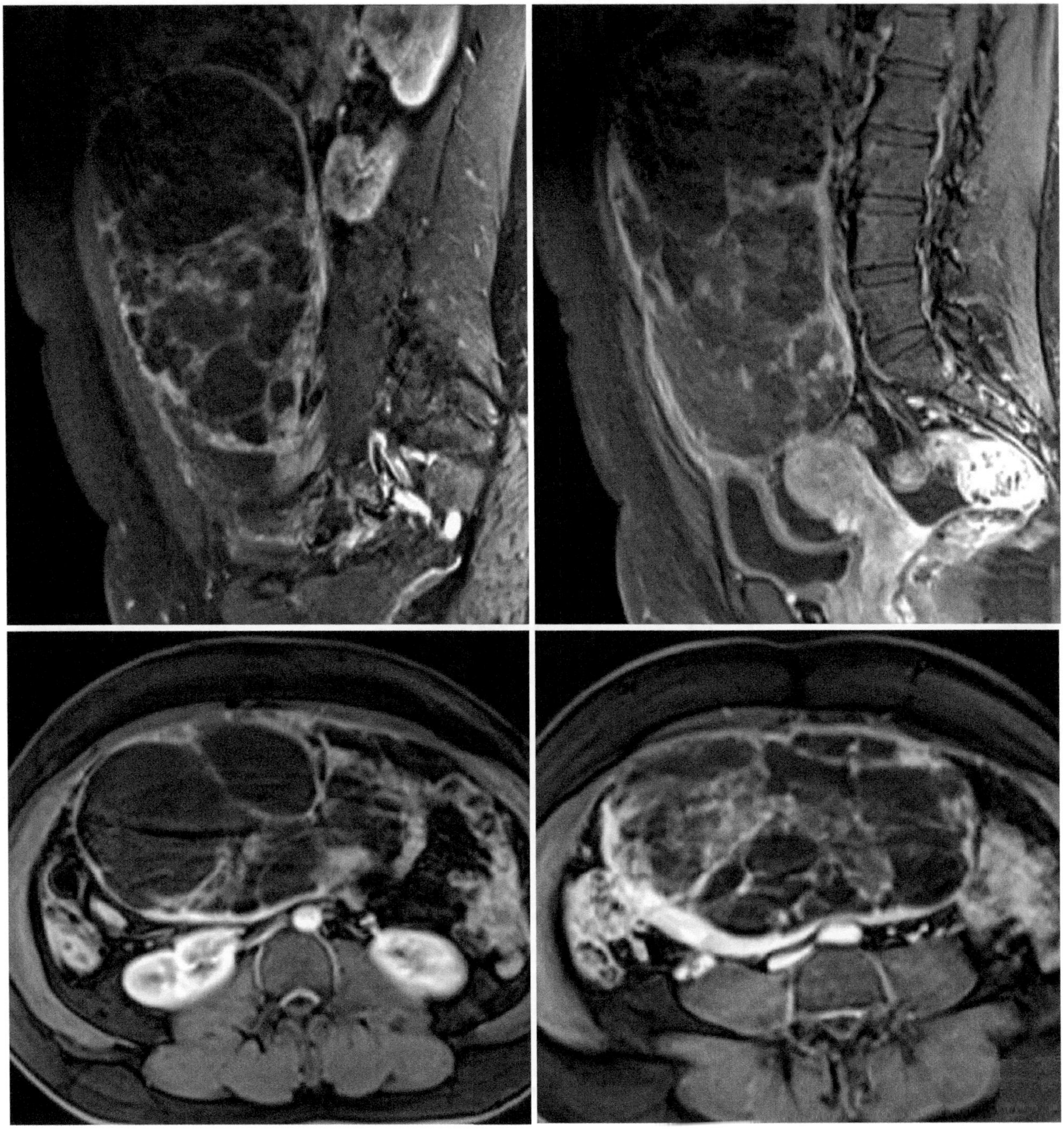

Figs. 28.7–28.10 Sagittal and axial contrast-enhanced T1WI: the cyst wall and septation were significantly enhanced

28.3 Differential Diagnosis

Ovarian yolk sac tumor is mainly distinguished from juvenile granulosa cell tumor, both of which occur in adolescents and young women. Juvenile granulosa cell tumor is associated with clinical symptoms such as precocious puberty or menstrual abnormalities due to estrogen secretion, and serum AFP is not elevated.

References

1. Dallenbach P, Bonnefoi H, Pelte MF, et al. Yolk sac tumours of the ovary: an update. Eur J Surg Oncol. 2006;32:1063–75.
2. Soslow RA, Tornos C. Diagnostic Pathology of Ovarian Tumors. 155.
3. Kurman RJ, Norris HJ. Endodermal sinus tumor of the ovary. A clinical and pathologic analysis of 71 cases. Cancer. 1976;38:2404–24.
4. de La Motte RT, Pautier P, Duvillard P, et al. Survival and reproductive function of 52 women treated with surgery and bleomycin, etoposide, cisplatin (BEP) chemotherapy for ovarian yolk sac tumor. Ann Oncol. 2008;19:1435–41.
5. Smith HO, Berwick M, Verschraegen CF, et al. Incidence and survival rates for female malignant germ cell tumors. Obstet Gynecol. 2006;107:1075–85.
6. Buy JN, Ghossain M. Gynecological Imaging 2013.
7. Kim SH. Radiology illustrated: Gynecologic imaging. (eBook).

29 Ovarian Lymphoma

Fenghua Ma

29.1 Clinical History

Female patient, 21 years old, with regular menstruation, menarche at the age of 10, 7/28–30, moderate menstrual bleeding, and mild dysmenorrhea. 10 days ago, she palpated a mass in her lower abdomen and went to the local hospital. Ultrasonography showed that there was a 160 mm*80 mm hypoechoic mass in the pelvic cavity, with a clear boundary, and the echo was not uniform, considered origin from the adnexa? CT showed solid space-occupying lesions in bilateral adnexa areas, and ovarian cancer was considered first; ascites and pelvic effusions were also showed. Examination of serum tumor markers: CA125: 56.1 U/mL, CA199: 56.1 U/mL. Physical examination at admission: bilateral adnexal masses with the size of about 4+ months pregnant and hard texture. The reexamination of ultrasonography showed large solid masses in front of the uterus, with ovarian origin, and ultrasonography diagnosis considered may be tumors.

MRI examination: solid masses in bilateral adnexa area, with irregular boundary; right size: 19.8 cm × 19.6 cm × 14.8 cm, left size: 6.9 cm × 6.8 cm × 5.8 cm, relatively uniform signal. The lesions showed iso-signal intensity on T1WI (Figs. 29.1 and 29.2), slightly high signal intensity on T2WI, and small patchy higher signal foci can be seen in the lesions on T2WI (Figs. 29.3–29.6). After contrast enhancement (Figs. 29.7–29.9), the lesions showed obvious inhomogeneous enhancement, and there were small round foci without enhancement in the lesions. A small amount of fluid was seen in the pelvic cavity.

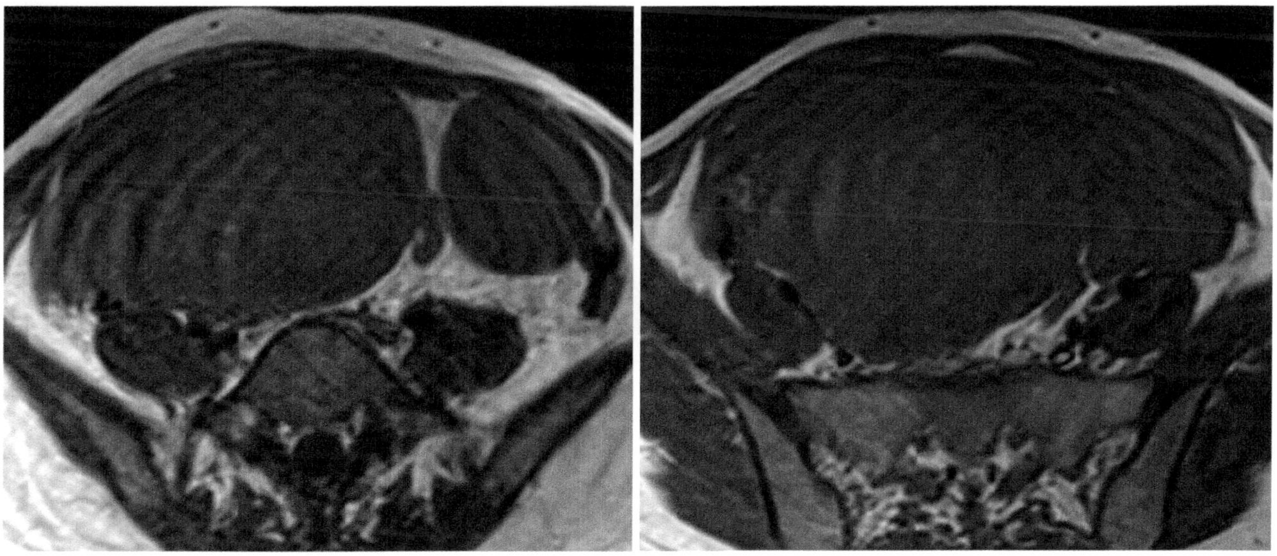

Figs. 29.1 and 29.2 Pre-contrast T1WI: Round solid masses were seen in bilateral adnexa area, isointense signal and the signal are homogeneous

F. Ma (✉)
Department of Radiology, Obstetrics and Gynecology Hospital, Fudan University, Shanghai, People's Republic of China

G. Zhang (ed.), *MRI of Gynaecological Diseases*, https://doi.org/10.1007/978-981-99-3644-1_29

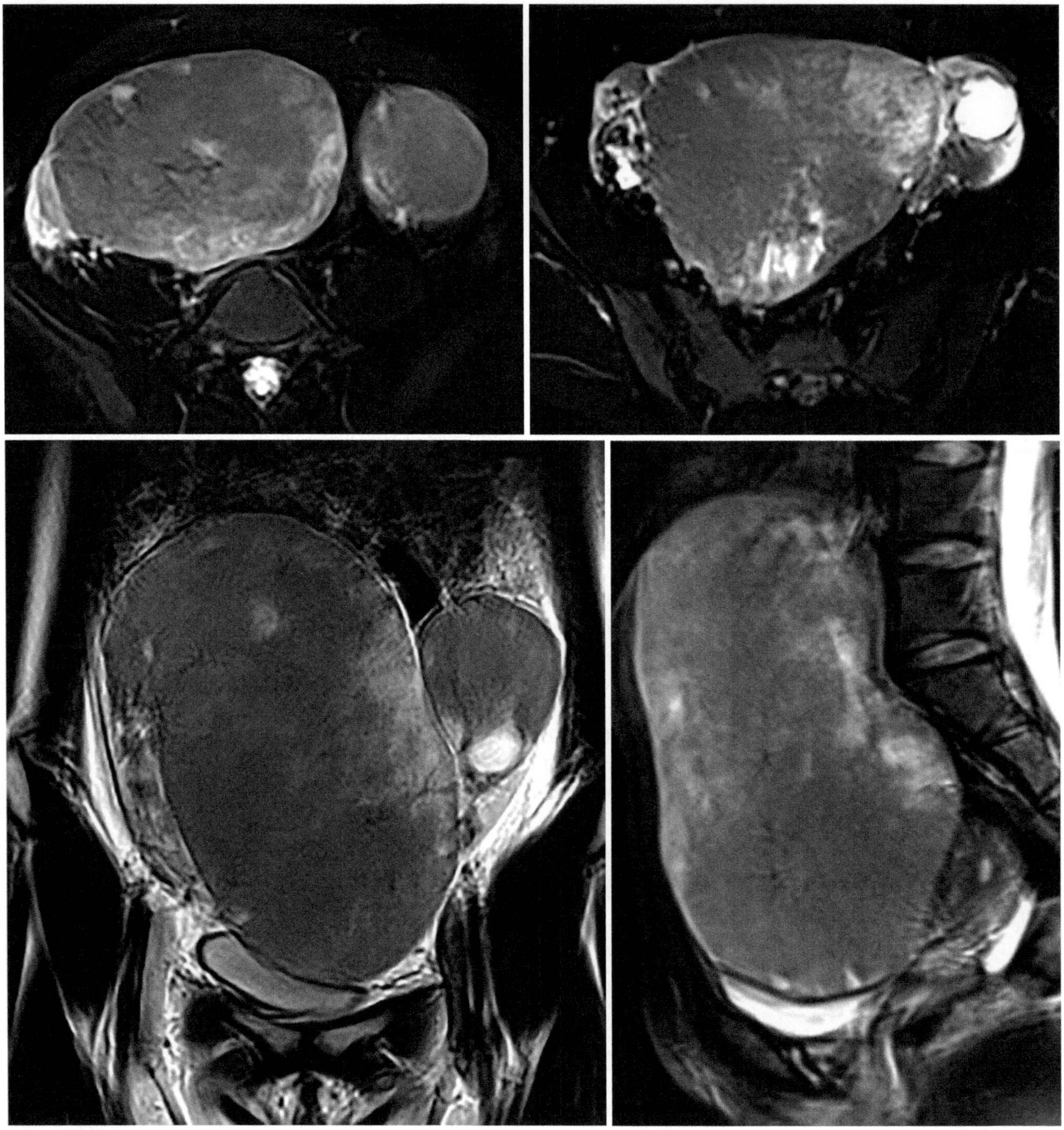

Figs. 29.3–29.6 Axial, coronal, and sagittal T2WI showed slightly hyperintense signal with homogeneous signal intensity, and small patchy higher signal foci can be seen in the lesions

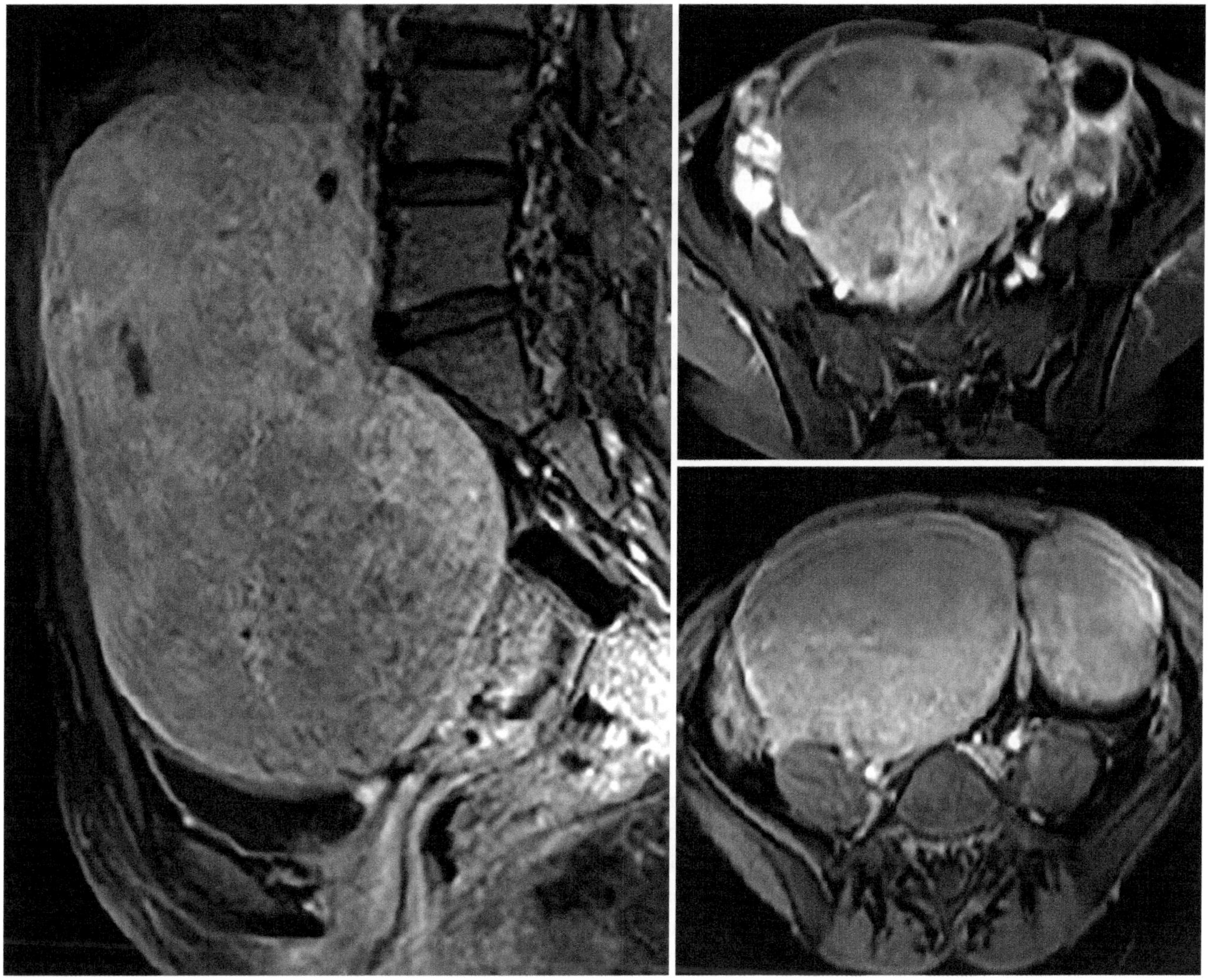

Figs. 29.7–29.9 Contrast-enhanced sagittal and axial T1WI images: the lesions showed obvious inhomogeneous enhancement, and there were small round foci without enhancement in the lesions

On the fourth day after admission, she underwent right salpingo-oophorectomy, left ovarian tumor resection, pelvic lymph node dissection, and greater omentum resection. Intraoperative findings: there were scattered enlarged lymph nodes seen in the greater omentum with a diameter of 1.5 cm. The uterus was in anterior position; shape and size were normal. The left ovarian tumor was 7 cm × 7 cm × 6 cm in size, and the ampulla of the left fallopian tube was thickened and hard; the right ovarian tumor was 20 cm × 20 cm × 15 cm in size, and the ampulla of the right fallopian tube was thickened and hard. No abnormalities were observed in the bladder and rectouterine pouch. Postoperative pathological result: B-cell lymphoma, involving bilateral ovaries, right fallopian tube, greater omentum, and right iliac lymph nodes. Immunohistochemical results: AE1/AE3(−), CD10(+), CD20(+), CD79α(+), Ki-67 (95%+), LCA(−), Vimentin(+), Inhibin-α(−).

29.2 Imaging Analysis

Primary ovarian lymphoma is rare and mostly non-Hodgkin lymphoma, accounting for 1.5% of all ovarian tumors [1]. Diffuse large B-cell lymphoma is the most common pathologic type, followed by Burkitt lymphoma, both of which are high-grade lymphomas [2, 3]. Because of the lack of lymphoid tissue in ovarian parenchyma, it is presumed that ovarian lymphoma originates from lymphocytes in the hilum of the ovary or corpus luteum vessels [4]. Most researchers consider that ovarian lymphoma is a local manifestation of lymphatic system diseases, with no specific clinical symptoms and may be accompanied by abdominal discomfort. CA125 can be elevated.

The incidence of ovarian lymphoma is low, and there are few reports in the literature. There are no characteristic imaging findings. Fox et al. [5] proposed the following diagnostic criteria for primary ovarian lymphoma: (1) the lesion was confined to the ovary with or without periovarian tissue infiltration, and there was no lesion in other sites; (2) no abnormalities in peripheral blood and bone marrow; (3) ovarian and para-ovarian lesions appeared first, and several months later lymphoma of an extra-ovarian site appeared. About 50% of the cases were bilateral lesions with smooth surface and nodular changes. Most of the lesions showed homogeneous low-density lesions with moderate enhancement on CT. On MRI, the lesions showed slightly low signal intensity on T1WI and slightly high signal intensity on T2WI. The signal was homogeneous, and moderate enhancement was shown after contrast enhancement [6–8].

29.3 Differential Diagnosis

Differential diagnosis includes epithelial ovarian tumors, metastatic tumor, etc. Malignant epithelial ovarian tumors rarely present as homogeneous solid masses, but are mostly cystic or solid and cystic. Cystic tumors with papillary mural nodules are typical manifestations. Ovarian serous carcinoma may appear as a solid mass with moderate hyperintensity on T2WI, with irregular boundary, and obvious enhancement was shown after contrast enhancement. Necrosis, hemorrhage, and cystic degeneration are common within the tumor. However, ovarian lymphomas are mostly solid homogeneous masses with relatively regular boundaries, and most of them are moderately enhanced after contrast enhancement. Ovarian lymphoma is difficult to distinguish from metastasis. Ovary is one of the most common sites of metastasis, and the most common primary sites include stomach and colon, followed by breast and genitourinary tract. Bilaterality is an important feature of ovarian metastasis. On CT and MR images, Krukenberg tumors typically appear as bilateral, lobulated, and solid tumors [9]. Although Krukenberg tumors are mainly solid tumors, about 33% of the tumors may be cystic predominant or completely cystic. Ovarian metastasis of colon cancer is often bilateral cystic tumor with solid components of different sizes [9]. Ovarian metastasis originating from the appendix is often bilateral ovarian mucinous tumors with pseudomyxoma peritonei, which is characterized by the presence of a large number of mucinous substances in the abdominal cavity. In patients with breast cancer, complex ovarian masses can be metastatic or coexisting primary ovarian tumors, especially in patients with BRCA mutations. Complex ovarian masses in patients with early-stage breast cancer are mostly primary, whereas metastatic tumors should be considered first in patients with advanced breast cancer if bilateral ovarian masses are found [10]. Different from those originating from the gastrointestinal tract, metastatic tumors originating from the breast are rarely seen with a pelvic mass as the initial presentation, and the gross appearance is characterized by bilateral, relatively small, solid, multinodular lesions, most of which are less than 7 cm in diameter [10]. In the case of known history of primary cancer, if small bilateral ovarian masses are found, the possibility of metastasis should be suspected.

References

1. Dimopoulos MA, Daliani D, Pugh W, et al. Primary ovarian non-Hodgkin's lymphoma: outcome after treatment with combination chemotherapy. Gynecol Oncol. 1997;64(3):446–50.
2. Monterroso V, Jaffe ES, Merino MJ, et al. Malignant lymphomas involving the ovary: a clinicopathologic analysis of 39 cases. Am J Surg Pathol. 1993;17(2):154–70.
3. Vang R, Medeiros LJ, Warnke RA, et al. Ovarian non-Hodgkin's lymphoma: a clinicopathologic study of eight primary cases. Mod Pathol. 2001;14(11):1093–9.
4. Crawshaw J, Sohaib SA, Wotherspoon A, et al. Primary non-Hodgkin's lymphoma of the ovaries: imaging findings. Br J Radiol. 2007;80(956):e155–8.
5. Fox H, Langley FA, Govan ADT, et al. Malignant lymphoma presenting as an ovarian tumour: a clinicopathological analysis of 34 cases. Br J Obstet Gynaecol. 1988;95(4):386–90.
6. Ferrozzi F, Catanese C, Uccelli M, et al. Ovarian lymphoma: findings with ultrasonography, computerized tomography and magnetic resonance [in Italian]. Radiol Med (Torino). 1998;95(5):493–7.
7. Buy JN. Gynecological imaging. https://doi.org/10.1007/978-3-642-31012-6.394-397.
8. Chang WC, Meux MD, Yeh BM, et al. CT and MRI of adnexal masses in patients with primary nonovarian malignancy. AJR Am J Roentgenol. 2006;186(4):1039–45.
9. Willmott F, Allouni KA, Rockall A. Radiological manifestations of metastasis to the ovary. J Clin Pathol. 2012;65(7):585–90.
10. Kondi-Pafiti A, Kairi-Vasilatou E, Iavazzo C, et al. Metastatic neoplasms of the ovaries: a clinicopathological study of 97 cases. Arch Gynecol Obstet. 2011;284(5):1283–8.

Ovarian Carcinosarcoma

30

Fenghua Ma

30.1 Clinical History

Female patient, 43 years old, with pelvic mass found on health checkup for 1 month. CT of the middle and lower abdomen in another hospital showed a left ovarian tumor, which was considered to be ovarian cancer. She went to the outpatient clinic of our hospital and underwent ultrasound examination: weak echo in the left pelvic cavity with a size of 63 mm × 65 mm × 45 mm, indicating left cystic mass, viscous, with possible ovarian origin. Physical examination on admission: a 6 cm mass was palpable in the left adnexa area, with moderate activity and no tenderness.

MRI examination: mixed solid and cystic mass in the left adnexa area, with oval shape and well-defined boundary, measuring 7.9 cm × 8.3 cm × 8.5 cm in size. The solid part showed isointense signal on T1WI and slightly hyperintense on T2WI; the cystic part showed hypointense signal on T1WI and hyperintense on T2WI. After contrast enhancement, the solid part was significantly inhomogeneous enhanced, and there was no obvious effusion in the pelvic cavity and no obvious enlarged lymph nodes.

She underwent laparoscopic total hysterectomy, bilateral salpingo-oophorectomy, pelvic lymph node dissection, and greater omentum resection. During the operation, the uterus was found in anterior position, 5 cm × 4 cm × 4 cm in size, with regular shape. The left ovary showed cystic enlargement, 6 cm × 6 cm × 5 cm in size, and dense adhesion to lateral peritoneum; part of the intestinal canal and the posterior wall of the uterus and the left fallopian tube was enlarged and adhered to the ovary. The size of right ovary was about 3 cm × 2 cm × 3 cm, and no obvious abnormality was observed in morphology. Postoperative pathological results: (1) in the left ovarian carcinosarcoma, epithelial component is poorly differentiated adenocarcinoma, and mesenchymal component contains heterologous chondrosarcoma; (2) poorly differentiated adenocarcinoma of bilateral fallopian tubes; (3) endometrial poorly differentiated adenocarcinoma, infiltrating the myometrium, and tumor thrombus can be seen in the vessel.

30.2 Imaging Analysis

Ovarian carcinosarcoma (OCS) is a rare, highly aggressive tumor composed of malignant epithelial and mesenchymal components, accounting for about 1–4% of all malignant ovarian tumors [1]. Since malignant cell lines originate from Müllerian nodules of mesoderm during embryonic development, it is also called malignant Müllerian tumor or malignant mixed mesodermal tumor (MMMT). OCS has a high degree of malignancy and poor prognosis. The median survival time is 8–16 months, and more than 70% of patients die within 1 year [2]. Histologically, MMMT contains epithelial and sarcoma components. According to the source of mesenchymal tissue, MMMT is divided into homologous and heterologous. Homologous MMMT or OCS contains malignant interstitial components of the ovary itself, such as spindle cells. Heterologous MMMT contains sarcomas of non-ovarian origin such as bone and cartilage components [2].

The histological origin of OCS has been controversial. At present, OCS is classified as a subtype of ovarian endometrioid adenocarcinoma by WHO [3], which is mixed epithelial and mesenchymal ovarian tumor. Three theories about its origin are proposed: (1) Collision tumor theory: tumors are formed by a mixture of two different groups of histological malignant cells, such as endometrium and mesenchyma; (2) Synthetic tumor theory: cancerous components in tumor tissue induce the transformation of mesenchymal cells into sarcoma; (3) Compound tumor theory: the tumor originates from epithelial pluripotent stem cells, which acquire abnormal differentiation ability during the proliferation process and eventually form a biphasic tumor, but its cancerous components dominate the biological behavior of the tumor. Current studies of cell culture, immunohistochemistry, and

F. Ma (✉)
Department of Radiology, Obstetrics and Gynecology Hospital, Fudan University, Shanghai, People's Republic of China

G. Zhang (ed.), *MRI of Gynaecological Diseases*, https://doi.org/10.1007/978-981-99-3644-1_30

molecular genetics have suggested that OCS is a theory of pluripotent stem cell origin [4].

The onset age of OCS varies from 18 to 86 years old. It mainly occurs in postmenopausal women with barren and low birth rate, with about 10% on both ovaries. The diameter of tumors ranges from 10 cm to 25 cm, most of which are more than 10 cm. It is macronodular or irregular in shape, and the section is solid and cystic, gray-white or yellowish-brown, fish flesh appearance, brittle, and uneven hardness. Obvious bone and cartilage may appear, accompanied by unequal hemorrhage or necrosis areas [5]. Since the gross and microscopic pathology of ovarian MMMT is similar to that of uterine MMMT, understanding the imaging features of uterine MMMT is helpful to understand the imaging manifestations of ovarian MMMT. Smith et al. [6] reported that CT features of uterine MMMT were large and heterogeneous tumors with a diameter > 30 cm and a low density area in the center. Bharwani et al. [7] analyzed the MR characteristics of 51 cases of uterine MMMTs. On T1WI, 71% of lesions showed higher signal intensity than myometrium, 33% showed heterogeneous signal intensity, and 27% showed intratumoral high signal intensity. On T2WI, 92% of lesions showed higher signal intensity than myometrium, and 82% of them were heterogeneous. 19 patients underwent contrast-enhanced examination, about 50% of the tumor showed early enhancement (less than 1 min of contrast agent injection), and the signal intensity was similar to or higher than that of myometrium; 62% of the tumor showed delayed enhancement (more than 4 min of contrast agent injection), 58% showed heterogeneous enhancement, and 42% showed homogeneous enhancement. Enlarged lymph nodes were seen in 40% of patients, with distant metastasis in about 8%. Cho et al. [8] analyzed 13 MMMTs from 8 patients and found that 5 cases were bilateral and 3 cases were unilateral. 2 MMMTs were multilocular cystic and 11 were mixed solid and cystic. 10 MMMTs were lager than 10 cm in diameter, and 11 tumors showed significant homogeneous enhancement. Ascites were observed in all eight patients. In our case, OCS was multilocular solid and cystic; the solid part showed iso-signal on T1WI (Figs. 30.1–30.3), and slightly high signal on T2WI (Figs. 30.4–30.6 and 30.7–30.9), with a slightly lower degree of enhancement than that of myometrium (Figs. 30.10–30.15). DWI (Figs. 30.16–30.18) showed significantly high signal, suggesting that it was malignant. Imaging features were non-specific, and it was difficult to distinguish from other ovarian malignant tumors only based on imaging findings. However, the possibility of OCS should be taken into account when bilateral, heterogeneous masses larger than 10 cm in diameter with high invasiveness are seen in the abdominal and pelvic cavity.

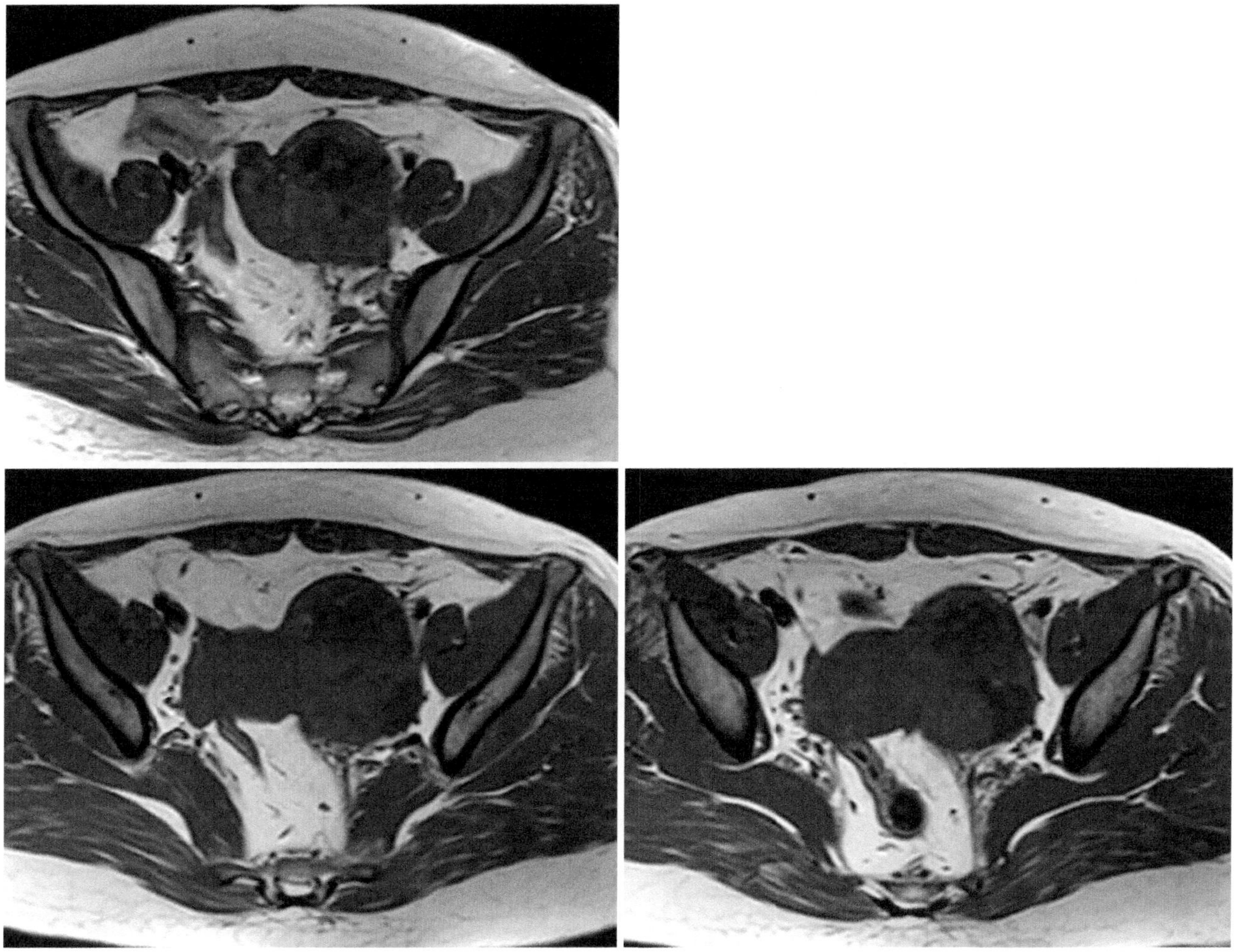

Figs. 30.1–30.3 Axial T1WI: The solid part showed iso-signal and the cystic part showed low signal

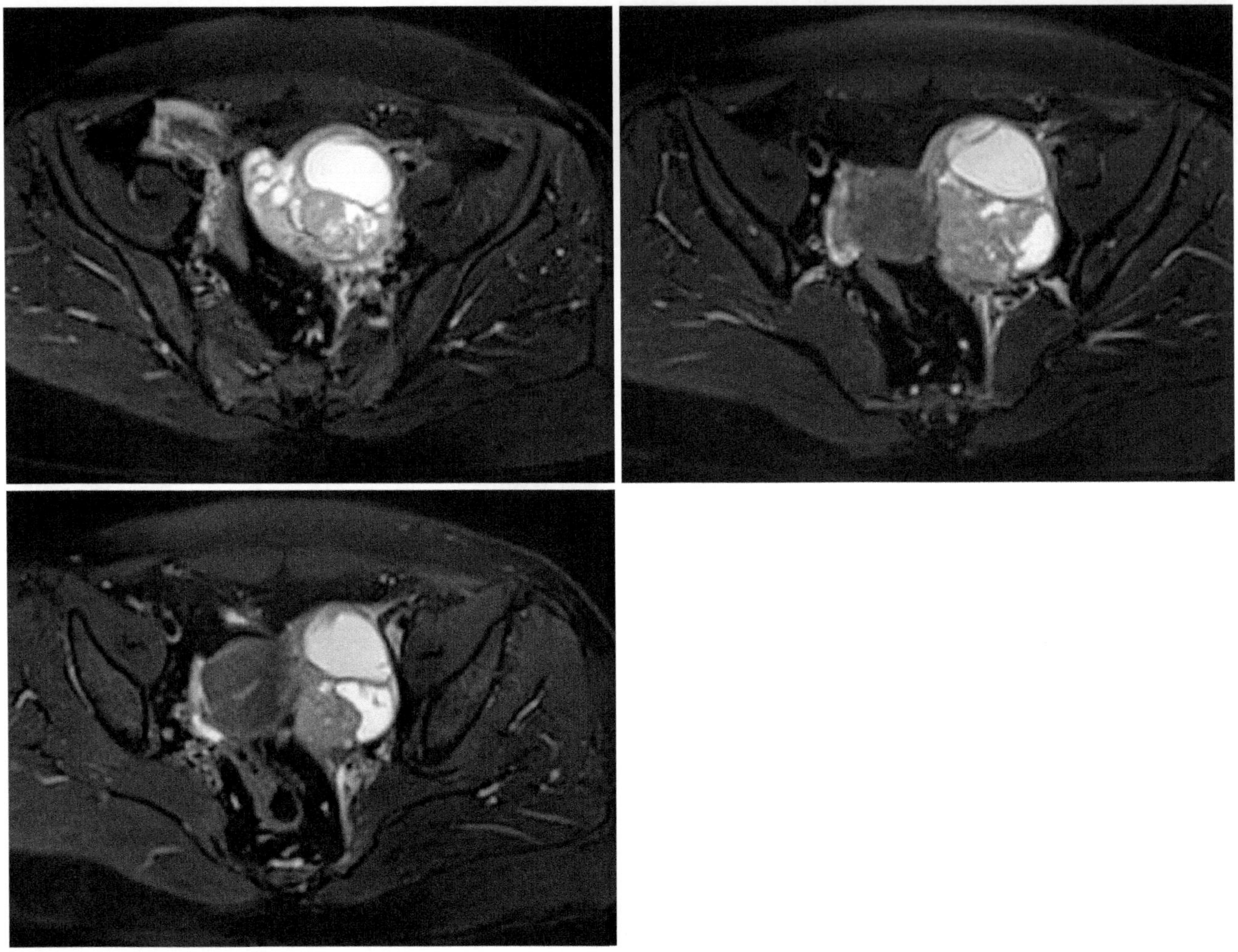

Figs. 30.4–30.6 Pre-contrast T2WI fat suppression: There is an irregular solid and cystic mass in the left adnexa area. The solid part showed slightly high signal, and the signal was homogeneous. The cystic part showed significantly high signal

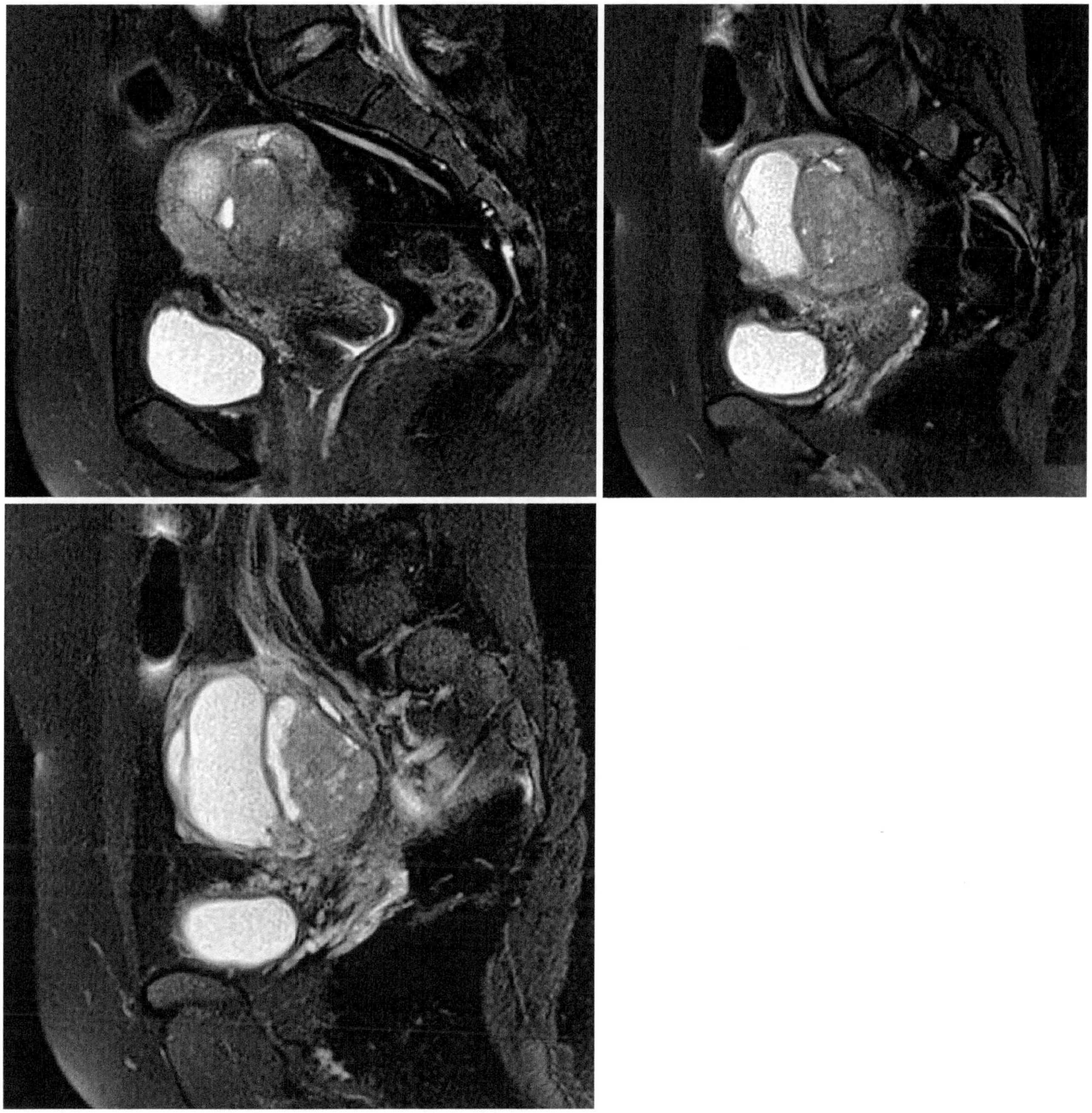

Figs. 30.7–30.9 Sagittal T2WI: The boundary between the lesion and myometrium was unclear

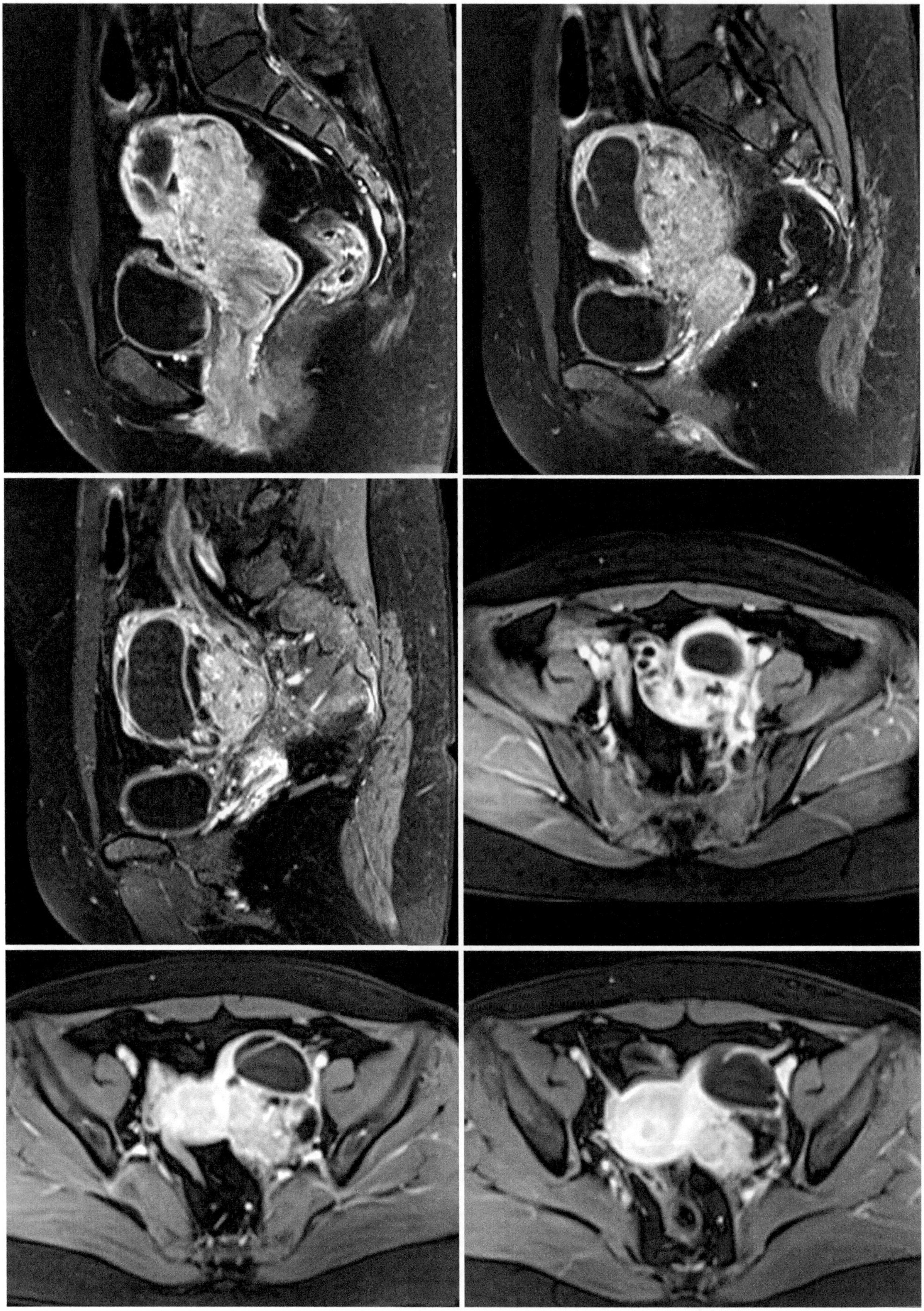

Figs. 30.10–30.15 Sagittal and axial T1WI contrast-enhanced images: The solid part of the lesion showed significantly inhomogeneous enhancement, the cystic part was not significantly enhanced, and the cystic wall was significantly enhanced

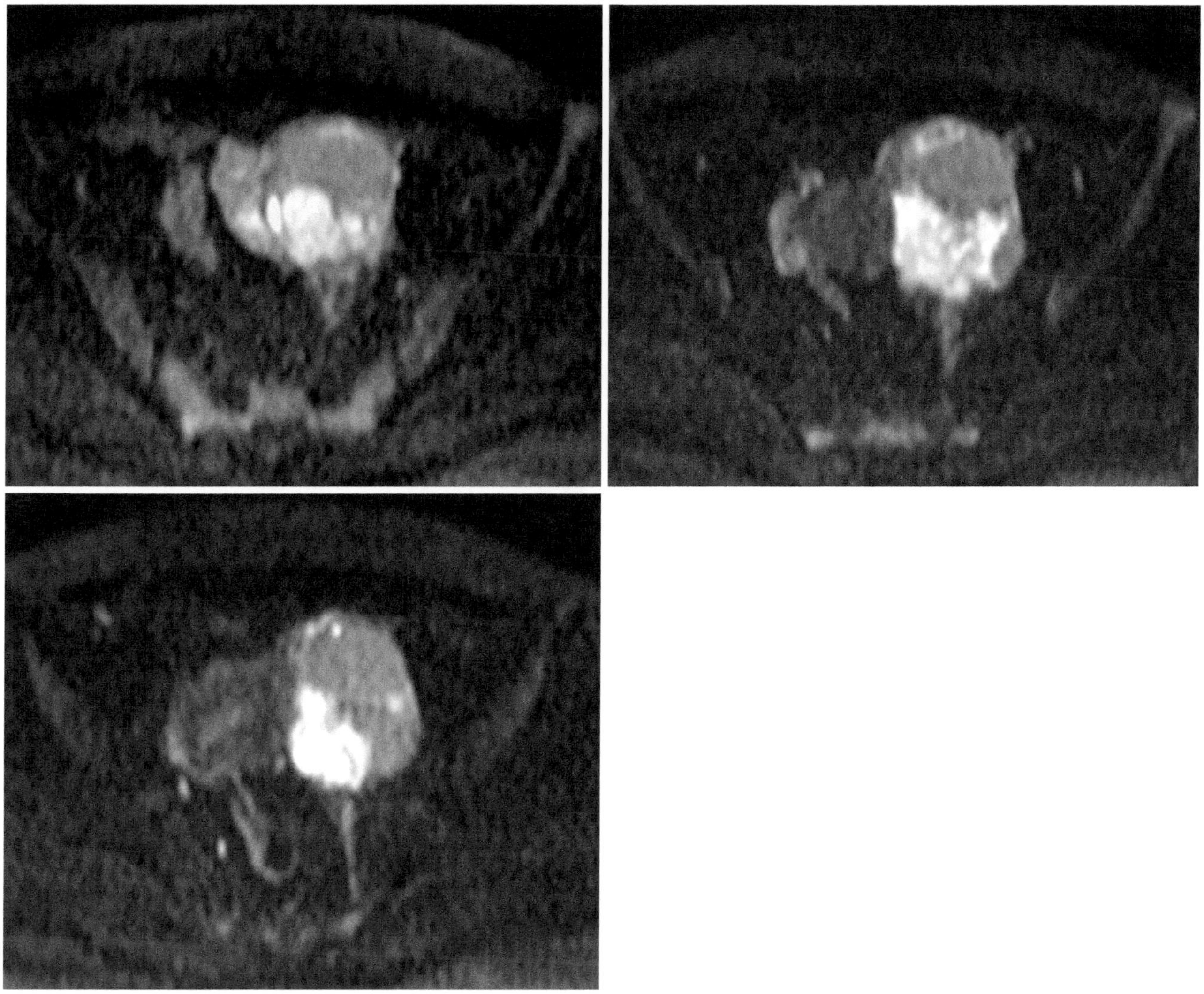

Figs. 30.16–30.18 Diffusion weighted imaging (DWI): The solid part showed significant high signal, and the cystic part showed low signal

References

1. del Carmen MG, Birrer M, Schorge JO. Carcinosarcoma of the ovary: a review of the literature. Gynecol Oncol. 2012;125(1):271–7.
2. Sit AS, Price FV, Kelley JL, et al. Chemotherapy for malignant mixed Müllerian tumors of the ovary. Gynecol Oncol. 2000;79:196–200.
3. Kaku T, Ogawa S, Kawano Y, et al. Histological classification of ovarian cancer. Med Electron Microsc. 2003;36:9–17.
4. Shen YM, Xie YP, Xu L, et al. Malignant mixed müllerian tumor of the fallopian tube: report of two cases and review of literature. Arch Gynecol Obstet. 2010;281:1023–8. Epub 2009 Dec 23. Review
5. Scully RE, Young RH, Clement PB. Tumors of the ovary, maldeveloped gonads, fallopian tubes and broad ligament. In: Rosai J, Sobin LH, editors. Atlas of tumor pathology, vol. 3. Washington, DC: Armed Force Institute of Pathology; 1998. p. 51–168.
6. Smith T, Moy L, Runowicz C. Müllerian mixed tumors: CT characteristics with clinical and pathologic observations. AJR. 1997;169:531–5.
7. Bharwani N, Newland A, Tunariu N, et al. MRI appearances of uterine malignant mixed müllerian tumors. AJR. 2010;195:1268–75.
8. Cho SB, Park CM, Park SW, et al. Malignant mixed müllerian tumors of the ovary: imaging findings. Eur Radiol. 2001;11:1147–50.

31 Ovarian Immature Teratoma

Mengwei Zhang

31.1 Clinical History

Female patient, 24 years old, was found to have a pelvic mass on health checkup for 3 days. She was conscious of a lower abdominal mass for nearly 2 months and had abdominal distension and pain during menstruation. Ultrasound examination showed an area of 129 mm × 75 mm × 75 mm with irregular echo above, colored blood flow in a punctate pattern on the right side of uterus, and medium hyperechoic area on the left side of uterus, 56 mm × 53 mm × 39 mm in size, and colored blood flow was not obvious.

She underwent transabdominal bilateral ovarian cystectomy. Intraoperative findings: the uterus was in anterior position, 5 cm × 5 cm × 4 cm in size and with normal shape. The right ovary showed cystic enlargement, with 13 cm × 8 cm × 8 cm in size, irregular shape, smooth surface, no obvious crevasse, and loose adhesion with part of the greater omentum. No abnormality was observed in the right fallopian tube. No abnormality was found in the left ovary and fallopian tube. No abnormality in the bladder and rectouterine pouch.

Postoperative pathological results: (1) right ovarian immature teratoma, grade I; (2) left ovarian cystic mature teratoma.

31.2 Imaging Analysis

Ovarian immature teratoma is the most common malignant germ cell tumor, accounting for about 20–35% of all germ cell tumors [1]. It is composed of derived tissues of three germ layers (ectoderm, mesoderm, and endoderm). Compared with mature teratoma, it contains different amounts of immature embryonic tissues [2]. Clinically, it occurs more common in young women aged 10–20 years old; the average age of onset is 20 years old and rarely in middle-aged or postmenopausal women. Clinical symptoms are nonspecific, mostly abdominal pain, abdominal distension, palpable abdominal mass, and occasionally teratoma rupture or torsion, with acute abdominal symptoms. AFP and CA125 are elevated in many patients with immature teratoma, although the level of CA125 is much lower than that of ovarian serous adenocarcinoma. In most patients, the mass is mostly confined to the ovary, 50–80% of which belongs to stage I, unilateral more common, and can invade the contralateral ovary in advanced patients. 10–15% of patients have contralateral benign cystic teratoma.

The gross pathological manifestations are mostly unilateral solid predominantly lobulated mass, with a large variation in diameter, with an average of 18 cm. Solid tissue is usually immature nerve tissue. Occasionally, it presents as unilocular or multilocular cystic predominantly with solid mural nodules. It has been reported that typical CT and MRI manifestations of immature teratoma are huge mixed masses, including solid components (containing multiple small cysts), scattered calcification, and small foci of fat [3, 4]. As for the predominantly solid mass, pre-contrast CT shows heterogeneous soft-tissue density, scattered calcification, and lipid droplets within the mass are highly suggestive of teratoma, dynamic contrast-enhanced CT shows tumor vessels in the arterial phase, and significant enhancement in the parenchymal phase indicates malignant tumor [5]. Most of the solid components on MRI show low signal intensity, and the signal of T2WI is equal to or slightly higher than that of myometrium. Fat foci are scattered in the solid components. Multiple low signal areas can be seen in the fat suppression image of T2WI, and solid components are obviously unevenly enhanced after contrast enhancement. In this case, a typical predominantly solid mass was seen in the right adnexa area, with mainly low signal on T1WI (Figs. 31.1 and 31.2), and scattered patchy high signal could be seen inside and heterogeneous high signal intensity on T2WI (Figs. 31.3–31.6).

M. Zhang (✉)
Department of Radiology, Obstetrics and Gynecology Hospital, Fudan University, Shanghai, P.R. China

G. Zhang (ed.), *MRI of Gynaecological Diseases*, https://doi.org/10.1007/978-981-99-3644-1_31

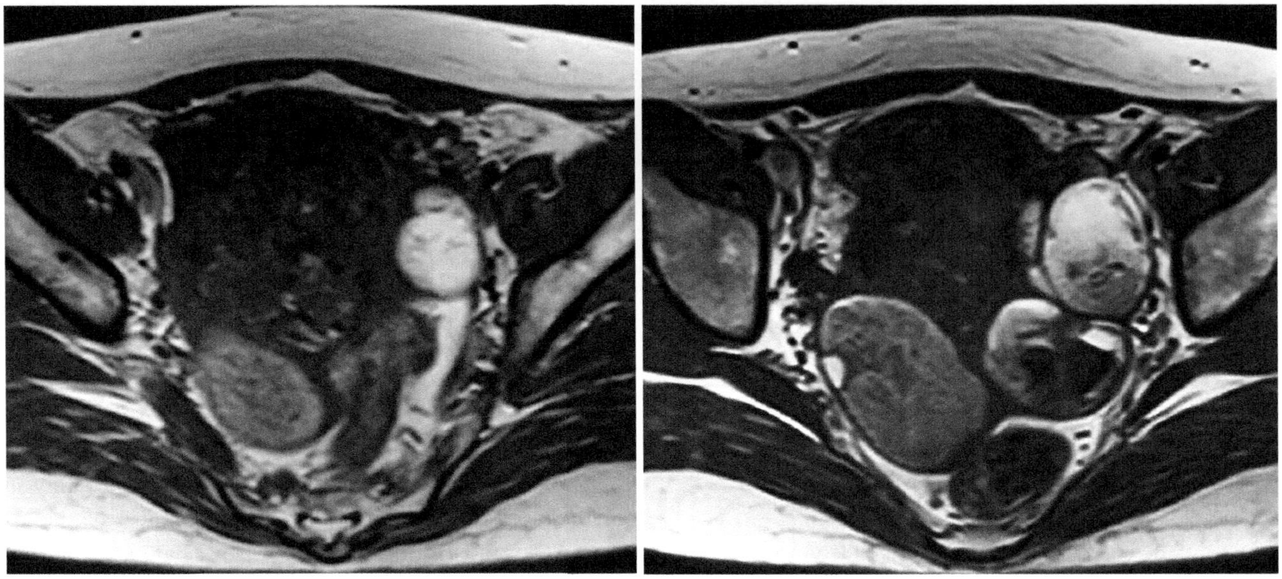

Figs. 31.1 and 31.2 An irregular solid and cystic mixed mass could be seen in the right adnexa area, mainly iso-hypointense on T1WI, and mixed high and low signal on T2WI fat suppression image. The cystic part showed moderate high signal, and the high signal on T2WI fat suppression image was not suppressed

After contrast enhancement, the solid component was obviously unevenly enhanced, and large fat foci could be seen inside the lesion, both presented with high signal on T1WI and T2WI and showed low signal on T1WI fat suppression after contrast enhancement (Figs. 31.7–31.9). Typical mature teratoma signals can be seen in the left adnexa area, and both T1WI and T2WI images showed predominantly high signal intensity and localized enhancement after contrast enhancement, and fat signal was suppressed on fat suppression images, which is different from the tumor mass in the right adnexa area, confirming coexistence of mature teratoma with immature teratoma in the same patient.

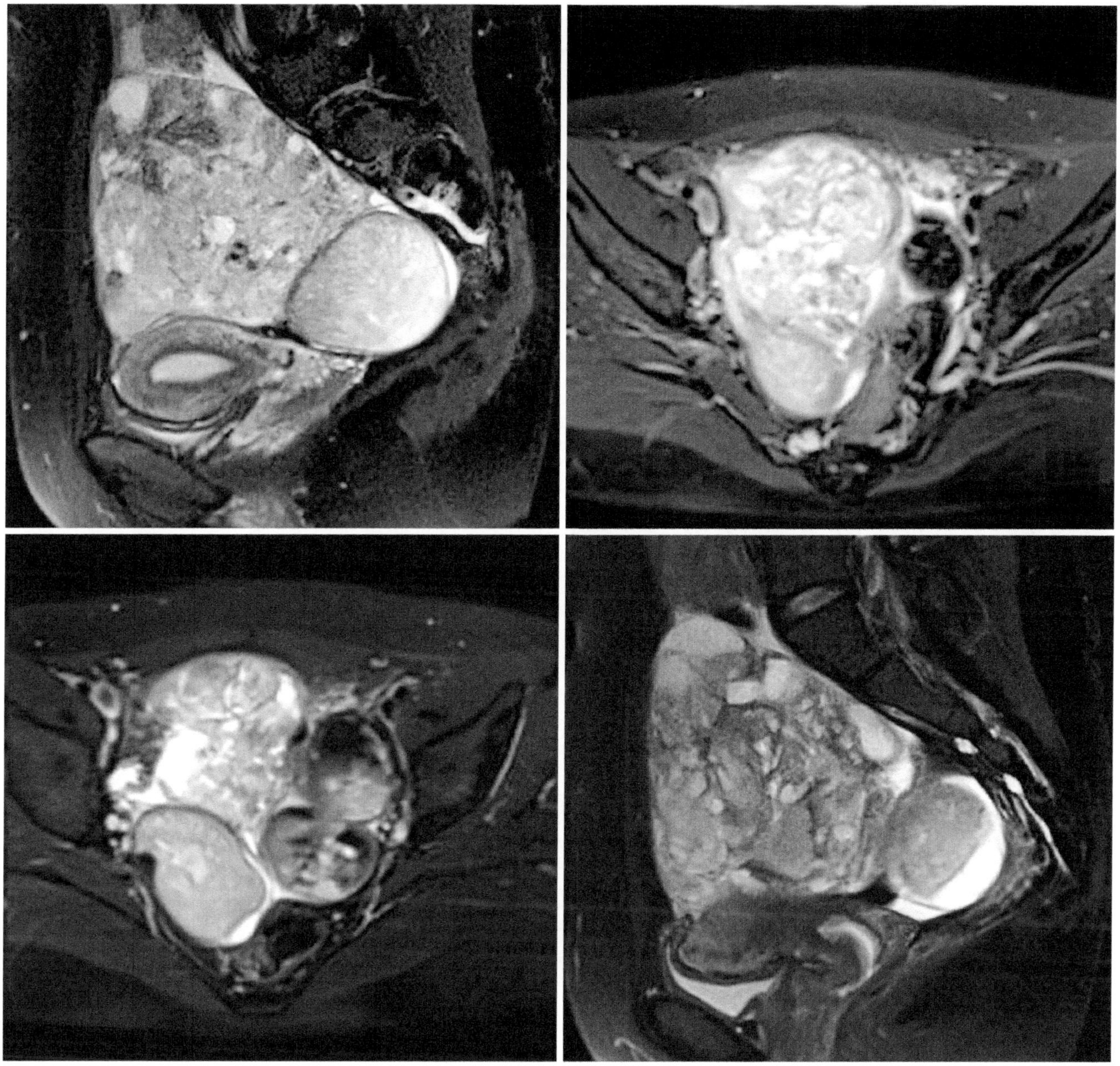

Figs. 31.3–31.6 A gourd-shaped mass was seen in the left adnexa area. On T1WI, it was predominantly high signal, and small patchy slightly low signal could be seen locally. On T2WI fat suppression image, it was high and low mixed signal, and the high signal area on the original T1WI was presented with low signal

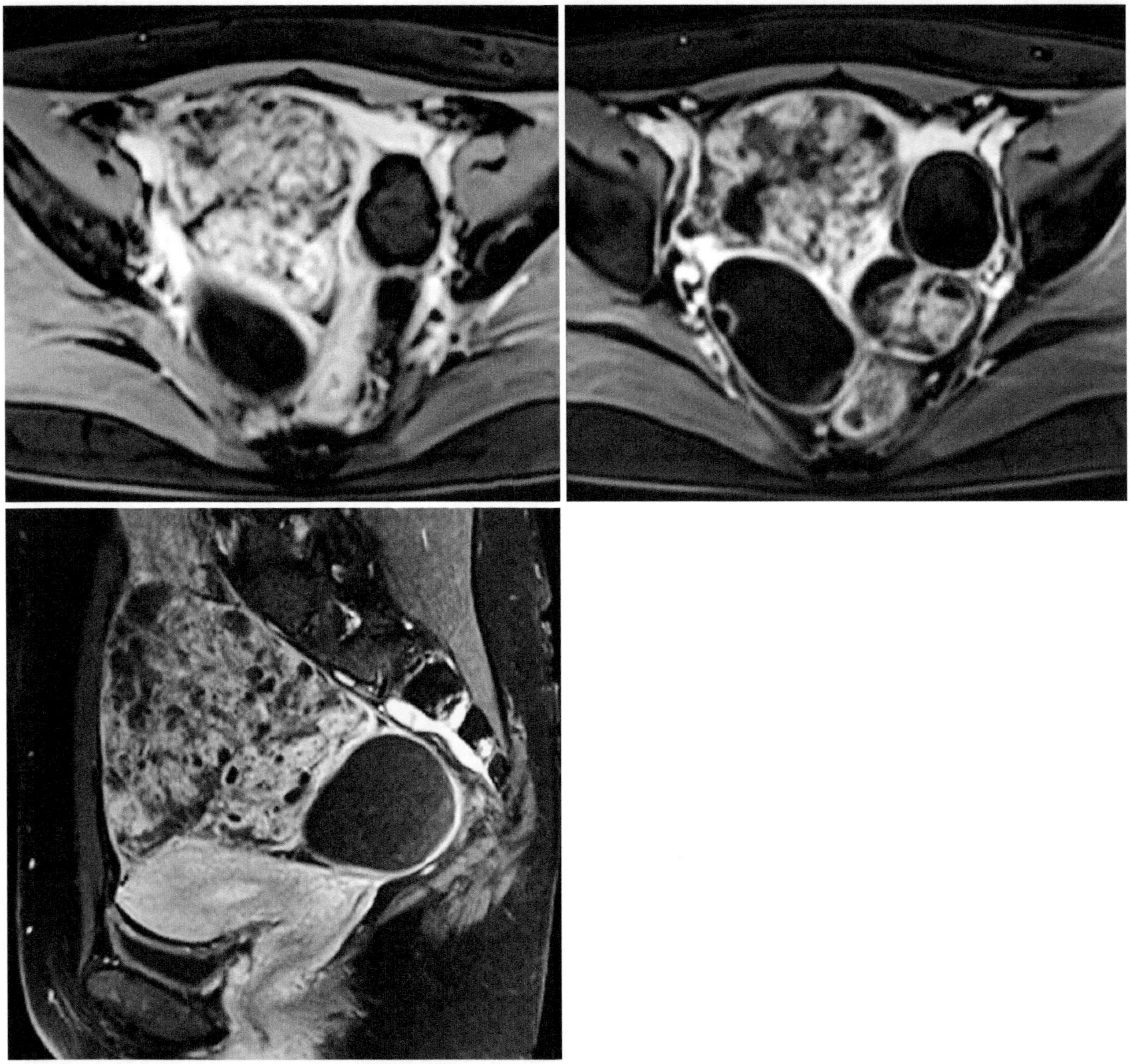

Figs. 31.7–31.9 Sagittal and axial T1WI contrast-enhanced images, the lesion in the right adnexa area was significantly unevenly enhanced, and there was no enhancement in the cystic area; small patchy mild enhancement was seen locally in the left lesion, and the high signal on the original T1WI was suppressed

31.3 Differential Diagnosis

It is not difficult to differentiate immature teratoma with a large amount of fat from other types of malignant tumors that are predominantly solid. Immature teratoma with a small amount of fat needs to be differentiated from malignant tumors that are predominantly solid. Some special MR sequences such as gradient echo chemical shift imaging can be used to determine the presence of a small amount of fat. Some immature teratoma presents as a predominantly cystic mass, which is difficult to distinguish from multilocular cystic borderline mucinous tumors or mucinous adenocarcinoma. However, the presence of fat foci within the tumor may help to differentiate.

References

1. Smith HO, Berwick M, Verschraegen CF, et al. Incidence and survival rates for female malignant germ cell tumors. Obstet Gynecol. 2006;107(5):1075–85.
2. Cho NH, Kim YT, Lee JH, et al. Diagnostic challenge of fetal ontogeny and its application on the ovarian teratomas. Int J Gynecol Pathol. 2005;24(2):173–82.
3. Bazot M, Cortez A, Sananes S, et al. Imaging of dermoid cysts with foci of immature tissue. J Comput Assist Tomogr. 1999;23:703–6.
4. Outwater EK, Siegelman ES, Hunt JL. Ovarian teratomas: tumor types and imaging characteristics. Radiographics. 2001;21:475–90.
5. Buy JN, Ghossain M. Gynecological imaging. 2013.

Part VI

Borderline Tumors of the Ovary

Borderline Epithelial Tumor of the Ovary

32

Shuhui Zhao

32.1 Clinical History

Case 1

Female patient, 37 years old, underwent routine health checkup, and bilateral cystic adnexal masses were incidental findings in an ultrasound examination. Regular menstruation, no abnormal vaginal bleeding and discharge, and leukorrhea with no abnormalities. No abdominal pain and no recent weight loss. Postoperative pathological result: bilateral borderline serous ovarian tumors.

Case 2

Female patient, 55 years old, had been experiencing menopausal for 2 years. The patient was diagnosed with thyroid cancer in June last year and underwent radical thyroidectomy. She was admitted to the nuclear medicine department of our hospital for radioisotope therapy in November last year. PET-CT indicated that there was a high metabolic low density mass in the right adnexa area, and adnexal source tumor was considered. She underwent gynecological ultrasound examination, and ultrasonography showed that bilateral ovaries were not shown, and a solid mass of 76 mm × 67 mm was found in the right pelvic cavity, with clear boundary, CDFI: obvious blood flow signal was seen. She underwent total hysterectomy and bilateral salpingo-oophorectomy. Postoperative pathological result: right ovarian borderline serous tumor and locally micropapillary subtype/noninvasive low-grade serous carcinoma; the tumor is mainly located on ovarian surface.

Case 3

Female patient, 29 years old, was found with adnexal mass 1.5 years after ovarian tumor surgery. The patient underwent laparoscopic left ovarian cyst removal surgery in our hospital 1.5 years ago, and postoperative pathology was mucinous borderline tumor of left ovary. One week ago, she had a small amount of intermittent vaginal bleeding without obvious inducement. Ultrasound examination showed that there was a medium-low mixed echo mass in the left adnexa area, 87 mm × 60 mm in size, with irregular morphology, mainly mass-like hyperechogenicity inside. CDFI: partially it had blood flow signals, and the rest were anechoic. She was diagnosed with left adnexal mass, left ovarian mucinous borderline tumor recurrence? She underwent laparoscopic left ovarian cyst removal, right ovarian biopsy, and multipoint peritoneal biopsy. Postoperative pathological result: mucinous borderline tumor of left ovary and biopsy of the right ovary and peritoneum showed no tumor involvement.

32.2 Imaging Analysis

Among all epithelial ovarian tumors, 4–14% tumors are low malignant. They are called borderline epithelial ovarian tumors. Atypical epithelial proliferation and moderate nuclear atypia can be seen in borderline epithelial ovarian tumors. There is no stromal invasion in borderline epithelial ovarian tumors. However, micro-invasion can be seen in about 10% cases. Borderline tumors may occur in all types of epithelial ovarian tumors. Serous and mucinous are the two most common types [1, 2]. Borderline epithelial ovarian tumors prevail in young women. Usually, they are early-stage disease at diagnosis. Peritoneal implants and lymphadenopathy are uncommon. They have excellent prognosis, even in patients with peritoneal implants. Relapse may occur in borderline epithelial ovarian tumors [3, 4].

Serous borderline tumor (Figs. 32.1 and 32.2) often occurs bilaterally (33–65%). Morphologically, they have various appearances. They can display as a cystic mass with papillary projections. Also, they can appear as an entirely solid mass. The solid lesion has high signal on T2WI and intense enhancement on contrast-enhanced images. Internal fibrous stalks are low signal on T2WI. Internal fibrous stalks have mild enhancement on contrast-enhanced images. In

S. Zhao (✉)
Department of Radiology, Xinhua Hospital, Medical College of Shanghai Jiao Tong University, Shanghai, P.R. China

G. Zhang (ed.), *MRI of Gynaecological Diseases*, https://doi.org/10.1007/978-981-99-3644-1_32

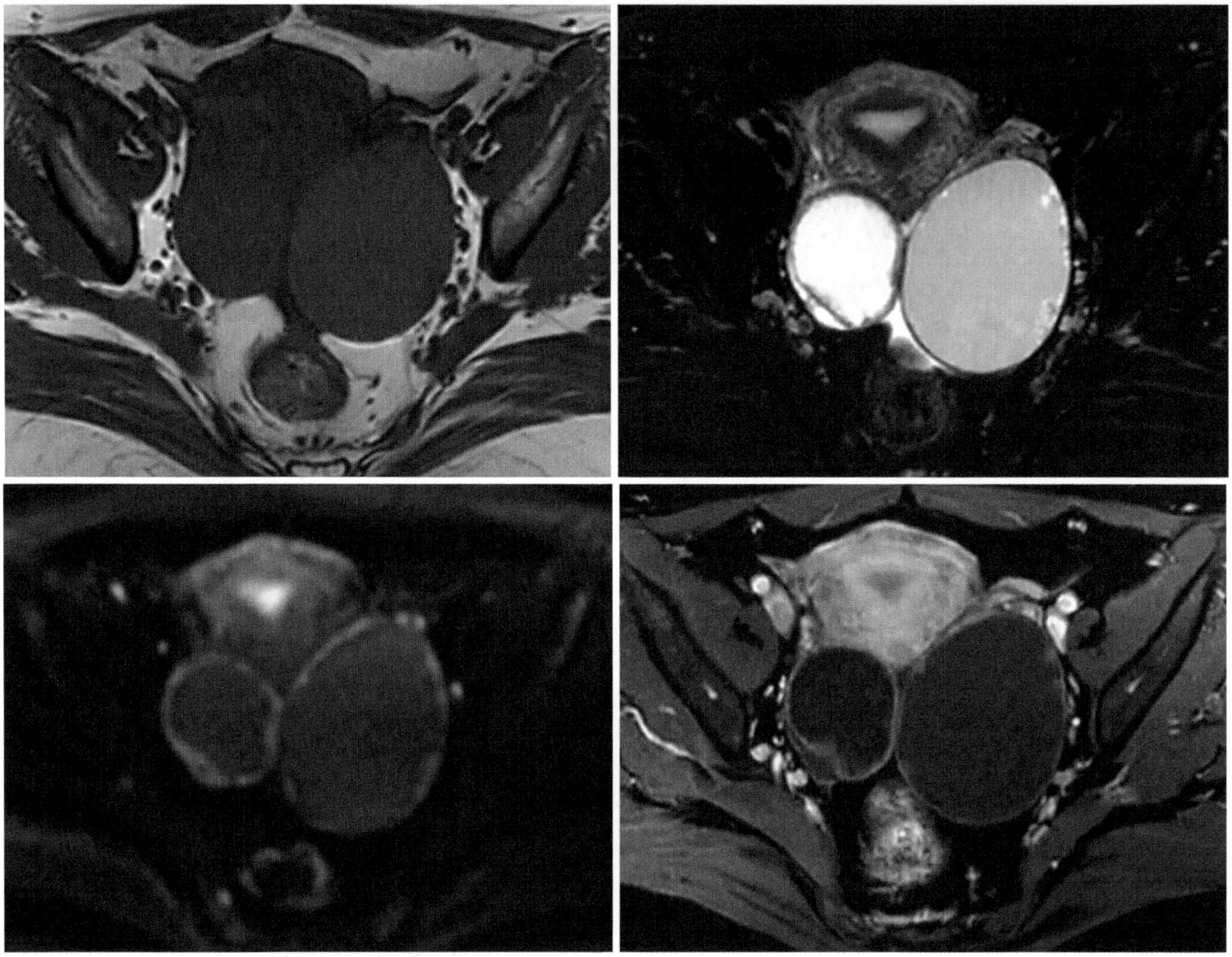

Fig. 32.1 A 37-year-old woman with bilateral borderline serous ovarian tumors. Axial T1-weighted image (**a**) showed bilateral ovarian lesions of low and slightly high signal intensity. T2-weighted with fat suppression image (**b**) showed the lesions had high signal intensity with multiple papillary projections from the cystic wall. The cystic wall and papillary projections showed restricted diffusion on DWI (**c**). T1-weighted contrast-enhanced image (**d**) showed the cystic wall and papillary projections had enhancement

addition, serous borderline tumor can display as a mixed solid and cystic lesion. Serous borderline tumor is characterized by papillary architecture with hypointense fibrous stalk on T2WI [4, 5].

Mucinous tumor (Fig. 32.3) often occurs unilaterally (96%). They often demonstrate as a huge multilocular cystic mass with a median diameter of 18.3 cm. In contrast to benign counterpart, borderline mucinous tumors have some distinguishing appearances. Honeycomb loculi, high signal intensity on T1WI, and low signal intensity on T2WI of the cystic content, thickened septation or wall (>5 mm), and vegetations (>5 mm) indicate a borderline mucinous tumor on MRI [6–8].

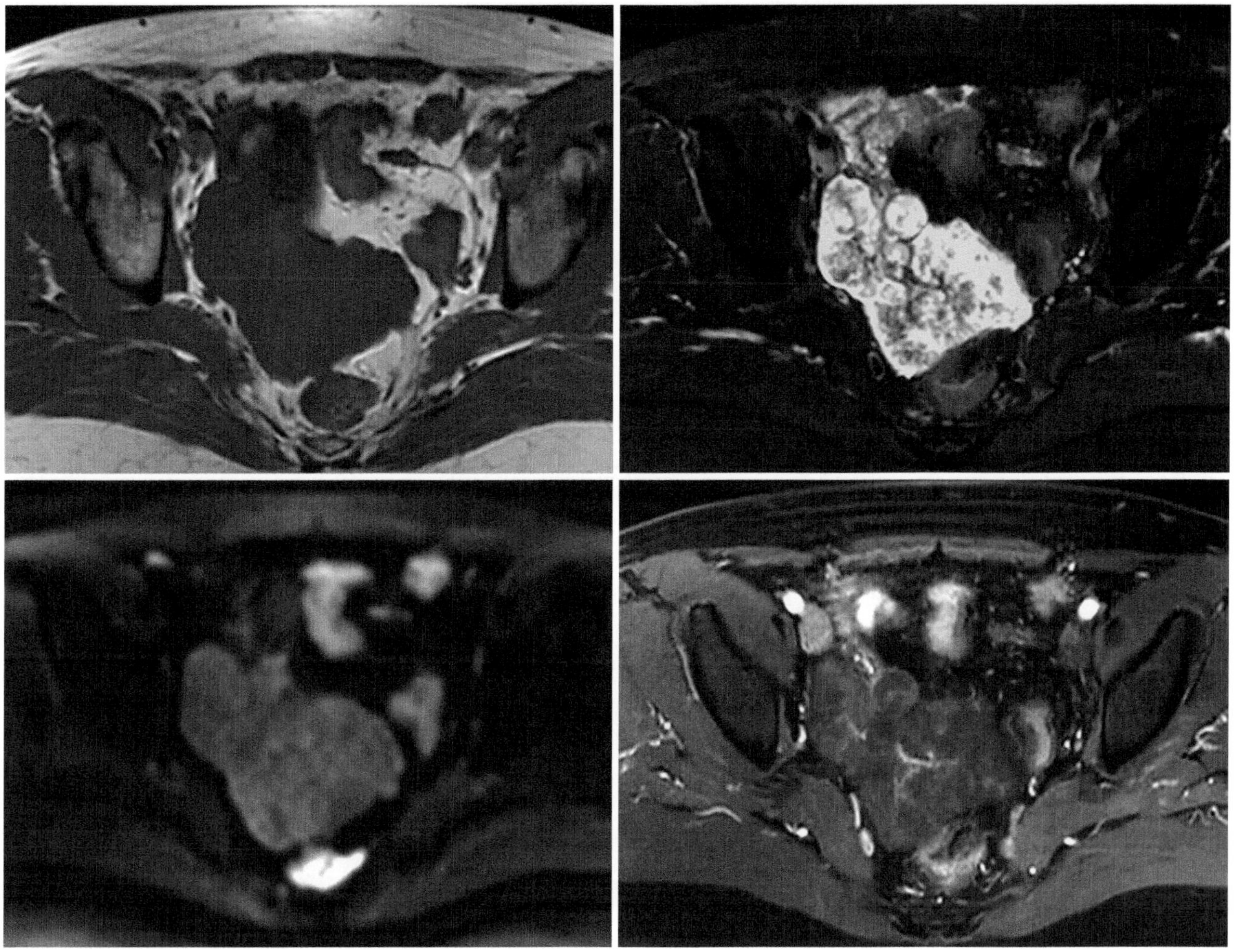

Fig. 32.2 A 55-year-old woman with right ovarian borderline serous tumor. Axial T1-weighted image (**a**) showed an ovarian lesion of low signal intensity. T2-weighted with fat suppression image (**b**) showed the lesion had high signal intensity. Internal branching fibrous stalks were low signal intensity. The lesion showed moderate signal intensity on DWI (**c**). T1-weighted contrast-enhanced image (**d**) showed the lesion had enhancement. Internal branching fibrous stalks had marked enhancement

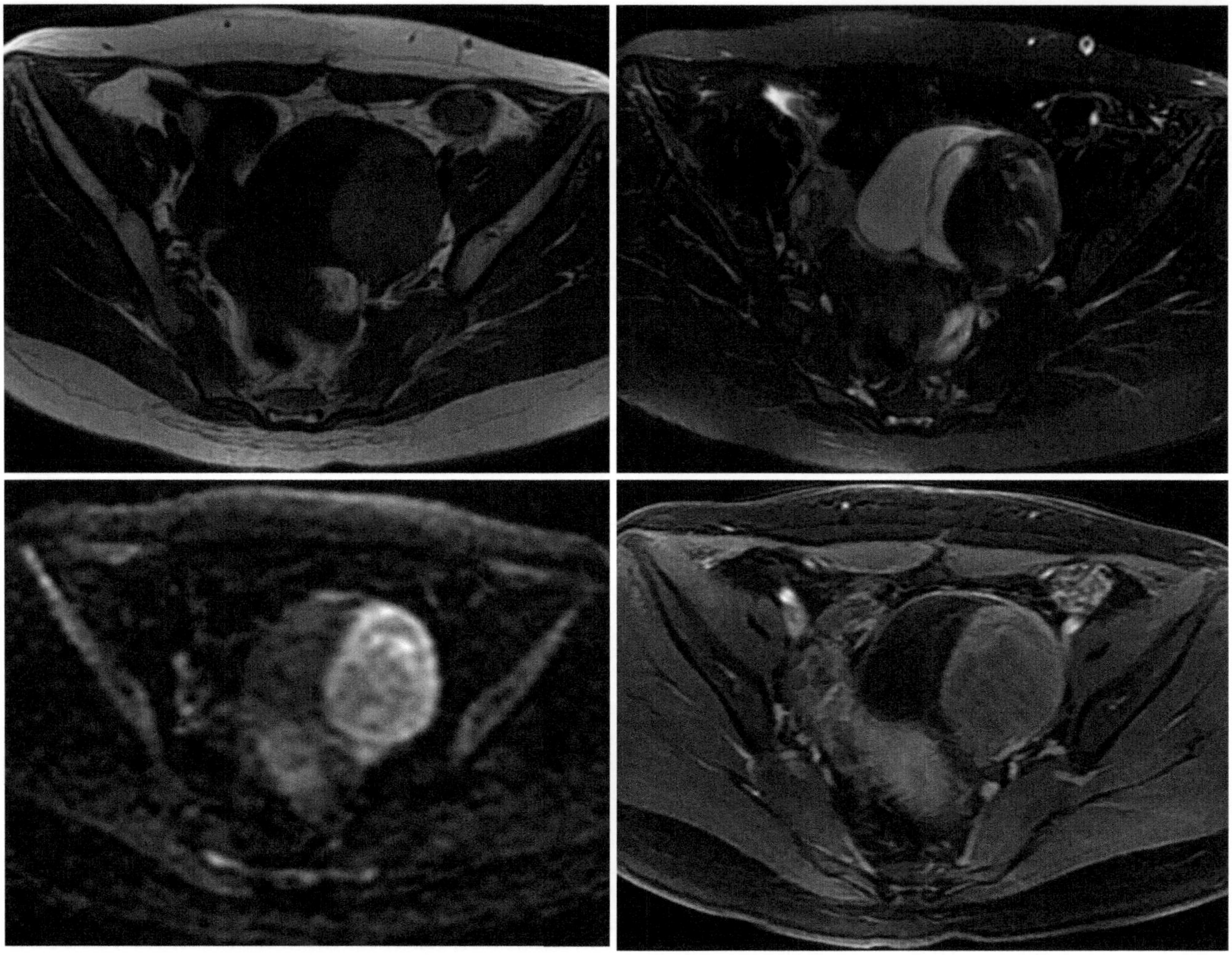

Fig. 32.3 A 29-year-old woman with mucinous borderline tumor of the left ovary. Axial T1-weighted image (**a**) and T2-weighted with fat suppression image (**b**) showed a multilocular cystic ovarian mass of heterogeneous signal intensity. Loculi with watery mucin had low signal intensity on T1WI and high signal intensity on T2WI. Loculi with thicker mucin had high signal intensity on T1WI and low signal intensity on T2WI. The lesion showed heterogeneous signal intensity on DWI (**c**). T1-weighted contrast-enhanced image (**d**) showed the cystic wall and septa had obvious enhancement

32.3 Differential Diagnosis

Ovarian serous borderline tumors need to be differentiated from ovarian cancer. Ovarian serous borderline tumors are variable in morphology, from mainly cystic to completely solid, characterized by papillary structures. Solid or solid and cystic serous borderline tumors have a typical branched papillary structure with dendritic internal fibrous branches and hypointense on T2WI. DWI is helpful to distinguish the two. The signal intensity of solid component on DWI is weaker than that of ovarian malignant epithelial tumors. Borderline ovarian tumors have a higher ADC value than ovarian cancer. When the b value is 1000 s/mm^2, the diagnostic cut-off value is 1.041×10^{-3} mm^2/s. In addition, the onset age of ovarian cancer is older than that of borderline ovarian tumors, and it is more prone to metastasize.

Ovarian mucinous borderline tumors need to be differentiated from benign mucinous cystadenoma. Both ovarian benign mucinous cystadenoma and mucinous borderline tumor are characterized by huge multilocular masses and lack of large solid components. The MRI signs suggestive of the diagnosis of ovarian mucinous borderline tumors are honeycomb loculi, T1WI high/T2WI low signal cystic fluid, irregular thickening of the cyst wall or septa, nodules, or papillary projections (≥5 mm).

References

1. Hart WR. Borderline epithelial tumors of the ovary. Mod Pathol. 2005;18(Suppl 2):S33–50.
2. Zhao S, Qiang J, Zhang G, Ma F, Cai S, Li H, et al. Diffusion-weighted MR imaging for differentiating borderline from malignant epithelial tumors of the ovary: pathological correlation. Eur Radiol. 2014;24(9):2292–9.
3. Bent CL, Sahdev A, Rockall AG, Singh N, Sohaib SA, Reznek RH. MRI appearances of borderline ovarian tumors. Clin Radiol. 2009;64(4):430–8.
4. Tanaka YO, Okada S, Satoh T, Matsumoto K, Oki A, Nishida M, et al. Ovarian serous surface papillary borderline tumors form sea anemone-like masses. J Magn Reson Imaging. 2015;33(3):633–40.
5. Zhao S, Qiang J, Zhang G, Boyko OB, Wang S, Cai S, et al. MRI appearances of ovarian serous borderline tumor: pathological correlation. J Magn Reson Imaging. 2014;40(1):151–6.
6. Ma F, Zhao S, Qiang J, Zhang G, Wang X, Wang L. MRI appearances of mucinous borderline ovarian tumors: pathological correlation. J Magn Reson Imaging. 2015;40(3):745–51.
7. Zhao S, Qiang J, Zhang G, Wang S, Qiu H, Wang L. MRI in differentiating ovarian borderline from benign mucinous cystadenoma: pathological correlation. J Magn Reson Imaging. 2014;39(1):162–6.
8. Okamoto Y, Tanaka YO, Tsunoda H, Yoshikawa H, Minami M. Malignant or borderline mucinous cystic neoplasms have a larger number of loculi than mucinous cystadenoma: a retrospective study with MR. J Magn Reson Imaging. 2007;26(1):94–9.

Seromucinous Borderline Tumor Derived from Endometriosis

33

Shouxin Gu

33.1 Clinical History

A 36-year-old woman underwent medical examination for occasional abdominal distension 1 month ago. Ultrasound examination revealed an ovarian cyst, which was considered as endometrioid cyst. There was no abnormal vaginal bleeding, nausea, vomiting, and other discomfort. Serum tumor markers showed elevated CA125 (81.17 U/mL) and CA199 (195.7 U/mL) and normal HE4 (43.93 pmol/L) and CEA (1.06 ng/mL). Intraoperative findings: solid and cystic enlargement of the right ovary, about 5 cm × 4 cm × 3 cm in size, with membranous adhesion to the right posterior wall of uterus and lateral pelvic wall. Postoperative pathological result: (right ovary) seromucinous borderline tumor, originating from endometriosis.

33.2 Imaging Analysis

In 2014, World Health Organization (WHO) classifications included the new pathological classification of seromucinous borderline tumor (SMBT), which combined previously diagnosed as endocervical-like mucinous borderline tumor/Müllerian mucinous borderline tumor (MMBT) and Müllerian mixed epithelial borderline tumor (MEBT) [1, 2]. SMBT is defined as a non-invasive, proliferative epithelial neoplasm with more than one epithelial cell type, usually serous and cervical mucinous components, but endometrioid and less commonly, clear cell, transitional cell, or squamous cell components can also be seen. The clinical features of SMBT are similar to those of serous borderline tumors, most of which are FIGO stage I and a few are advanced stage, with implantation and/or lymph node involvement. Histogenesis is considered to be associated with endometriosis, with at least 1/3 associated with endometriosis and frequently occurring in endometriotic cyst. SMBT is a kind of borderline ovarian tumor, and the characteristics of serum tumor markers in borderline ovarian tumor are helpful for reference. Overall, tumor markers are of little significance in the diagnosis of borderline ovarian tumor. In our case, serum CA125 and CA199 were elevated; CEA and HE4 were normal.

The most commonly used imaging modality of SMBT is ultrasonography, but the overall accuracy of ultrasonography is not high, and the consistency between ultrasound examiners is also low. Although CT can show the complex structure of the tumor, it has limited effect in differentiating borderline from benign and malignant tumors. MRI is the best imaging modality of SMBT.

The characteristic MR imaging features of SMBT are ovarian cystic mass, unilocular, or multilocular, with papillary mural nodules (Figs. 33.1 and 33.2). The MR imaging features of SMBT are similar to those of serous borderline tumor (SBT), and it is difficult to distinguish SMBT from SBT on MRI. However, there are still some clues for identification. Higher contrast enhancement ratio of the solid portion and exophytic growth were imaging findings suggesting SBT. Higher intracystic fluid signal intensity on T1WI (Figs. 33.3 and 33.4) and lower signal intensity on T2WI (Figs. 33.5 and 33.6) suggested SMBT. MRI findings suggesting endometriosis favored the diagnosis of SMBT.

S. Gu (✉)
Department of Radiology, Obstetrics and Gynecology Hospital, Fudan University, Shanghai, P.R. China

G. Zhang (ed.), *MRI of Gynaecological Diseases*, https://doi.org/10.1007/978-981-99-3644-1_33

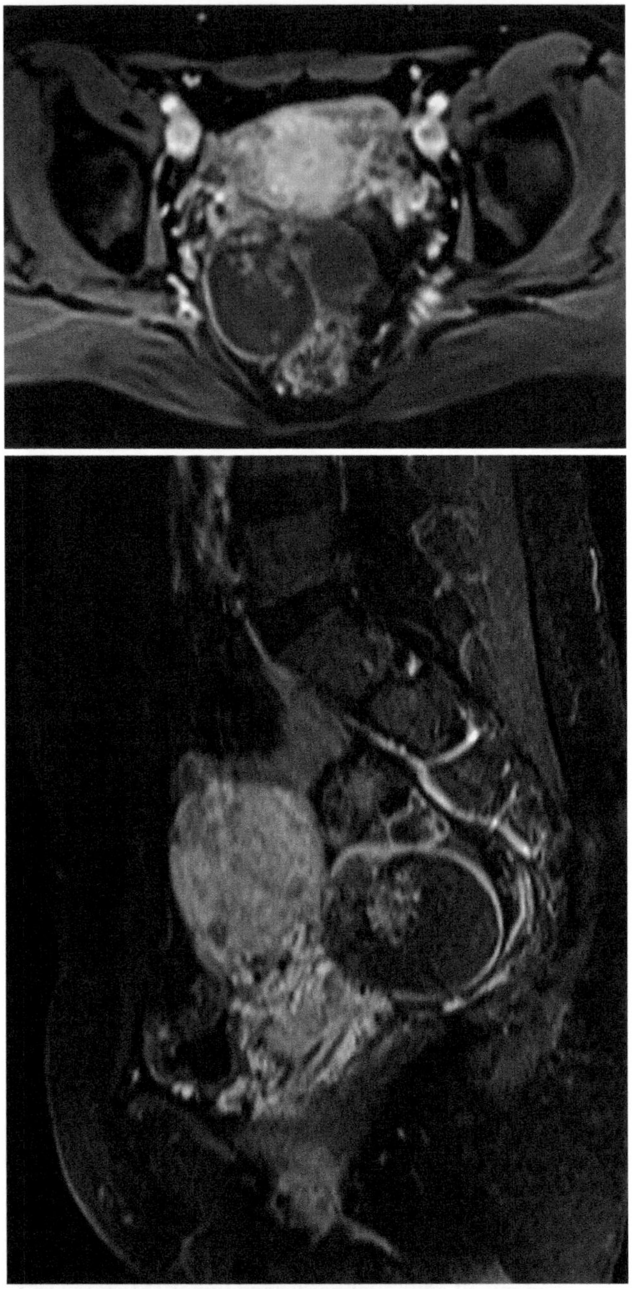

Figs. 33.1 and 33.2 Axial contrast-enhanced T1WI fat suppression image showed significant papillary nodule enhancement. Sagittal delayed contrast-enhanced fat-suppressed T1-weighted image showed significant papillary nodule enhancement similar to that of the myometrium

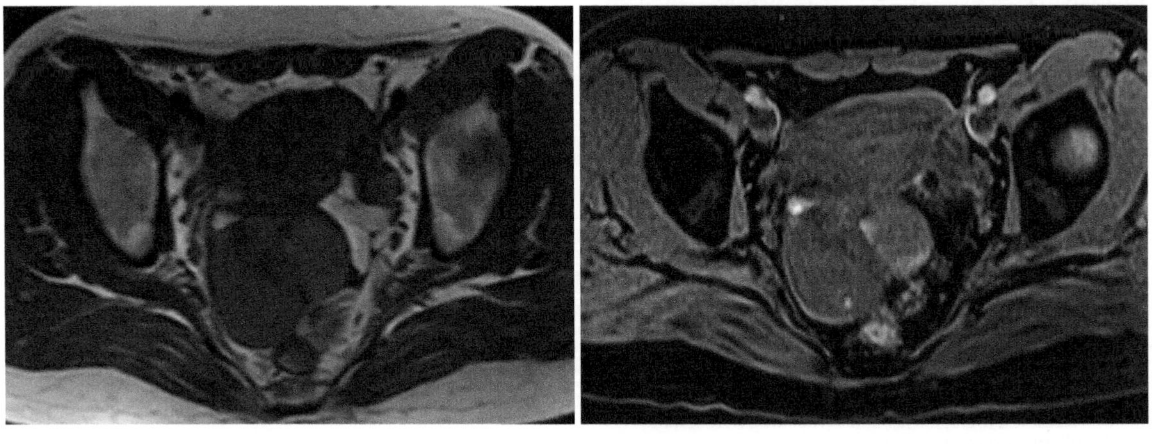

Figs. 33.3 and 33.4 MRI showed an ovarian tumor consisted of a cyst with mural nodules. The cystic portion showed slightly high signal intensity on T1WI. Mural nodules showed slightly low signal intensity on T1WI. On T1WI fat suppression image, the cystic fluid mainly showed low signal intensity, and patchy high signal intensity was observed locally

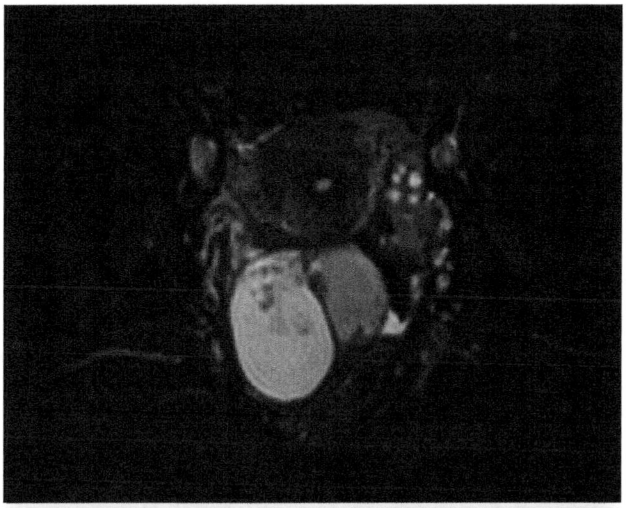

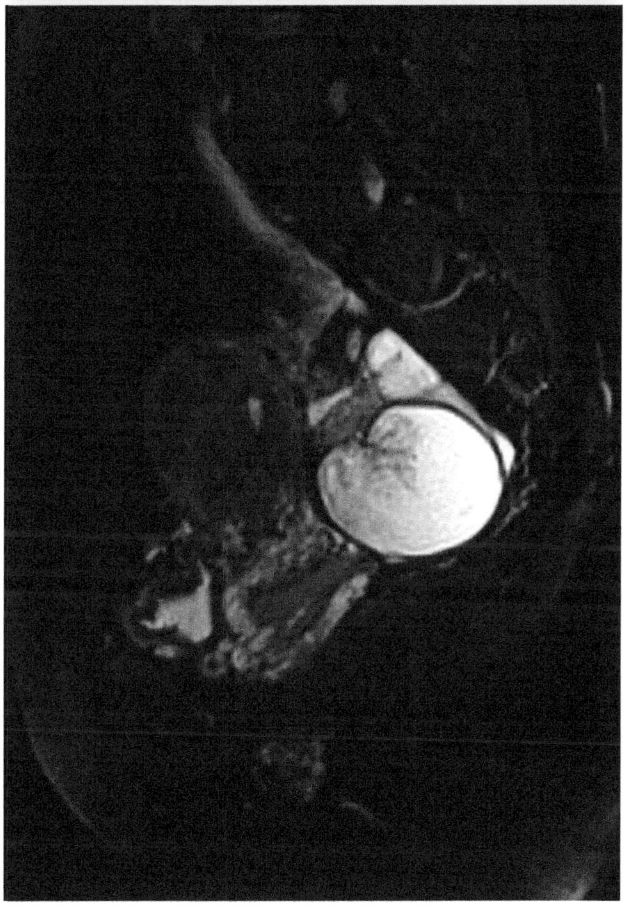

Figs. 33.5 and 33.6 MRI showed an ovarian tumor consisted of a cyst with mural nodules. The cystic portion showed high or slightly low signal intensity on T2WI fat suppression image. The papillary shaped nodule consists of a peripheral slight high signal intensity portion and central low signal intensity portion on sagittal T2-weighted image with fat suppression

33.3 Differential Diagnosis

SMBT is thought to be an endometriosis-related ovarian neoplasm and probably a precursor lesion of a malignant tumor, along with clear cell carcinoma (CCC) and endometrioid carcinoma (EC), which are malignant tumors often arising from endometriotic cysts. Mean ADC value (Figs. 33.7 and 33.8) of SMBT was significantly higher than that of a malignant ovarian tumor [3]. In terms of differentiation of SMBT from serous borderline tumor, higher intracystic fluid signal intensity on T1WI and lower signal intensity on T2WI suggested SMBT [1].

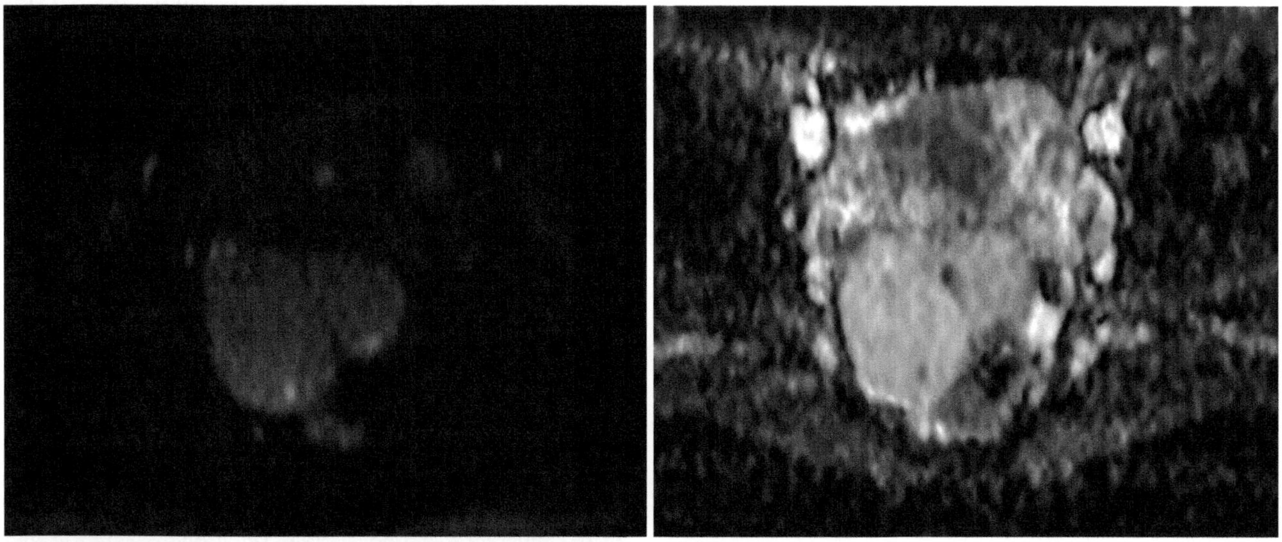

Figs. 33.7 and 33.8 The diffusion restriction of the solid component is normal on DWI and the corresponding ADC map

References

1. Kurata Y, Kido A, Moribata Y, et al. Differentiation of seromucinous borderline tumor from serous borderline tumor on MR imaging. Magn Reson Med Sci. 2018;17(3):211–7.
2. Ando T, Kato H, Kawaguchi M, et al. MR findings for differentiating decidualized endometriomas from seromucinous borderline tumors of the ovary. Abdom Radiol (NY). 2020;45(6):1783–9.
3. Kurata Y, Kido A, Moribata Y, et al. Diagnostic performance of MR imaging findings and quantitative values in the differentiation of seromucinous borderline tumour from endometriosis-related malignant ovarian tumour. Eur Radiol. 2017;27(4):1695–703.

Part VII

Gestational Trophoblastic Diseases

34 Hydatidiform Mole

Jielin Xie and Yan Ning

34.1 Clinical History

Female patient, 49 years old, had amenorrhea for 10 months and irregular vaginal bleeding for 2 months. Laboratory results showed urine pregnancy test was positive, and serum HCG was 144886.6 mIU/mL. Ultrasonography showed hyperechoic masses in uterine cavity. After 3 days, serum HCG was higher (176307.8 mIU/mL); ultrasonography indicated hyperechogenicity in uterine cavity, showing honeycomb like heterogeneous, which was considered hydatidiform mole. The patient went to our hospital for further diagnosis and treatment. Ultrasonography showed dense cystic structures in uterine cavity, about 2–4 mm in diameter. The patient underwent curettage of uterine cavity guided by ultrasound.

Postoperative pathological result: complete hydatidiform mole (Figs. 34.1 and 34.2).

J. Xie (✉)
Department of Radiology, Obstetrics and Gynecology Hospital, Fudan University, Shanghai, P.R. China

Y. Ning
Department of Pathology, Obstetrics and Gynecology Hospital, Fudan University, Shanghai, P.R. China

G. Zhang (ed.), *MRI of Gynaecological Diseases*, https://doi.org/10.1007/978-981-99-3644-1_34

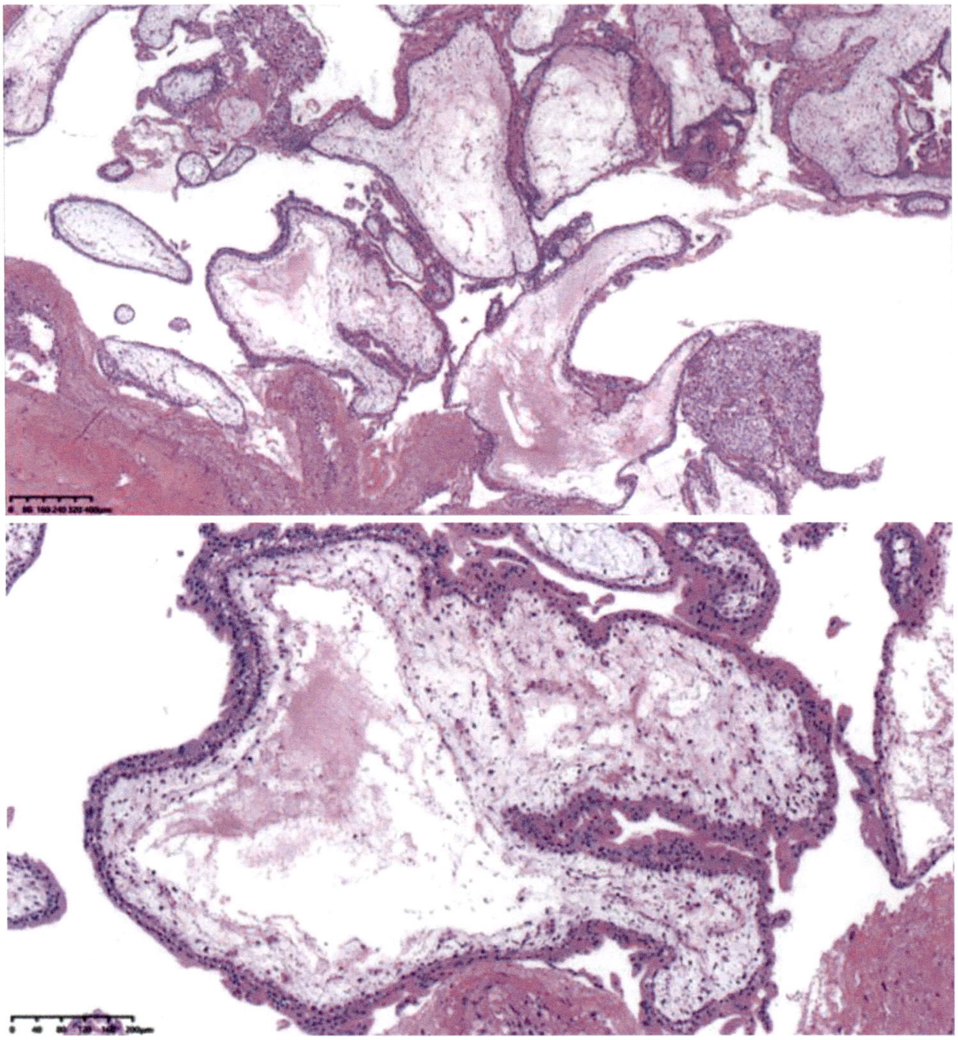

Figs. 34.1 and 34.2 Hydropic villi with cistern formation, abnormally shaped, "cauliflower-like" villi and branching and budding architecture (HE×40). Villi had myxoid stroma with small canalicular vessels and karyorrhectic nuclear debris, circumferential trophoblastic hyperplasia. No definitive fetal vessels or red blood cells were present (HE×100)

34.2 Imaging Analysis

Hydatidiform mole is an abnormal proliferation of placental villous trophoblast cells after pregnancy, and the terminal villi turn into vesicles, which are strung together in clusters, shaped like grapes. Hydatidiform mole is divided into complete and partial [1]. The cause of hydatidiform mole is not yet clear. It usually occurs in patients older than 40 years or younger than 20 years, and is mainly related to fertilization defects. The most common clinical symptoms are vaginal bleeding after menopause, accompanied by abnormal uterine enlargement and softening. Other symptoms include ovarian luteinized cysts, hyperemesis gravidarum, and pregnancy-induced hypertension syndrome. Clinically, ultrasonography is usually used as the main examination method of this disease, which can be diagnosed in combination with abnormal elevation of serum HCG and the patient's symptoms. MRI has excellent soft tissue resolution and is more and more widely used in the diagnosis of hydatidiform mole. MRI manifestations of hydatidiform mole mainly include (1) uterine enlarged and uterine cavity expands and may be accompanied by local thickening of myometrium. (2) Intrauterine lesions are honeycomb-like or grape-like soft tissue masses with uneven hyperintensity on T2WI (Fig. 34.3). (3) Multiple homogeneous compartments can be seen inside the mass, and the cystic part shows hypointense on T1WI (Fig. 34.4) and hyperintense on T2WI. (4) The lesion capsule is intact, and uterine junctional zone is continuous. No invasion of myometrium is observed. (5) On contrast-enhanced images, only mild or moderate prolonged enhancement is observed of compartments, with no enhancement of the cystic part (Figs. 34.5 and 34.6). (6) No obvious thickening and tortuous vessels are observed in myometrium [2, 3].

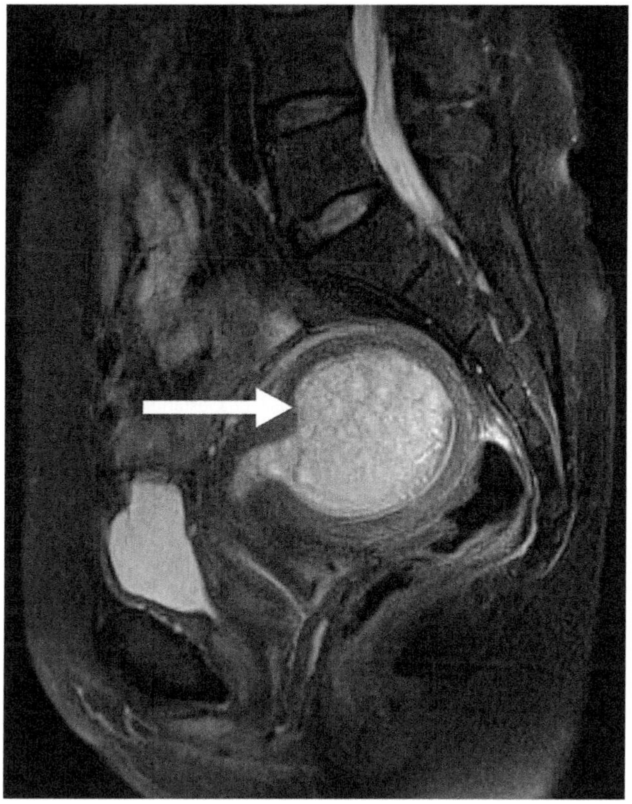

Fig. 34.3 Sagittal fat-suppressed T2WI image showed the uterus was enlarged, and intrauterine cavity was full of heterogeneous hyperintense lesion, and the boundary between the lesion and myometrium was clear

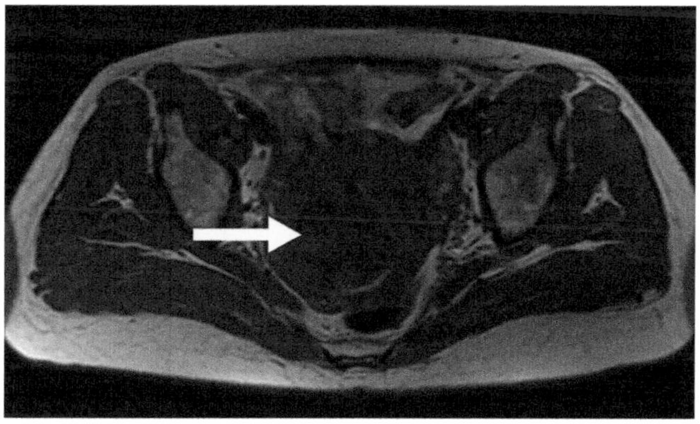

Fig. 34.4 Axial pre-contrast T1WI showed intrauterine cavity was full of heterogeneous hypointense

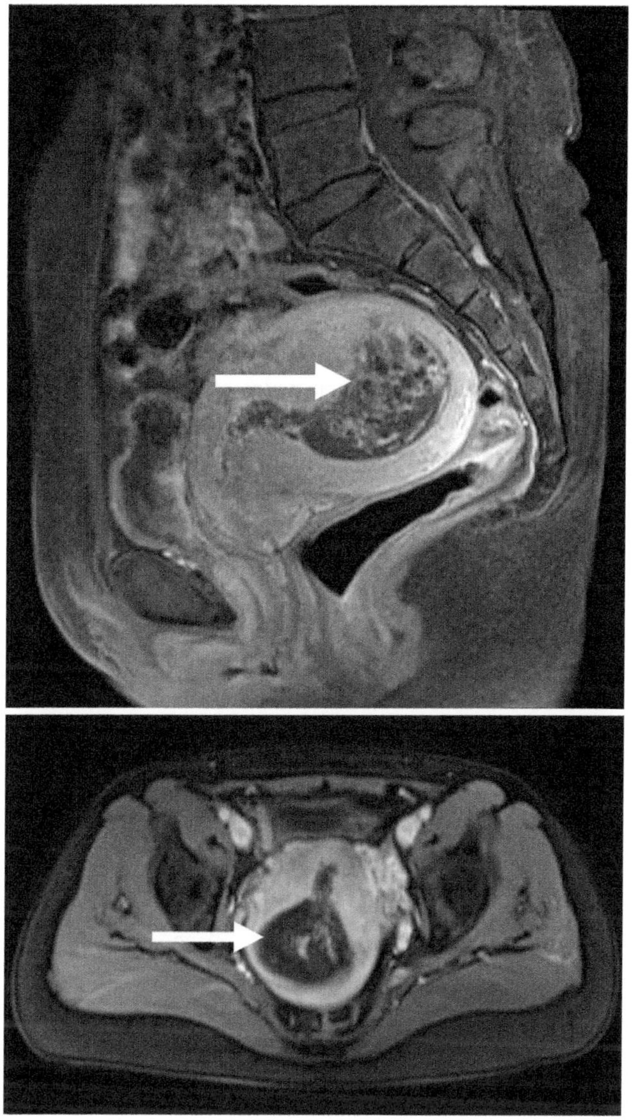

Figs. 34.5 and 34.6 Sagittal contrast-enhanced fat-suppressed T1WI image showed intrauterine lesion with heterogeneous honeycomb-like enhancement and multiple septations enhancement. Axial contrast-enhanced fat-suppressed T1WI image showed the cystic part of intrauterine lesion was unenhanced, and septations were enhanced

34.3 Differential Diagnosis

It is mainly differentiated from other gynecological benign and malignant tumors, including endometrial cancer and multiple endometrial polyps. Endometrial cancer masses are mostly located in uterine cavity, presenting hypointense on T1WI and medium hyperintense on T2WI. The signal of the mass is lower than normal endometrial signal, which can invade myometrium. In addition, most patients have postmenopausal vaginal bleeding, which is significantly different from the reproductive age of patients with hydatidiform mole. MRI manifestations of multiple endometrial polyps are similar to those of hydatidiform mole, showing abnormal intrauterine honeycomb-like hypointense on T1WI and hyperintense on T2WI with visible septations, but the septation of the former was more uniform. According to pregnancy history, vaginal bleeding and other symptoms, as well as the absence of abnormal serum HCG can be identified [4–6].

References

1. Monchek R, Wiedaseck S. Gestational trophoblstic disease: an overview. J Midwifery Womens Health. 2012;57(3):255–9.
2. Fonseca EKUN, Rodrigues MAS, Yamauchi FI, et al. "Bunch of grapes" in complete hydatidiform mole. Abdom Radiol. 2017;42(5):1606–7.
3. Imafuku H, Miyahara Y, Ebina Y, et al. Ultrasound and MRI findings of twin pregnancies with complete Hydatidiform mole and coexisting Normal fetus: two case reports. Kobe J Med Sci. 2018;64(1):E1–5.
4. Lok C, Frijstein M, van Trommel N. Clinical presentation and diagnosis of gestational trophoblastic disease. Best Pract Res Clin Obstet Gynaecol. 2021;74:42–52.
5. Shanbhogue AK, Lalwani N, Menias CO. Gestational trophoblastic disease. Radiol Clin N Am. 2013;51(6):1023–34.
6. Bajaj SK, Misra R, Gupta R, et al. Complete hydatidiform mole with coexisting twin fetus: usefulness of MRI in management planning. J Obstet Gynaecol India. 2014;64(Suppl 1):9–13.

35 Invasive Hydatidiform Mole

Jielin Xie

35.1 Clinical History

Female patient, 22 years old, had amenorrhea for 65 days. The patient self-measured urine HCG (+) after 40 days of menopause, no vaginal bleeding during pregnancy, and occasional vague pain in the lower abdomen. After 65 days of menopause, ultrasonography showed mixed structure in uterine cavity, which was full of small honeycomb-like anechoic areas. Serum HCG (dilute): >200,000 mIU/mL. Uterine curettage under the guidance of ultrasound was performed, and a small amount of vaginal bleeding continued after operation. Re-examination of ultrasonography showed mixed intrauterine structure, abundant cord-like color blood flow was observed in the interior and basement, and blood supply was from the posterior wall of myometrium. Ultrasound-guided uterine curettage was performed again, and postoperative serum HCG continued to fluctuate.

Postoperative pathological reult: (Uterine cavity) hydatidiform mole with moderate trophoblast proliferation.

35.2 Imaging Analysis

Invasive hydatidiform mole refers to the invasion of hydatidiform mole mass into myometrium and minority metastasis to the outside of uterus; most of metastasis occur within 6 months after uterine curettage. Clinical diagnostic criteria [1]: (1) Patient had a history of hydatidiform mole, and serum HCG level did not fall to normal level 8–12 weeks after the second uterine curettage. Imaging examination showed that the mass invaded myometrium or there was lung metastasis. (2) After uterine curettage, serum HCG has decreased to normal level, and then there were symptoms, and serum HCG increased rapidly or there was metastasis in the lung. The main clinical symptom is irregular vaginal bleeding, with varying amounts. Other symptoms include delayed uterine involution after hydatidiform mole curettage and persistence of ovarian luteinized cysts. The most common site of invasive hydatidiform mole metastasis is the lung, followed by vagina and parametrium, and brain metastasis is rare. MRI manifestations mainly include (1) enlarged uterine volume and soft tissue mass can be seen in uterine cavity or myometrium, without capsule, and a few can be honeycomb or grape shape. (2) The mass usually showed heterogeneous hyperintensity on T2WI, and there may be hemorrhagic signal foci at the edge or inside of the mass (Fig. 35.1). (3) Uterine junctional zone was discontinuous and the mass invaded myometrium (Fig. 35.2). (4) Contrast-enhanced images showed marked prolonged enhancement of septations or solid parts (Figs. 35.3 and 35.4). (5) Significantly thickening and tortuous vessels can be seen in myometrium or parametrium. (6) Hematogenous metastasis is common and rarely pelvic and inguinal lymph node metastasis [2–4].

J. Xie (✉)
Department of Radiology, Obstetrics and Gynecology Hospital, Fudan University, Shanghai, P.R. China

G. Zhang (ed.), *MRI of Gynaecological Diseases*, https://doi.org/10.1007/978-981-99-3644-1_35

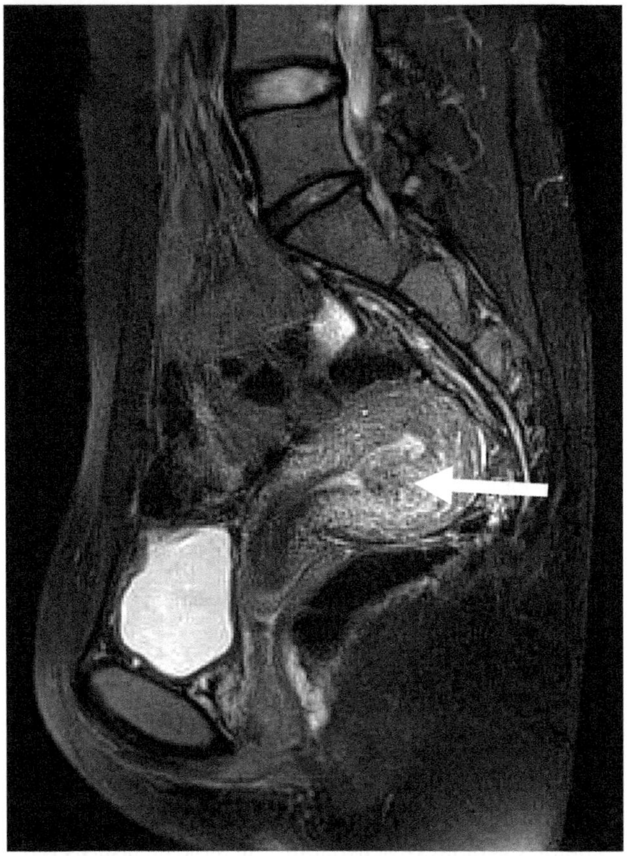

Fig. 35.1 Sagittal fat-suppressed T2WI image showed slightly enlarged uterus and intrauterine heterogeneous hyperintense mass with unclear boundary between the mass and myometrium and invasion of superficial myometrium of posterior wall of uterus

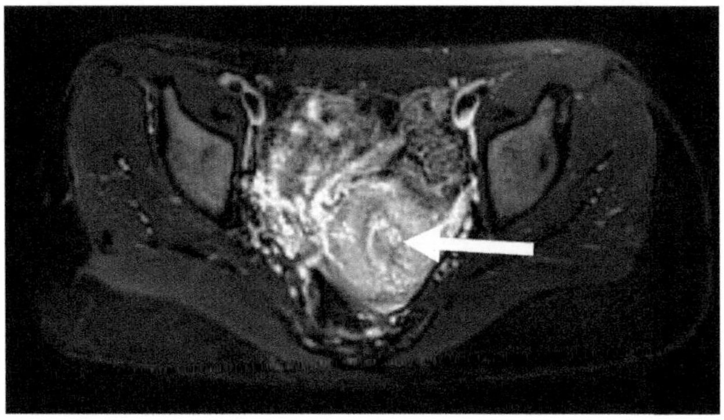

Fig. 35.2 Axial pre-contrast fat-suppressed T2WI image showed intrauterine heterogeneous hyperintense mass

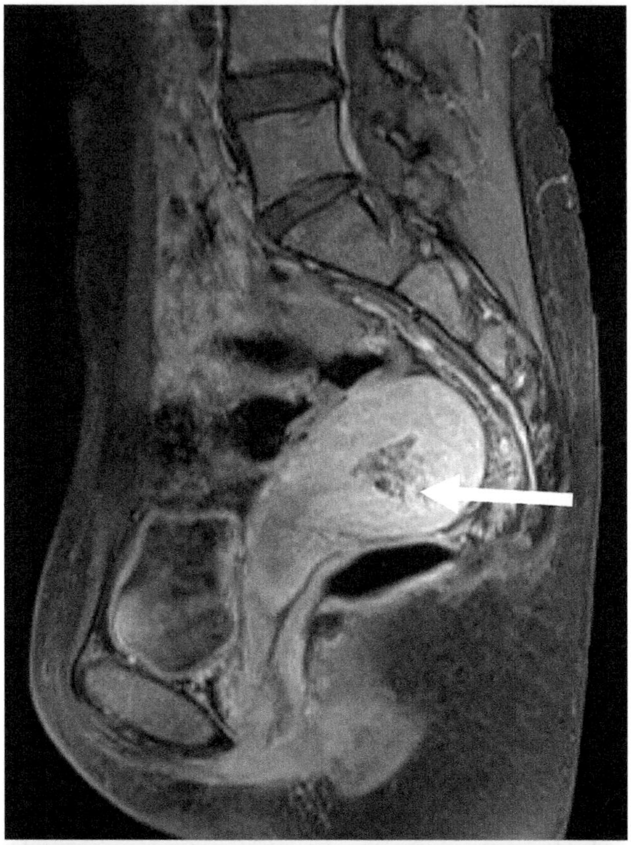

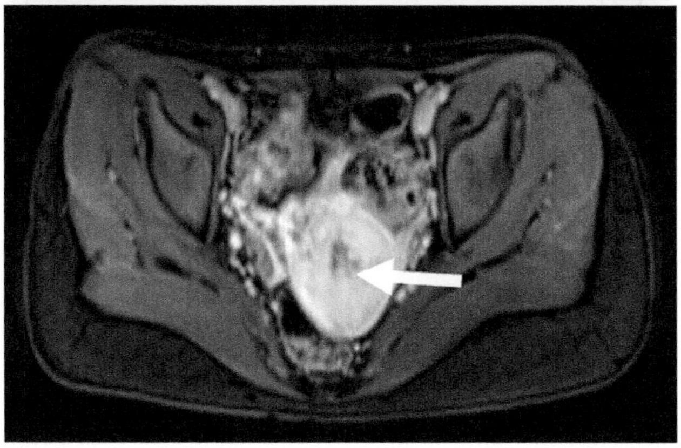

Figs. 35.3 and 35.4 Sagittal contrast-enhanced T1WI image showed heterogeneous honeycomb-like enhancement of intrauterine mass, invading superficial myometrium. Axial contrast-enhanced T1WI image showed heterogeneous enhancement of intrauterine lesion

35.3 Differential Diagnosis

Invasive hydatidiform mole is mainly differentiated from endometrial cancer, residual pregnancy, and adenomyosis. Endometrial cancer masses are mostly located in uterine cavity, which can invade myometrium, presenting hypointense on T1WI and medium hyperintense on T2WI, and the signal intensity of the mass is lower than normal endometrial signal. Clinical symptoms of patients are mostly postmenopausal vaginal bleeding, which can be easily identified according to clinical history, physical signs, and age of onset. MRI findings of residual pregnancy are similar to those of invasive hydatidiform mole, which is difficult to distinguish, and can be diagnosed according to clinical manifestations. After uterine curettage, serum HCG of residual pregnancy can return to normal level. Adenomyosis can be characterized by significant enlargement of the uterus with high-signal hemorrhagic foci in myometrium, which overlaps with MRI findings of invasive hydatidiform mole to some extent. However, MRI findings of adenomyosis are mainly characterized by widening of uterine junctional zone, and diffuse spotted hemorrhagic foci in myometrium, which is different from discontinuous of uterine junctional zone of invasive hydatidiform mole [4–6].

References

1. Ngan HY, Seckl MJ, Berkowitz RS, et al. Update on the diagnosis and management of gestational trophoblastic disease. Int J Gynaecol Obstet. 2015;131(Suppl 2):S123–6.
2. Bynum J, Murphy KM, DeScipio C, et al. Invasive complete Hydatidiform moles: analysis of a case series with genotyping. Int J Gynecol Pathol. 2016;35(2):134–41.
3. Shaaban AM, Rezvani M, Haroun RR, et al. Gestational trophoblastic disease: clinical and imaging features. Radiographics. 2017;37(2):681–700.
4. Tambe SG, Goel K, Sambharam K. Gestational trophoblastic neoplasia: a unique challenge in caesarean scar pregnancy. Eur J Obstet Gynecol Reprod Biol. 2021;264:381–2.
5. Lok C, Frijstein M, van Trommel N. Clinical presentation and diagnosis of gestational trophoblastic disease. Best Pract Res Clin Obstet Gynaecol. 2021;74:42–52.
6. Lin LH, Polizio R, Fushida K, et al. Imaging in gestational trophoblastic disease. Semin Ultrasound CT MR. 2019;40(4):332–49.

36 Choriocarcinoma

Jielin Xie

36.1 Clinical History

Female patient, 32 years old, 3 years after hydatidiform mole curettage had irregular vaginal bleeding for 2 months. The patient underwent uterine curettage in a local hospital 3 years ago due to hydatidiform mole. Postoperative menstrual cycle was regular, and there was no irregular vaginal bleeding, without cough, hemoptysis, chest pain, and other symptoms. Serum HCG was not followed up after operation. Vaginal bleeding has not been stopped since 2 months ago, and ultrasound examination in our hospital indicated that mixed structure in the anterior uterine wall of myometrium and trophoblastic disease should be excluded according to medical history. Serum HCG (dilute): >200,000 mIU/mL. Intramyometrium lesion resection was performed laparoscopically after 6 cycles of chemotherapy.

Postoperative pathological result: (Myometrial lesion) extensive necrotic, hyperproliferative trophoblast cells, no villus, clinically consistent with choriocarcinoma.

36.2 Imaging Analysis

Choriocarcinoma is a highly malignant tumor that can hematogenous metastasis to the whole body at an early stage, most commonly to the lung. 50% of choriocarcinoma secondary to hydatidiform mole (mostly more than 1 year after uterine curettage), 25% to abortion, 22.5% to term pregnancy, and a few to ectopic pregnancy [1]. Histologically, invasive hydatidiform mole was diagnosed in patients with villi or degenerated villi in myometrium or metastases, and choriocarcinoma was diagnosed in patients with trophoblast infiltration and necrotic hemorrhage but no villi. Since most of the patients are women of reproductive age, and histological results could not be obtained due to lesions are unresectable, the diagnosis can also be made by combining clinical manifestations with serum HCG [2]. Clinical manifestations are mainly vaginal bleeding, the amount of which is variable. If the primary uterine lesion has disappeared and metastasis develops, there will be no vaginal bleeding. Patients with lung metastasis often have cough, bloody sputum, or repeated hemoptysis and other symptoms. MRI findings of choriocarcinoma mainly include the following:

1. The uterus is enlarged, with soft tissue mass in myometrium, no capsule, and unclear boundary with myometrium (Figs. 36.1 and 36.2).
2. The mass is usually heterogeneous hyperintense on T2WI, and there may be hemorrhagic signal at the edge or inside of the mass (Fig. 36.3).
3. Contrast-enhanced image showed significant nodular or strip-like enhancement within the mass (Fig. 36.4).
4. Obvious thickening and tortuous vessels can be seen in the myometrium or parametrium (Fig. 36.3).
5. It is prone to hematogenous metastasis at the early stage, and corresponding metastases may occur [3–5].

J. Xie (✉)
Department of Radiology, Obstetrics and Gynecology Hospital, Fudan University, Shanghai, P.R. China

G. Zhang (ed.), *MRI of Gynaecological Diseases*, https://doi.org/10.1007/978-981-99-3644-1_36

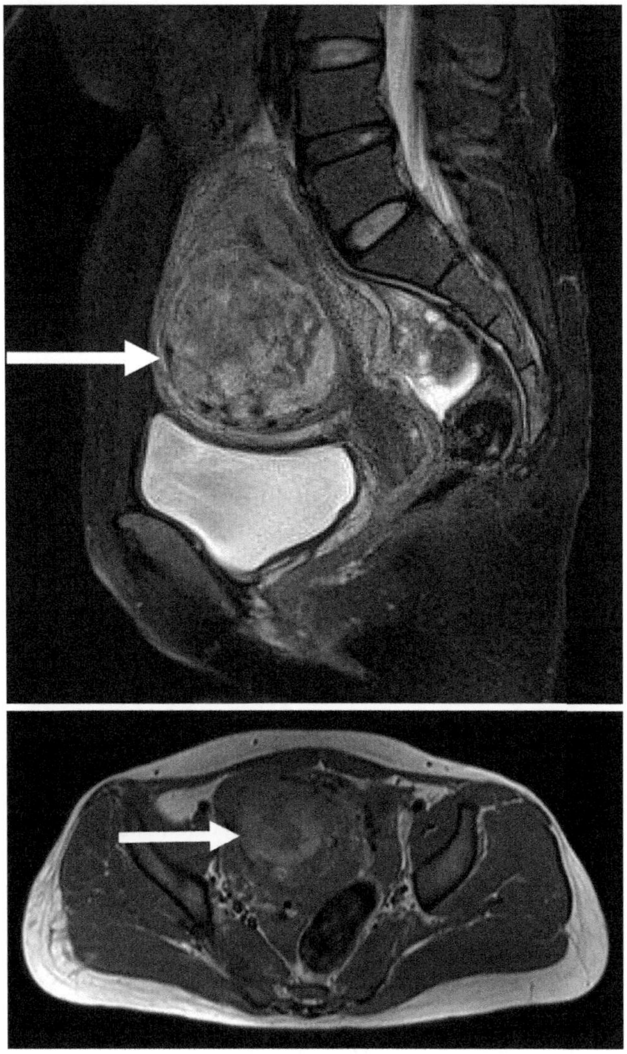

Figs. 36.1 and 36.2 Sagittal T2WI image showed enlarged uterus with a mass of heterogeneous hyperintense in the anterior uterine wall of myometrium. The boundary between the mass and myometrium is unclear. Axial T1WI image showed hemorrhagic signal in the mass, presenting heterogeneous hyperintense

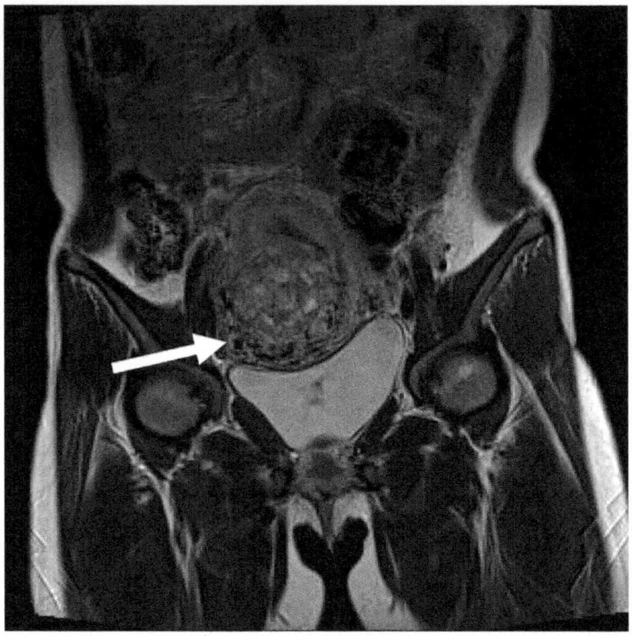

Fig. 36.3 Coronal T2WI image showed multiple tortuous vessels in myometrium around the mass

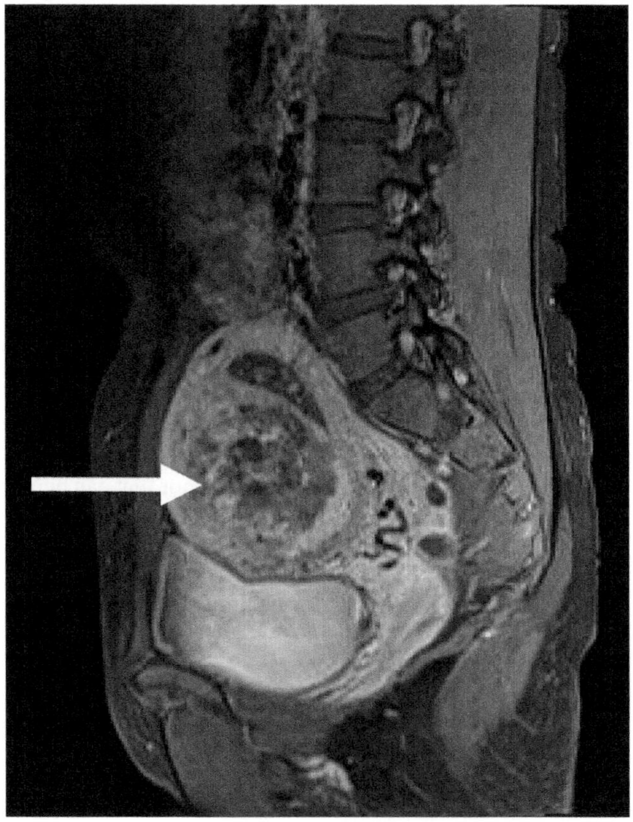

Fig. 36.4 Most of the mass did not enhance on sagittal contrast-enhanced T1WI, with nodular and strip-like significant internal enhancement

36.3 Differential Diagnosis

MRI manifestations of choriocarcinoma are similar to those of invasive hydatidiform mole and cannot be identified. The differentiation is mainly based on clinical history and histological findings. Uterine fibroids can be accompanied by thickening vessels around the body of uterus, and the uterus is enlarged. However, uterine fibroids are mostly hypointense on T1WI and T2WI with clear boundaries, and their parenchymal part is hypointense on T2WI, which is obviously different from choriocarcinoma. The signal of placenta implantation or residual on pre-contrast MRI is similar to that of choriocarcinoma, but after contrast enhancement, it has a clear boundary with surrounding myometrium, and the degree of enhancement is mild. At the same time, there is a clinical history of abortion or full-term labor, and serum HCG is generally not continuously increased, which can be identified [6, 7].

References

1. Silva ALMD, Monteiro KDN, Sun SY, et al. Gestational trophoblastic neoplasia: novelties and challenges. Placenta. 2021;116:38–42.
2. Kani KK, Lee JH, Dighe M, et al. Gestatational trophoblastic disease: multimodality imaging assessment with special emphasis on spectrum of abnormalities and value of imaging in staging and management of disease. Curr Probl Diagn Radiol. 2012;41(1):1–10.
3. Lima LL, Parente RC, Maestá I, et al. Clinical and radiological correlations in patients with gestational trophoblastic disease. Radiol Bras. 2016;49(4):241–50.
4. Shaaban AM, Rezvani M, Haroun RR, et al. Gestational trophoblastic disease: clinical and imaging features. Radiographics. 2017;37(2):681–700.
5. Lin LH, Polizio R, Fushida K, et al. Imaging in gestational trophoblastic disease. Semin Ultrasound CT MR. 2019;40(4):332–49.
6. Jha P, Paroder V, Mar W, et al. Multimodality imaging of placental masses: a pictorial review. Abdom Radiol (NY). 2016;41(12):2435–44.
7. Marusik C, Frykholm C, Ericson K, et al. Diagnosis of placental mesenchymal dysplasia with magnetic resonance imaging. Ultrasound Obstet Gynecol. 2017;49(3):410–2.

Part VIII

Other Pelvic Tumors

37 Ovarian Metastatic Cancer

He Zhang

37.1 Clinical History

Case 1
A 48-year-old woman complained of abdominal distention and increased frequency of defecation several days ago. No obvious abdominal pain or vaginal bleeding was found. Ultrasonography revealed solid masses in bilateral adnexa areas. The final pathological result was Krukenberg tumor. MRI images are shown in Fig. 37.1.

Case 2
A 25-year-old woman complained of serious abdominal pain nearly a couple of weeks ago. No abnormal vaginal bleeding or discharge was found. Ultrasonography revealed solid masses in bilateral adnexa areas. Serum tumor markers were as follows: CEA: 16.5 ng/mL, CA125: 283 U/mL, and CA199: 38.8 U/mL. The final pathological result was ovarian metastatic tumor from sigmoid colon. MRI images are shown in Fig. 37.2.

H. Zhang (✉)
Department of Radiology, Obstetrics and Gynecology Hospital, Fudan University, Shanghai, P.R. China
e-mail: zhanghe1790@fckyy.org.cn

G. Zhang (ed.), *MRI of Gynaecological Diseases*, https://doi.org/10.1007/978-981-99-3644-1_37

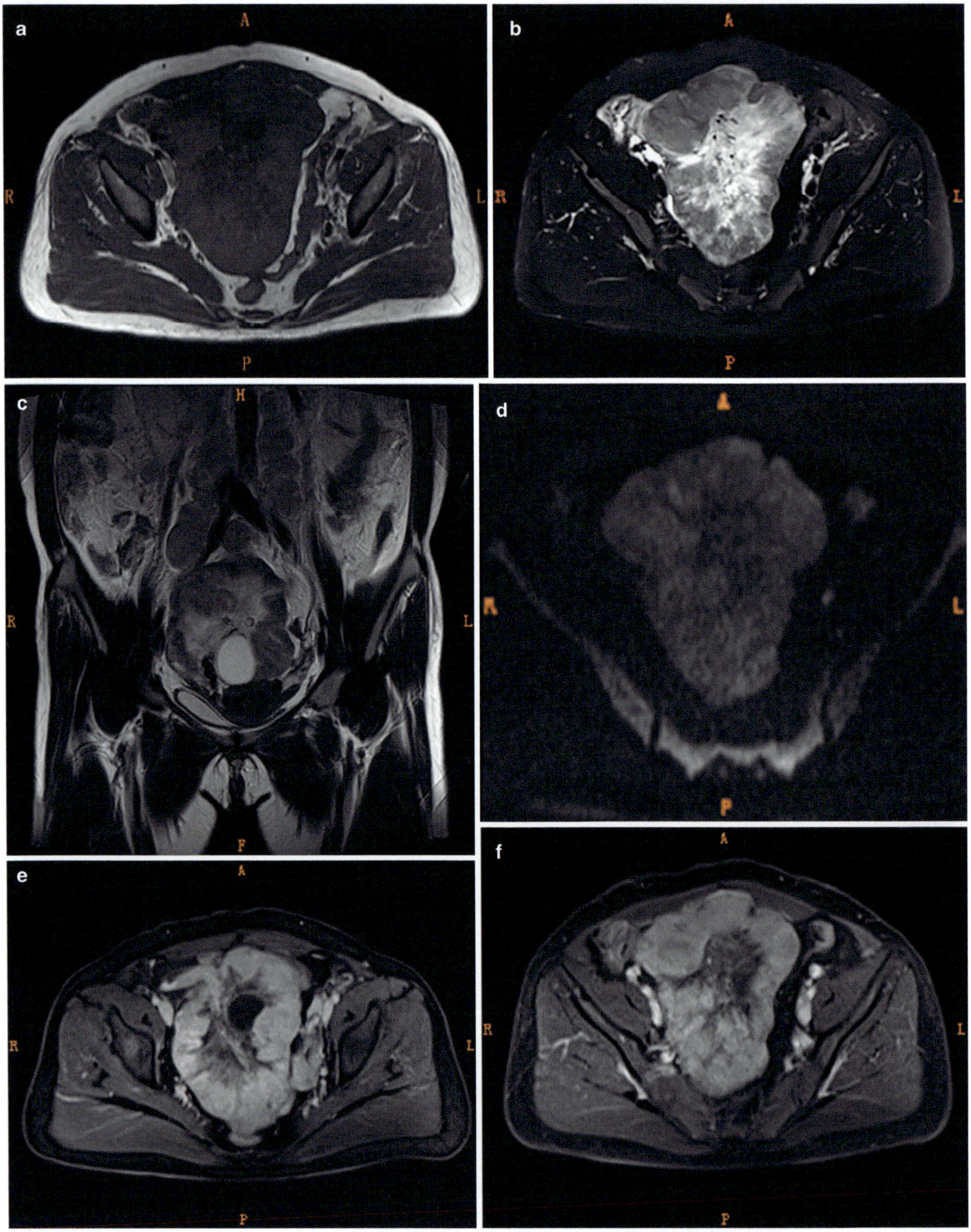

Fig. 37.1 **Case 1.** Krukenberg tumor. The giant solid mass occupied the whole abdominal and pelvic cavity with isointense signal on both T1WI (**a**) and T2WI (**b**). A chain of enlarged lymph nodes (**c**) besides the aorta were seen on coronal MRI. On DWI (**d**), the tumor displayed as relatively high signal and enhanced heterogeneously (**e**, **f**) with no enhancement within the necrotic area after contrast enhancement

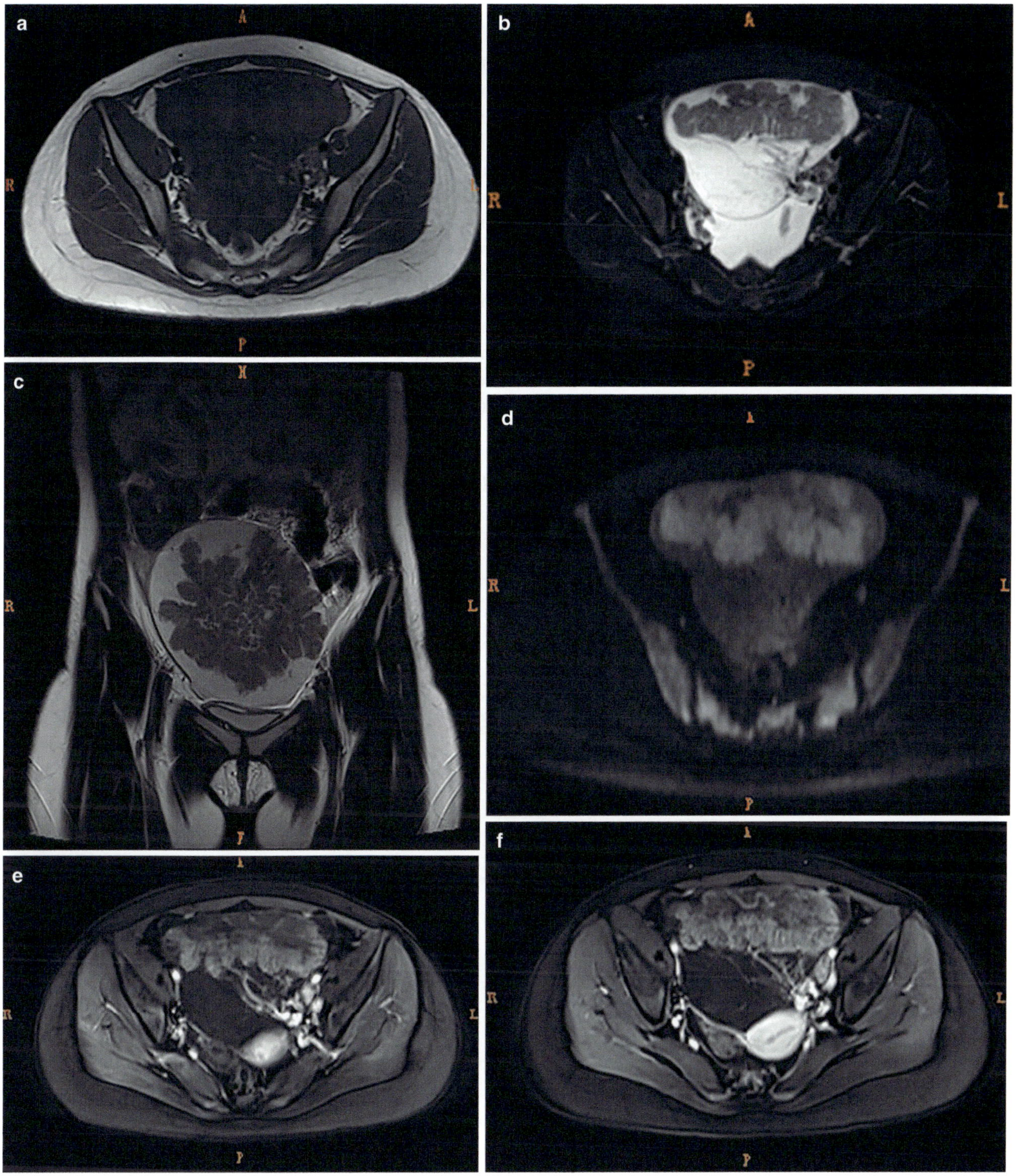

Fig. 37.2 **Case 2.** Krukenberg tumor (ovarian metastatic tumor from sigmoid colon). The giant solid mass occupied the whole abdominal and pelvic cavity, in which solid components displayed as isointense signal on both T1WI (**a**) and T2WI (**b**). On coronal T2WI (**c**), a segmental thickness of the colon was also seen on the top of the mass accidentally. On DWI (**d**), the tumor displayed as relatively high signal and enhanced heterogeneously (**e**, **f**) with no enhancement within the necrotic area after contrast enhancement

37.2 Imaging Analysis

Ovarian metastatic tumors (OMTs) account for approximately 5–10% of all ovarian cancers. Imaging features of OMTs are variable depending on primary tumors, which generally have similar imaging manifestations with OMTs [1, 2]. Clinical symptoms are mainly pelvic complaints, with less than 25% cases have coexistent stomach or intestinal complaints [3]. The most common OMT is metastasized from the colon followed by gastric, breast, lung, and contralateral ovarian cancer. Other rare tumors such as endometrial cancer, melanoma, pancreatic cancer, and carcinoid can also metastasize to ovary and fallopian tubes. It is a challenge to discriminate between primary ovarian cancer and OMTs. Typically, OMTs manifest as bilateral solid, lobulated masses in the adnexa areas [4]. Histologically, ovarian metastatic tumors originating from gastrointestinal tract are signet-ring cell carcinoma, showing small round, closely-arranged cells. These tumors are known as "Krukenberg tumor," most commonly originating from gastric cancer. OMTs arising from colon or rectum cancer (2–13%) have similar imaging features with primary ovarian cancer. On MRI, the tumors always show heterogeneous signal mass with inhomogeneous enhancement after contrast enhancement.

37.3 Differential Diagnosis

OMTs should be distinguished from ovarian cystadenoma, ovarian fibroma/fibrothecoma, and ovarian granulosa cell tumor. Ovarian cystadenomas always are multilobular cystic mass with intact capsule. Among cystic mass, vegetations can be seen beneath cystic wall. For solid OMTs, ovarian sex cord-stromal tumors should be included into differential diagnoses. Ovarian fibroma/fibrothecoma are benign tumors that can be seen as solid masses with hypointense signal on MRI images. Meigs syndrome could help to establish this diagnosis. Ovarian granulosa cell tumor (GCT), a low malignant potential ovarian tumor, is the most common of ovarian malignant sex cord-stromal tumor [5]. Sometimes, GCT can be shown as bilateral solid masses and should be differentiated with OMT.

References

1. Vargas HA, Barrett T, Sala E. MRI of ovarian masses. J Magn Reson Imaging. 2013;37(2):265–81.
2. Imaoka I, Wada A, Kaji Y, Hayashi T, Hayashi M, Matsuo M, et al. Developing an MR imaging strategy for diagnosis of ovarian masses. Radiographics. 2006;26(5):1431–48.
3. Davidson B, Tropé CG. Ovarian cancer: diagnostic, biological and prognostic aspects. Womens Health. 2014;10(5):519–33.
4. Rajkotia K, Veeramani M, Macura KJ. Magnetic resonance imaging of adnexal masses. Top Magn Reson Imaging. 2006;17(6):379–97.
5. Tanaka YO, Tsunoda H, Kitagawa Y, Ueno T, Yoshikawa H, Saida Y. Functioning ovarian tumors: direct and indirect findings at MR imaging. Radiographics. 2004;24(suppl 1):S147–66.

Pseudomyxoma Peritonei

38

Mengwei Zhang

38.1 Clinical History

Female patient, 69 years old, had been menopause more than 20 years ago and had no abnormal vaginal bleeding after menopause. The patient palpated the lower abdominal mass half a month ago, without abdominal pain and distension, abnormal vaginal discharge, fever, and fatigue. Color Doppler ultrasonography showed that there was a giant solid and cystic mixed mass at the back of the uterus, with a size of 19.6 cm × 16.5 cm × 13.4 cm. There was a moderate echogenic zone inside, and the boundary with the posterior wall of uterus was unclear. The patient underwent laparoscopic exploration, total hysterectomy, bilateral salpingo-oophorectomy, appendectomy, greater omentum resection, and complex intestinal adhesion decomposition.

Postoperative pathological results: the lumen of appendix tissue was dilated with local myxoepithelial hyperplasia. The morphology was consistent with low-grade mucinous tumor with pseudomyxoma peritonei formation. Bilateral ovaries, bilateral salpinx interstitium, uterine seromuscular layer, broad ligament, greater omentum, and rectouterine pouch were involved.

38.2 Imaging Analysis

Pseudomyxoma peritonei (PMP) is a malignant clinical syndrome characterized by the accumulation and redistribution of mucus produced by mucinous tumor cells in abdominal cavity. The clinical manifestations are mucinous ascites, peritoneal implantation, omental cake, and ovarian involvement [1, 2]. The incidence of PMP is about 2–4/1 million [1, 2]; the ratio of male to female is about 1:1.2–3.4; the median age of onset is 43–63 years [3–5]. PMP has a wide range of sources, mainly from appendix. So far, the largest case study was reported by Carr et al., a total of 274 cases, of which 257 cases (94%) were from appendix [6]. A small number of PMP arises from primary mucinous tumors of abdominal organs such as the ovaries, stomach, colon, pancreas, gallbladder, urachus, and teratoma [4].

The pathological classification of PMP is related to prognosis and is very important for the selection of treatment strategies. In 1995, Ronnett et al. [7] reported a pathological classification method of PMP: low-grade or disseminated peritoneal adenomucinosis (DPAM), high-grade or peritoneal mucinous carcinomatosis (PMCA) including signet ring cell adenocarcinomas (PMCA-S), and an intermediate group characterized by the presence of discordant cells derived from a well-differentiated mucinous appendicular or intestinal adenocarcinoma or atypical appendicular adenomas with or without an associated appendicular carcinoma (PMCA-I). In 2010, the fourth edition of the World Health Organization (WHO) classification of digestive system tumors divides PMP into low-grade PMP and high-grade PMP [8]. In 2016, the Peritoneal Surface Oncology Group International (PSOGI) classification divides PMP into three groups and excludes acellular mucinous type lesions from its definition. These three groups are defined as PMP with low-grade histologic characteristics (LG-PMP), PMP with high-grade histology (HG-PMP), and PMP with the presence of signet ring cells (SC-PMP) [2]. In 2014, PSOGI recommended cytoreductive surgery (CRS) combined with hyperthermic intraperitoneal chemotherapy (HIPEC) as the standard treatment for PMP at the ninth International Congress on Peritoneal Cancer in the Netherlands [9].

Typical MR manifestations of PMP: (1) There is a cystic or solid and cystic mass in the right lower abdomen that may be accompanied by calcification (Fig. 38.1). (2) There is a large amount of mucinous effusion in the abdominal and pelvic cavity, and multiple compartments can be seen, which can be cystic, separated, encapsulated, and solid and cystic. (3) There is extensive implantation metastasis, mainly liver and spleen subcapsular parenchyma, with varying degrees of indentation, showing characteristic scalloping sign. (4) The

M. Zhang (✉)
Department of Radiology, Obstetrics and Gynecology Hospital, Fudan University, Shanghai, P.R. China

G. Zhang (ed.), *MRI of Gynaecological Diseases*, https://doi.org/10.1007/978-981-99-3644-1_38

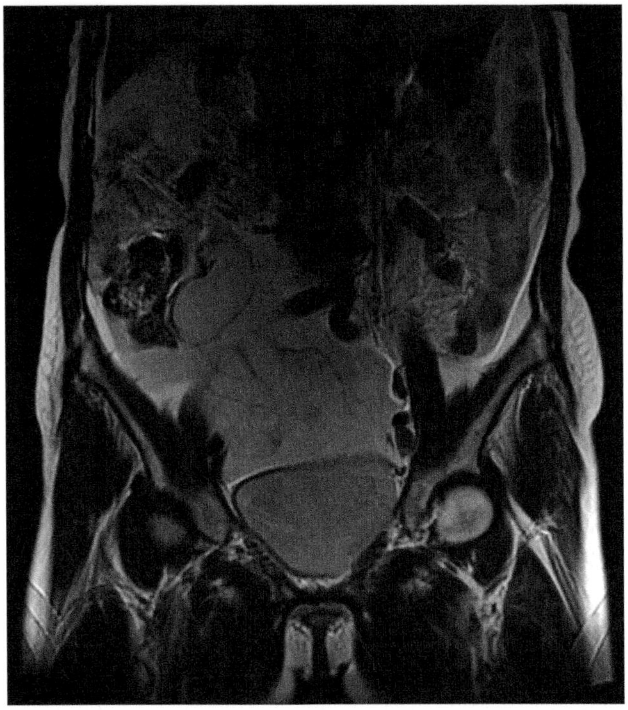

Fig. 38.1 A giant solid and cystic mixed mass was seen on the right side of the abdominal and pelvic cavity, with a size of about 16.8 cm × 8.5 cm × 18.1 cm, and the cystic wall was partially discontinuous

greater and lesser omentum and mesentery often show infiltrative and diffuse thickening and enhancement, and the omental cake sign can be seen. (5) The intestine is asymmetrically thickened and converged to the center, and the lumen becomes compressed and flattened. (6) There are signs of calcification, abdominal wall invasion, lymph node metastasis, and retroperitoneal or thoracic invasion.

38.3 Differential Diagnosis

MR findings are helpful in differentiating pseudomyxoma peritonei from common ascites and tuberculous peritonitis [10]. Pseudomyxoma peritonei generally has a wall, with small septation in it (Figs. 38.2 and 38.3). The intestinal canal is compressed and converges to the center, rather than floating toward the anterior abdominal wall. Reticular and branched fatty spaces can be seen in the mesentery, and it is difficult to extract ascites, or the ascites are bloody mucus jelly-like substances. MR signal on T2WI was slightly lower than that of common ascites (Figs. 38.4 and 38.5). Multiple "scalloping" or "nodular" indentations are common at the edges of liver and spleen. There is a solid and cystic mass in abdominal cavity, and MR signal of the solid part of the mass on T2WI is slightly higher than the solid mass in abdominal cavity. However, the MR signal of common ascites is significantly high intensity on T2WI, and intestinal canal is floating to the anterior abdominal wall, and there is generally no septation within it. There is no solid and cystic mass and no "scalloping" or "nodular" indentations at the edges of liver and spleen. Tuberculous peritonitis has kneading sensation and tenderness in the abdomen, and the mass is relatively limited. There is no solid and cystic mass in abdominal cavity and no "scalloping" or "nodular" indentations at the edges of liver and spleen. Sometimes PMP should be distinguished from peritoneal metastasis, lymphangioma, teratoma, pancreatic cysts, and primary peritoneal mesothelioma.

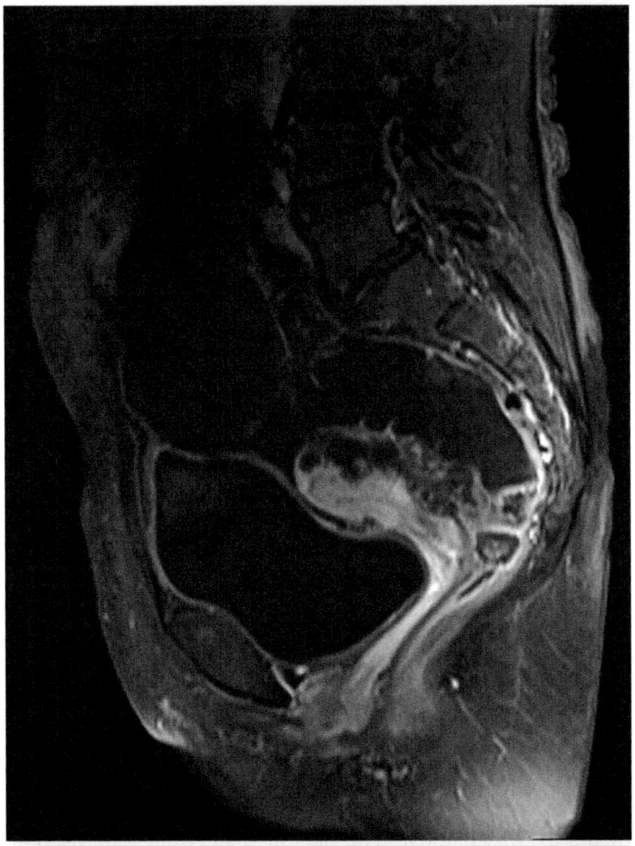

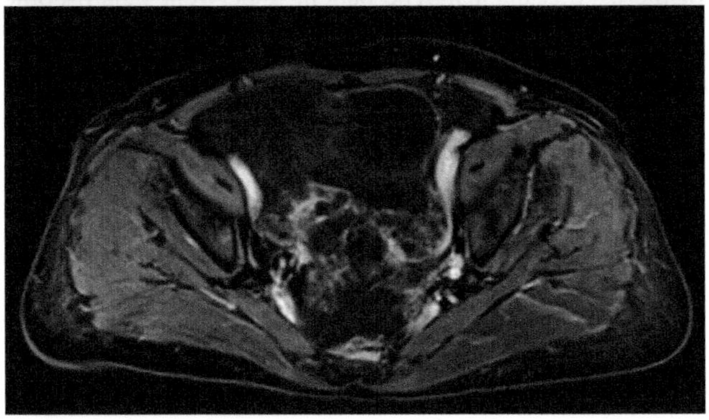

Figs. 38.2 and 38.3 The cystic wall and internal septation were slightly enhanced after contrast enhancement. There are many effusions in the abdominal and pelvic cavity, and the range is unclear

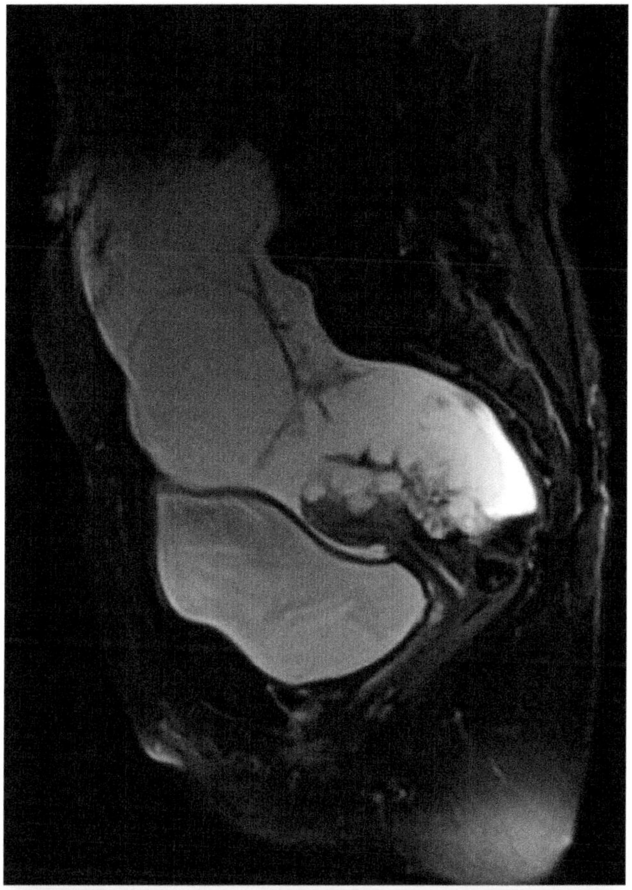

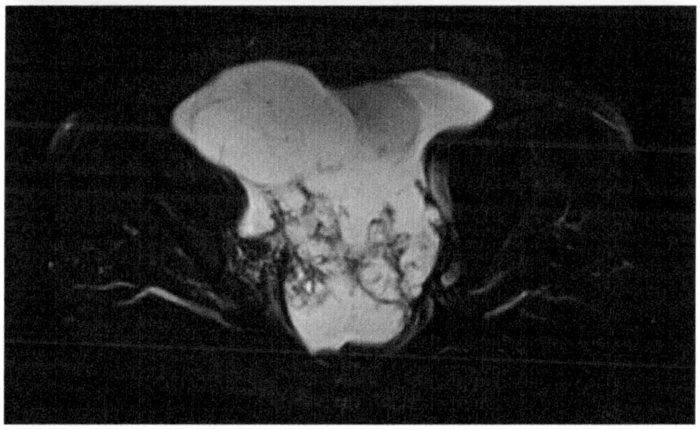

Figs. 38.4 and 38.5 The upper end reached upper edge of the fourth lumbar vertebra, and the lower end reached rectouterine and vesicouterine pouch. The appendix was tortuous and thickened, up to 3.5 cm × 6.6 cm × 3.3 cm in size, and showed low signal intensity on T1WI and high signal intensity on T2WI, and the cystic wall was enhanced after contrast enhancement

PMP is lack of specific clinical manifestations, but its imaging features have relatively specific manifestations. CT and MRI can display the location of the lesion, show the invasion of abdominal organs and blood vessels, and be helpful for surgeons to fully understand the range of tumor before operation, formulate surgical plans, and improve surgical resection rate and quality of life of patients.

References

1. Rizvi SA, Syed W, Shergill R. Approach to pseudomyxoma peritonei. World J Gastrointest Surg. 2018;10(5):49–56.
2. Carr NJ, Cecil TD, Mohamed F, et al. A consensus for classification and pathologic reporting of pseudomyxoma peritonei and associated appendiceal neoplasia: the results of the peritoneal surface oncology group international (PSOGI) modified Delphi process. Am J Surg Pathol. 2016;40(1):14–26.
3. Smeenk RM, van Velthuysen ML, Verwaal VJ, et al. Appendiceal neoplasms and pseudomyxoma peritonei: a population based study. Eur J Surg Oncol. 2008;34(2):196–201.
4. Mittal R, Chandramohan A, Moran B. Pseudomyxoma peritonei: natural history and treatment. Int J Hyperth. 2017;33(5):511–9.
5. Hinson F, Ambrose N. Pseudomyxoma peritonei. Br J Surg. 1998;85:1332–9.
6. Carr NJ, Finch J, Ilesley IC, et al. Pathology and prognosis in pseudomyxoma peritonei: a review of 274 cases. J Clin Pathol. 2012;65(10):919–23.
7. Ronnett BM, Zahn CM, Kurman RJ, et al. Disseminated peritoneal adenomucinosis and peritoneal mucinous carcinomatosis: a clinicopathologic analysis of 109 cases with emphasis on distinguishing pathologic features, site of origin, prognosis, and relationship to "pseudomyxoma peritonei". Am J Surg Pathol. 1995;19(12):1390–408.
8. Bosman FT, Cameiro F, Hruban RH, et al. World Health Organization classification of tumours of the digestive system. Lyon: IARC Press; 2010.
9. Li Y, Yu Y, Liu Y. Report on the 9(th) international congress on peritoneal surface malignancies. Cancer Biol Med. 2014;11(4):281–4.
10. Qiu QD, Xu CY, Xiang SF. MR diagnosis of peritoneal pseudomyxoma (report of 17 cases). J Med Imaging. 2008;18(4):380–3.

Part IX

Post-embolization Manifestations

39 Interventional Treatment of Uterine Fibroids

Mengwei Zhang and Guofu Zhang

39.1 Clinical History

Female patient, 42 years old, had regular menstruation; menarche at the age of 16, 7/30, with heavy menstrual bleeding; and mild dysmenorrhea. Uterine fibroids were found in health checkup 10 years ago, and laparoscopic myomectomy was performed 5 years ago. In recent years, the reexamination suggested the recurrence of uterine fibroids, gradually increased, and showed multiple growth, consciously palpable mass in the abdomen, frequent urination, and anemia symptoms such as dizziness and weakness after fatigue. The patient resisted hysterectomy and expected to retain the uterus.

Uterine artery embolization (UAE) was performed by interventional radiologist. Bilateral uterine arteries were superselected (Fig. 39.1), and polyvinyl alcohol (PVA) microspheres with diameters of 300–500 μm were used as embolization agents.

MRI examination: The uterus was in neutral position and the size of uterine body was about 8.5 cm × 5.8 cm × 7.2 cm. There was no obvious thickening of the endometrium and no obvious signal abnormality. Multiple round nodular abnormalities in the myometrium showed isointense on T1WI and hypointense on T2WI (Figs. 39.2 and 39.3), with well-defined boundary and capsule. The maximum diameter was about 3.7 cm, and significant enhancement was observed after contrast enhancement (Fig. 39.4). There was no obvious abnormality in bilateral adnexa areas.

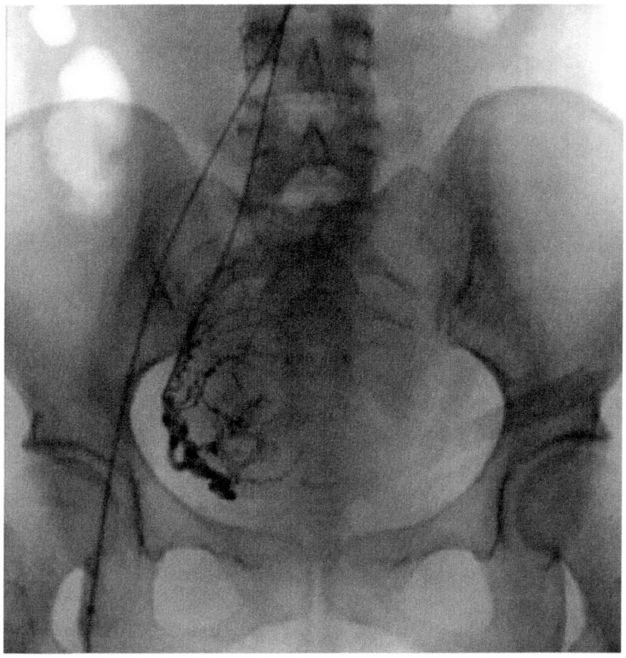

Fig. 39.1 Multiple uterine fibroids before interventional therapy. DSA-guided uterine artery angiography was performed to observe the course of uterine arteries and the staining of lesions, and then appropriate embolization agents were used to completely embolize bilateral uterine arteries in turn

M. Zhang (✉) · G. Zhang
Department of Radiology, Obstetrics and Gynecology Hospital, Fudan University, Shanghai, P.R. China

G. Zhang (ed.), *MRI of Gynaecological Diseases*, https://doi.org/10.1007/978-981-99-3644-1_39

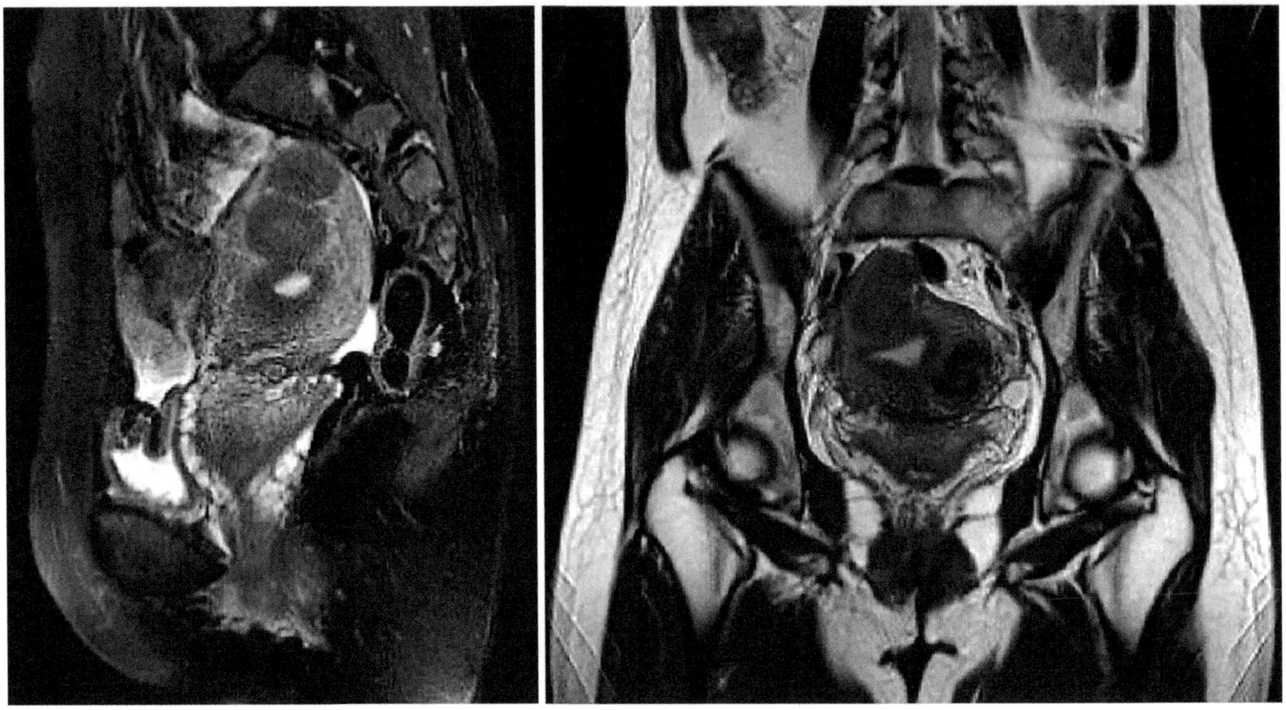

Figs. 39.2 and 39.3 Multiple uterine fibroids before interventional therapy. The uterus was enlarged. Sagittal and coronal T2WI images showed multiple round nodular hypointensity lesions in the myometrium, with well-defined boundary and capsule

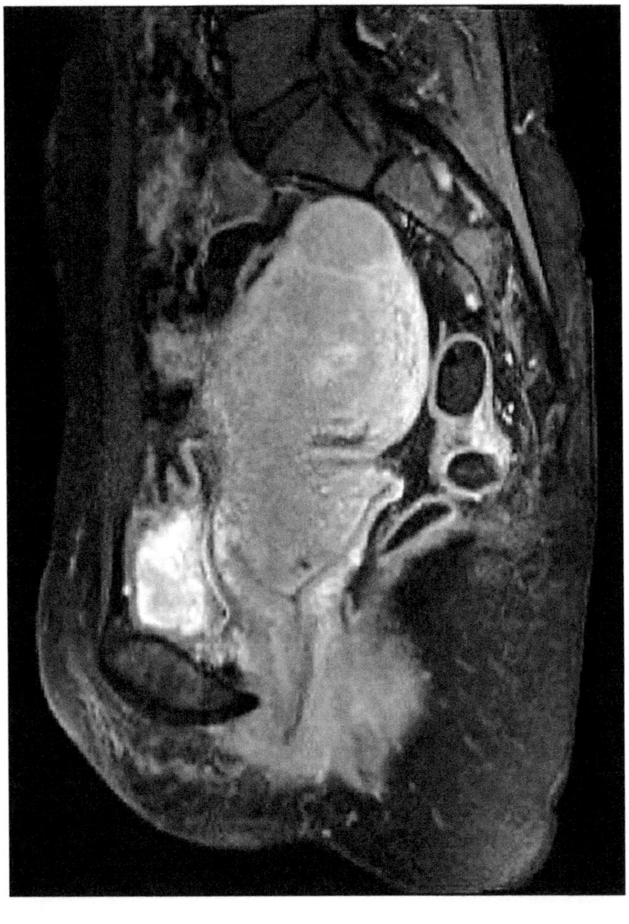

Fig. 39.4 Multiple uterine fibroids before interventional therapy. The lesions were uniformly enhanced after contrast enhancement

39.2 Imaging Analysis

Uterine myomas, also known as uterine fibroids, are the most common benign tumors of the female genital tract, composed of smooth muscle and connective tissue. They are common in women between 30 and 50 years old and rarely seen under 20 years old. According to autopsy statistics, about 20% of women over 30 years old have uterine fibroids. Because uterine fibroids are mostly asymptomatic or rarely symptomatic, the clinical reported incidence is far lower than the real incidence of fibroids [1]. The causes of the disease are complex, the specific pathogenesis is not clear, and there is a correlation with sex hormones and myometrial cell mutations. Clinically, the treatment option for the disease should be comprehensively analyzed according to patient's reproductive needs, age, location and size of fibroids, etc. and finally determines the treatment plan.

The traditional treatment is mainly surgery, such as hysterectomy and myomectomy. Hysterectomy is considered the definitive treatment, but it is not suitable for the treatment of young patients of childbearing age. The need to preserve uterus and adnexa led to the development of less-invasive techniques such as myomectomy, which was the standard treatment until uterine artery embolization technique was developed. Uterine artery embolization was introduced in the 1970s, initially used for postpartum hemorrhage hemostasis [2], and then used for pelvic perfusion chemotherapy for gynecological malignant tumors. In 1995, Ravina JH first used UAE in clinical treatment of uterine fibroids instead of surgery and achieved 16 successful cases [3]. The emergence of UAE provides a new and less invasive method for the treatment of uterine fibroids. The mechanism of UAE is through interventional embolization of blood supply of fibroids, causing the absorption of hypoxic-ischemic necrosis of fibroids, resulting in fibroid atrophy, so as to alleviate or eliminate clinical symptoms. Normal myometrium rapidly establishes a new blood supply through collateral vessels of ovarian and vaginal circulation, making it less likely to cause permanent adverse effects. At present, polyvinyl alcohol microspheres are mostly used as embolization agents in clinical practice, and the diameter of 300–500 μm is better. Indications for UAE are symptomatic uterine fibroids and desire for uterus preservation and/or refusal of surgery. Patients with current pregnancy, contrast agent allergy, current or recent pelvic inflammatory disease, or pelvic malignancy are excluded. Chinese guidelines suggest that UAE is most suitable for hypervascular fibroids [4], and other treatments should be considered for fibroids with low enhancement on preoperative contrast-enhanced images. The effect of embolization on ovarian function should be considered for the feasibility of UAE for uterine fibroids supplied by ovarian artery [4]. Surgical treatment is usually preferred for fibroids with pedicle, that is, submucosal fibroid with pedicle and subserosal fibroid with pedicle. A study by Kim et al. in 2012 found that there was only a 20% rate of complete infarction of cervical fibroids after UAE [5]. Cervical fibroids were found to have poor vascularity on angiography, suggesting that UAE for the treatment of cervical fibroids may not be effective.

Advantages of uterine artery embolization described in the literature include treatment of a larger number of fibroids in a single intervention, shorter duration of surgery, and faster recovery after the procedure, with consequent earlier return to activities, shorter length of hospital stay, and reduced incidence of complications and need for blood transfusion. Conversely, the most common complications were expulsion of the fibroid and amenorrhea. The latter may be caused by decreased ovarian function. Studies have shown a decrease in ovarian function after UAE that is similar to hysterectomy, but is more frequent in older women, which may be an asset for perimenopausal women seeking relief from heavy menstrual bleeding (HMB) [6]. The relatively high reintervention rates on mid- to long-term follow-up have been considered a major limitation of UAE. Reintervention rates are estimated at 9% at 1 year and 28% at 5 years from randomized controlled trials of UAE versus surgery [7, 8].

UAE has been shown to be a safe and effective treatment for symptomatic uterine fibroids, with over 25 years of supporting data. MRI of the patient in this case before treatment

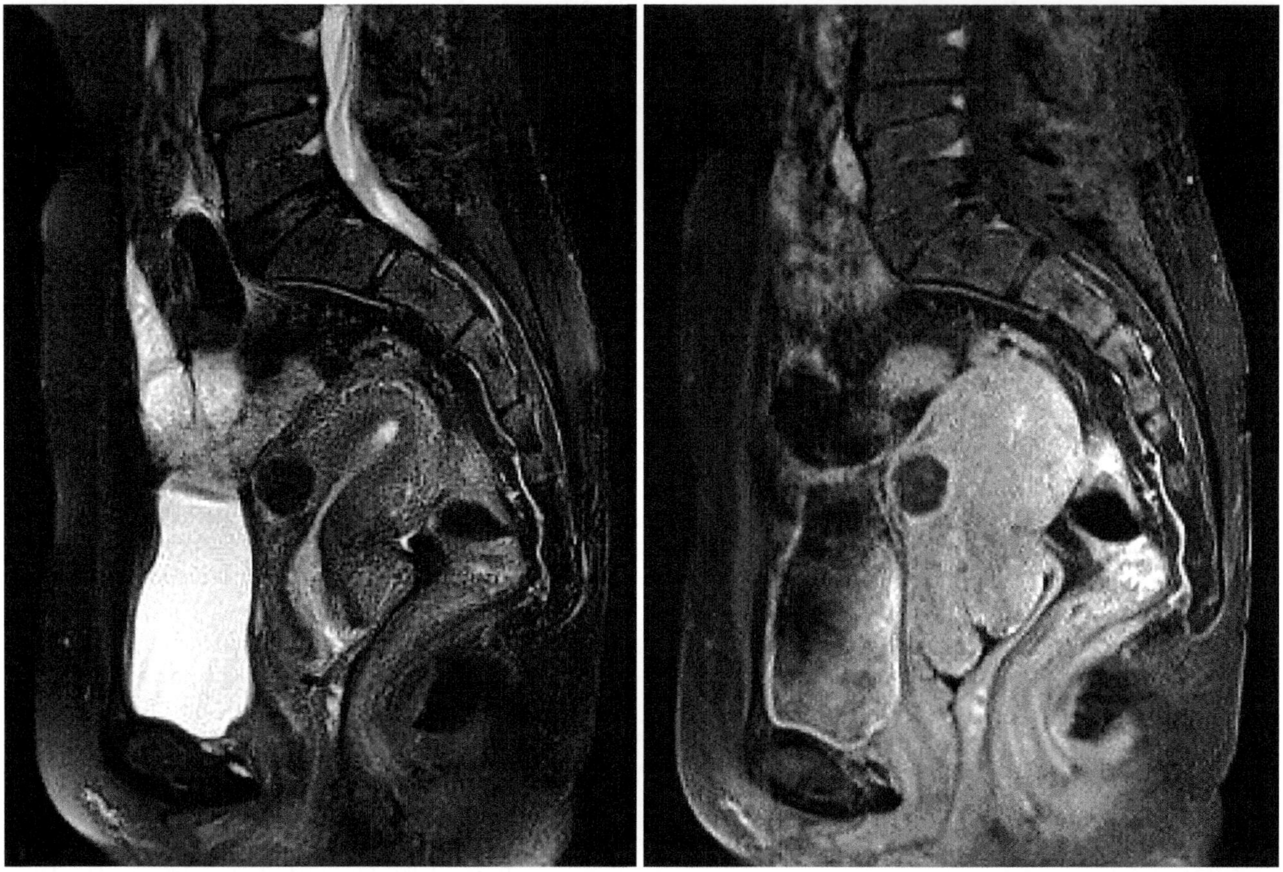

Figs. 39.5 and 39.6 Uterine fibroids after interventional therapy. MRI reexamination 6 months after uterine artery embolization showed that uterine volume was significantly decreased and some small fibroids disappeared. On T2WI, round low signal intensity lesion was shown in the myometrium, and there was no obvious enhancement after contrast enhancement

showed increased uterine volume and multiple intramural fibroids, and the diameter of the larger one was greater than 3 cm. Six months after UAE, MRI (Figs. 39.5 and 39.6) showed that the uterine volume was significantly decreased, the number of fibroids was reduced, and necrosis of intramural fibroids was shown. MRI reexamination 1.5 years (Figs. 39.7 and 39.8) after UAE showed no significant change in uterine volume and no recurrence compared with 1 year ago.

Compared with hysterectomy and myomectomy, UAE has unique advantages such as preserving the uterus and minimally invasive, but UAE also has its limitations. It is necessary for gynecologists and interventional radiologists to grasp the indications and select appropriate patients for UAE treatment of uterine fibroids.

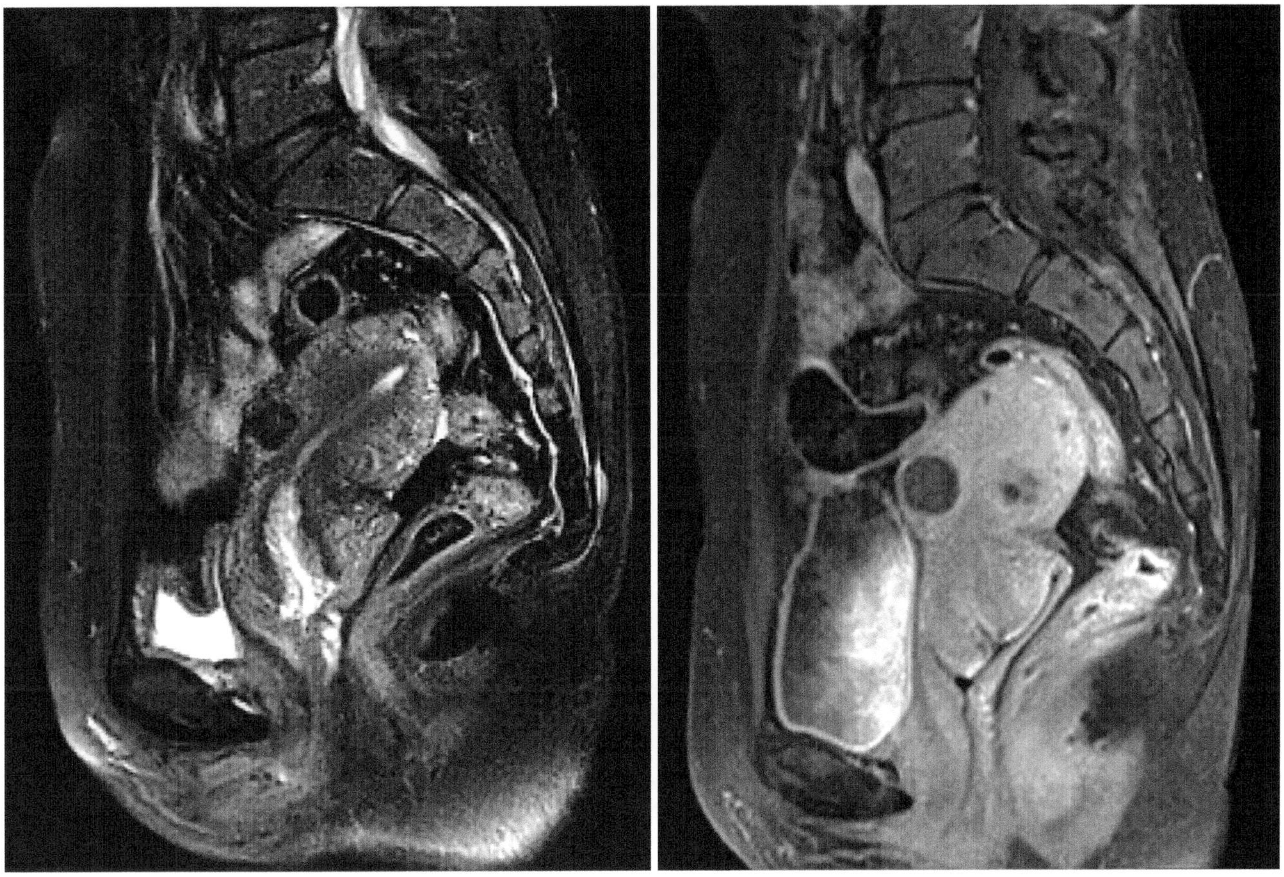

Figs. 39.7 and 39.8 Uterine fibroids after interventional therapy. MRI reexamination 1.5 years after uterine artery embolization showed that uterine volume was significantly decreased compared with 1 year ago and returned to nearly normal size. There was no significant change in the necrotic area of intramural fibroids, and no new recurrence was observed

References

1. Xing X, Beihua K, Tao D, et al. Obstetrics and gynecology. 9th ed. Beijing: People's Medical Publishing House; 2018.
2. Farrer-Brown G, Beilby JO, Tarbit MH. The vascular patterns in myomatous uteri. J Obstet Gynaecol Br Common Wealth. 1970;77:967–75.
3. Ravina JH, Herbreteau D, Ciraru-Vigneron N, et al. Arterial embolisation to treat uterine myomata. Lancet. 1995;346(8976):671–2.
4. Consensus for diagnosis and treatment of uterine myoma. Chin J Obstet Gynecol. 2017;52(12):793–800.
5. Kim MD, Lee M, Jung DC, et al. Limited efficacy of uterine artery embolization for cervical leiomyomas. J Vasc Interv Radiol. 2012;23:236–40.
6. Katsumori T, Kasahara R, Tsuchida Y, et al. Amenorrhea and resumption of menstruation after uterine artery embolization for fibroids. Int J Gynaecol Obstet. 2008;103:217–21.
7. van der Kooij SM, Hehenkamp WJ, Volkers NA, et al. Uterine artery embolization vs hysterectomy in the treatment of symptomatic uterine fibroids: 5-year outcome from the randomized EMMY trial. Am J Obstet Gynecol. 2010;203(105):e1–13.
8. Edwards RD, Moss JG, Lumsden MA, et al. Uterine-artery embolization versus surgery for symptomatic uterine fibroids. N Engl J Med. 2007;356:360–70.

Interventional Treatment of Adenomyosis

40

Mengwei Zhang and Guofu Zhang

40.1 Clinical History

Female patient, 42 years old, had dysmenorrhea for 5 years, progressive aggravation for 3 years, increased menstrual volume, prolonged menstrual period, and fatigue. She still felt obvious pain with oral painkillers during menstrual period, which seriously affected her life and work. She went to gynecology outpatient department of our hospital a few years ago, and ultrasonography showed adenomyosis. She was treated conservatively with medication, but relapsed after drug withdrawal and had liver and kidney function damage. The patient resisted hysterectomy and expected to retain the uterus. She visited the interventional radiology department to consult uterine artery embolization.

Uterine artery embolization (UAE) was performed by interventional radiologist. Bilateral uterine arteries were superselected, and Embosphere microspheres with diameters of 300–500 μm were used as embolic agents (Fig. 40.1).

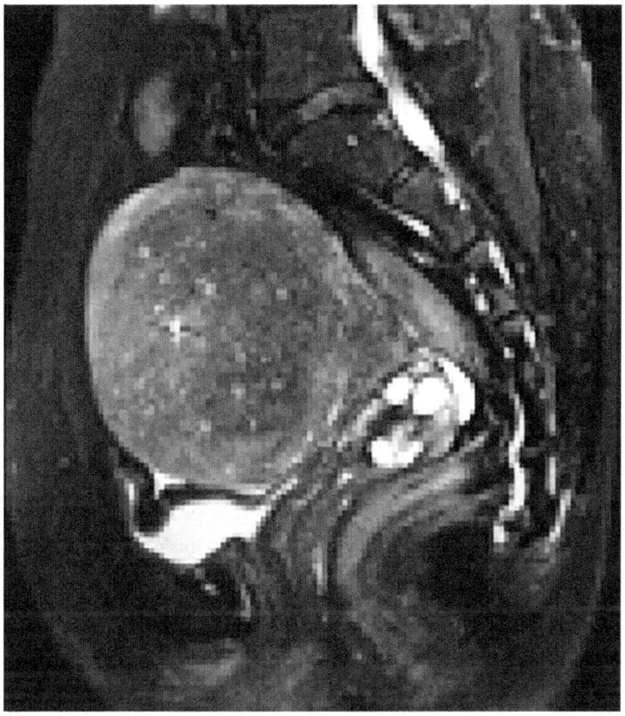

Fig. 40.1 Adenomyosis before interventional therapy. DSA-guided uterine artery angiography was performed to observe the course of uterine arteries and the staining of lesions, and then appropriate embolic agents were used to completely embolize bilateral uterine arteries in turn

M. Zhang (✉) · G. Zhang
Department of Radiology, Obstetrics and Gynecology Hospital, Fudan University, Shanghai, P.R. China

G. Zhang (ed.), *MRI of Gynaecological Diseases*, https://doi.org/10.1007/978-981-99-3644-1_40

40.2 Imaging Analysis

Adenomyosis is a diffuse or localized lesion of endometrial glands and stroma invading the myometrium, which is a common gynecological disease [1]. It is more common in women of childbearing age, especially in multiparous women of 30–50 years old. In recent years, the age of onset is getting younger, which may be related to the increase of cesarean section, abortion, and other gynecological operations. The main clinical manifestations are enlarged uterus, dysmenorrhea, prolonged menstrual period, and heavy menstrual bleeding (HMB). Traditional treatment methods include hysterectomy and drug treatment. Hysterectomy is the definitive cure, but it is not easy to be accepted by patients with fertility requirements and desire to preserve uterus. Drug treatment has poor curative effect, is easy to relapse, and has side effects. For young patients or those who have the desire to preserve uterus, UAE can effectively treat dysmenorrhea and menstrual disorders and other symptoms while preserving uterus. UAE is to inject appropriate embolic agent into uterine artery with the help of medical imaging technique and directly block the blood supply of the lesion, so that the lesion will shrink or even disappear, so as to achieve the purpose of treatment. UAE has the advantages of minimally invasive, short hospital stay, reduced complication incidence, and blood transfusion need and can preserve the uterus of patients. It has achieved good curative effect in many gynecological and obstetric diseases, such as special types of ectopic pregnancy, placenta previa, postpartum hemorrhage, uterine fibroids, adenomyosis, cervical cancer, and so on. The mechanism of UAE in the treatment of adenomyosis may be direct obstruction of small blood vessels in ectopic endometrial area and cause secondary intravascular thrombosis, resulting in ischemia, atrophy, and necrosis of ectopic endometrium. However, secondary microthrombi can also lead to gradual recanalization of blocked small blood vessels through autolysis, or the formation of collateral microcirculation around the lesion, resulting in the continued survival of small lesions of ectopic endometrium, which is manifested as the recurrence of clinical symptoms after a period of time [2]. The short-term clinical efficacy of UAE in the treatment of adenomyosis is clear [3–5], but the long-term efficacy is controversial. Kim et al. [5] reported that 54 patients with symptomatic adenomyosis treated by UAE were followed up for 3 years. According to the recurrence of clinical symptoms, the failure rate of UAE was 42.6%. Yao et al. [2] reported that clinical symptoms of patients with diffuse adenomyosis treated by UAE were significantly alleviated within 24 months, the pain degree of dysmenorrhea was significantly reduced, amount of menstruation was significantly decreased, and the symptoms of anemia were improved or even eliminated. However, 36.84% (7/19) of patients had a recurrence trend after 24 months. The diameter of embolic agent particles is another important factor affecting the effect of UAE. For adenomyosis, the inner vascular network is small and the outer vascular network is not obvious. Studies [6] have shown that embolization effect is closely related to the size of embolic agent. In order to achieve better embolization effect, the embolic agent particles with smaller diameter (300–500 μm) can be appropriately selected. In our hospital, Embosphere microspheres with diameter of 300–500 μm are generally used as embolic agent. Embosphere microspheres were approved by the US Food and Drug Administration (FDA) for the treatment of uterine fibroids embolization as early as 2002, with advantages of good histocompatibility, low complication rate, and mild pain after UAE [7].

The main adverse reactions and postoperative complications after UAE are post-embolization syndrome that appeared 1–3 days after UAE: fever, body temperature of 37.5–38.5 °C, abdominal pain, lumbosacral pain, nausea, vomiting, etc. We generally use symptomatic treatment such as analgesia. Most patients can be relieved within 1–2 weeks, which will not have a great impact on the mid- and long-term health of patients. Clinical studies [8] have also reported amenorrhea and decreased sexual desire after UAE, indicating that a certain proportion of patients' ovarian and uterine functions are affected after UAE. However, according to our experience, the effects of UAE on ovarian and uterine function are reversible, especially for women younger than 40 years old. Kulshrestha et al. [9] reported a 28-year-old woman with adenomyosis associated abnormal uterine bleeding (AUB) who was pregnant after UAE and delivered a healthy baby boy. Notably, the patient underwent UAE twice, using 500–700 μm particle size for the first time, but did not achieve therapeutic effect. A month later she had another episode of acute AUB for which a repeat session of emergency UAE was performed with smaller PVA particles of size 100–300 μm initially, followed by 300–500 μm diameter. The second UAE achieved therapeutic effect, and her urine pregnancy test confirmed pregnancy after 9 months. There are very limited cases of UAE in our hospital for nulliparous patients with adenomyosis, and many of them have not been followed up regularly in our hospital after UAE treatment. However, we also followed up a 35-year-old woman with adenomyosis who had never been pregnant. She became pregnant 6 months after UAE and delivered a healthy baby girl.

MRI of this case (Figs. 40.2–40.4) showed that the uterus was diffusely enlarged, thickening of myometrium, and uterine junctional zone, and there were punctate and cystic endometrioid high signal foci in myometrium. MRI reexamination 3 days after UAE (Figs. 40.5 and 40.6) showed that blood flow of myometrium was decreased and blood supply of the lesion

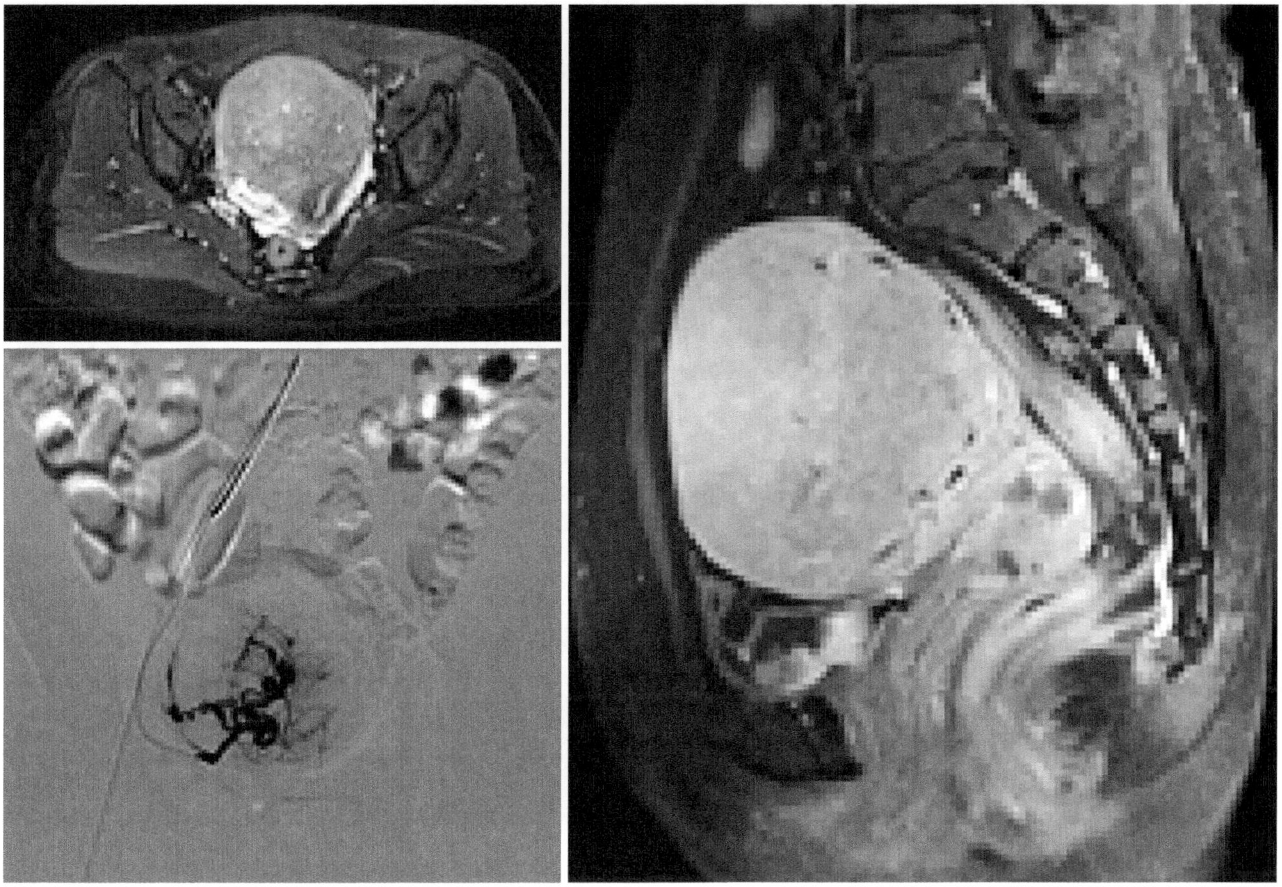

Figs. 40.2–40.4 Adenomyosis before interventional therapy. The uterus was diffusely enlarged, with thickening of myometrium and uterine junctional zone, punctate endometrioid high signal foci were seen on T2WI, and the boundary between uterine junctional zone and myometrium is unclear. Heterogeneous enhancement of myometrium was shown after contrast enhancement

was blocked. After UAE, the symptoms of dysmenorrhea and menorrhagia were significantly relieved. After 6 months, the patient underwent MRI examination again (Figs. 40.7 and 40.8). The volume of uterus was significantly reduced, myometrium and uterine junctional zone were decreased, the lesion was significantly smaller than before, and there was no obvious enhancement after contrast enhancement.

In conclusion, UAE for adenomyosis is a minimally invasive, safe, and effective treatment with fewer complications and fast recovery, retaining the uterus so as to retain reproductive function. However, UAE also has its limitations. It is necessary for gynecologists and interventional radiologists to grasp the indications and select appropriate patients for UAE treatment of adenomyosis.

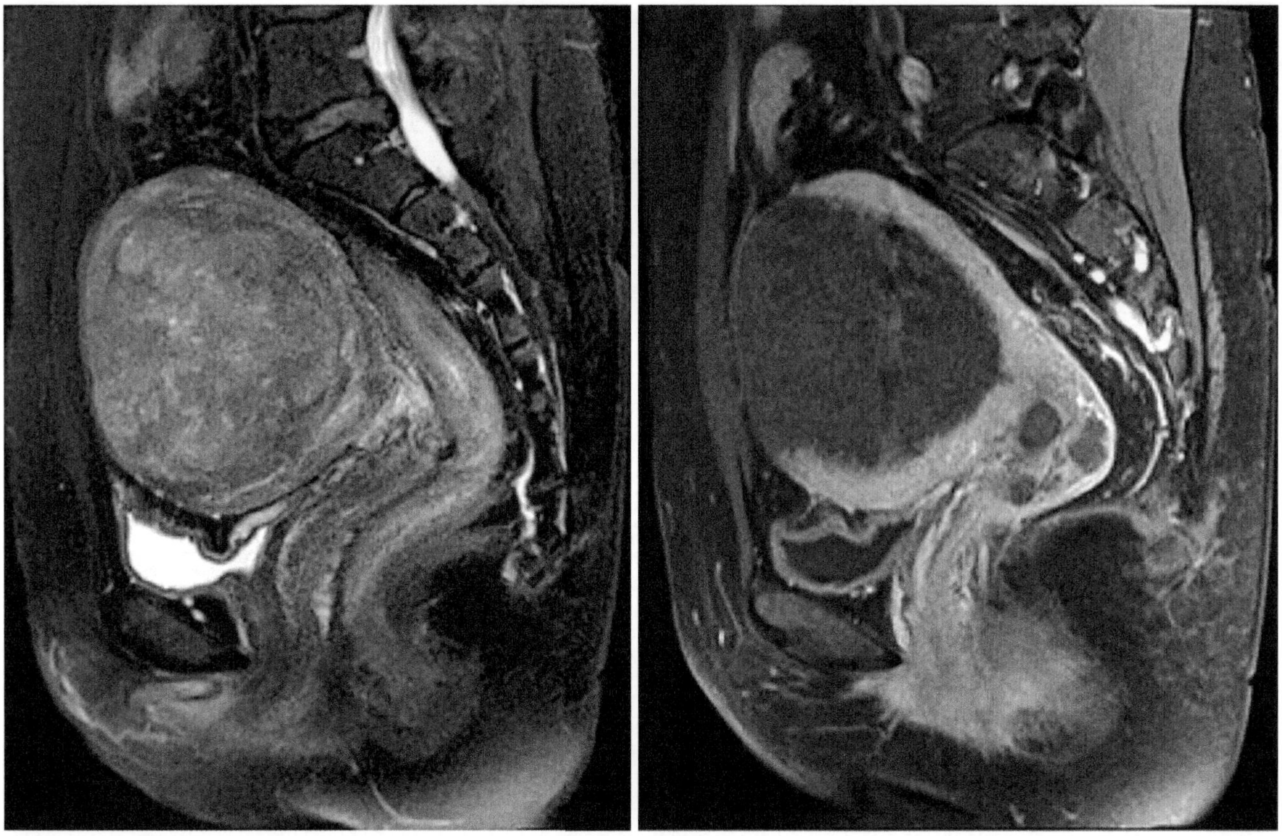

Figs. 40.5 and 40.6 Adenomyosis after interventional therapy. MRI reexamination 3 days after uterine artery embolization showed that the uterus was enlarged, and a mass-like T2WI slightly high signal foci were seen at uterine fundus, no obvious enhancement was observed after contrast enhancement, and blood flow of myometrium was significantly reduced

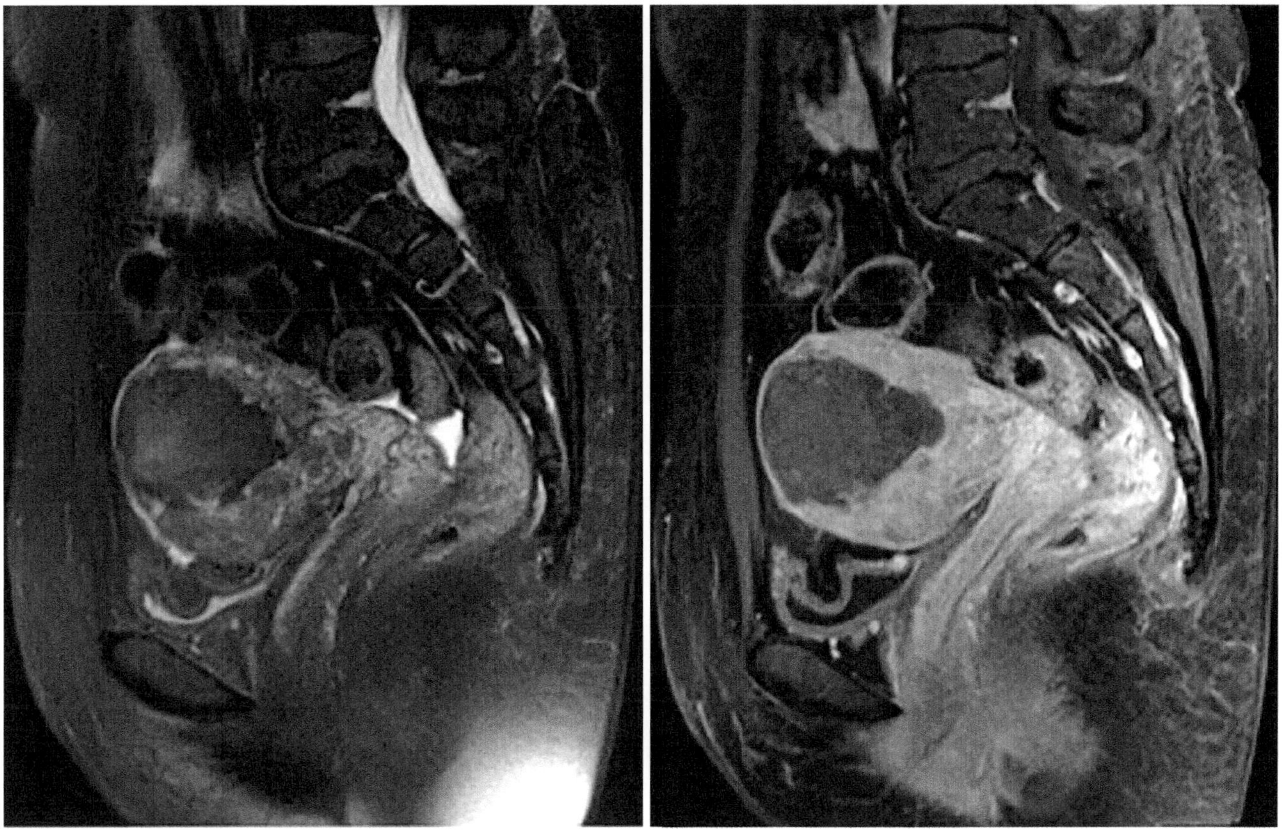

Figs. 40.7 and 40.8 Adenomyosis after interventional therapy. MRI reexamination 6 months after UAE showed that uterine volume was significantly smaller than before, and there was no obvious enhancement in the lesion area after contrast enhancement

References

1. Youji F. Obstetrics and gynecology. 2nd ed. Beijing: People's Medical Publishing House; 2010.
2. Qunli Y, Jiandong L, Xiangrong X, et al. Uterine artery embolization for the treatment of diffuse adenomyosis: long-term follow-up analysis. J Interv Radiol. 2013;22:896–9.
3. Popovic M, Puchner S, Berzaczy D, et al. Uterine artery embolization for the treatment of adenomyosis: a review. J Vasc Interv Radiol. 2011;22:901–9.
4. Smeets AJ, Nijenhuis RJ, Boekkooi PF, et al. Long-term follow-up of uterine artery embolization for symptomatic adenomyosis. Cardiovasc Intervent Radiol. 2012;35:815–9.
5. Kim MD, Kim S, Kim NK, et al. Long-term results of uterine artery embolization for symptomatic adenomyosis. Am J Roentgenol. 2007;188:176–81.
6. Jun Z, Bingyang J, Chunlin C, et al. Effect of different embolic agents on prognosis of uterine artery embolization in the treatment of uterine fibroid. Chinese J Pract Gynecol Obstet. 2015;10(31):951–5.
7. Ruifeng Z, Xuyao Z, Binbin W. Efficacy analysis of Embosphere microspheres in the treatment of uterine fibroids. Chinese J Health Care Med. 2016;18(3):230–1.
8. Dariushnia SR, Nikolic B, Stokes LS, et al. Society of Interventional Radiology Standards of practice committee. Quality improvement guidelines for uterine artery embolization for symptomatic leiomyomata. J Vasc Interv Radiol. 2014;25(11):1737–47.
9. Kulshrestha V, Yadav R, Malla S, et al. Successful pregnancy outcome in refractory adenomyosis treated with two sessions of uterine artery embolization: a case report and brief review. J Gynecol Obstet Hum Reprod. 2021;50(7):102132.

Part X

Gynaecological Diseases in Young Women

41 Gynecological Diseases in Young Women

He Zhang and Xiang Tao

The ovarian disease spectrum of young women (children, adolescent) includes lots of etiologies, for example, epithelial tumors, sex cord-stromal tumors, and germ cell tumors. Although some specific ovarian tumors occur in their own peak age, however, almost all kinds of ovarian tumors can be seen in young girls. In this chapter, based on our experiences and cases, we will discuss gynecological diseases in this specific population.

Epithelial ovarian cancer (Figs. 41.1, 41.2 and 41.3) generally develops in women at the average age between 40 and 60 years old, but it still can be found in young girls or adolescent. In our institution, this etiology still accounts a large part of the whole data; some of cancer pathological diagnoses are reported with an accompanying borderline tumor. For radiologists, it is necessary to be considered cancer diagnosis into the differential diagnoses.

Ovarian sex cord-stromal tumors (Figs. 41.4, 41.5, and 41.6), relatively, are rare according to the prevalence in women. Compared with epithelial tumors, sex cord-stromal tumors are commonly seen in young girls [1]. On MRI, it is more difficult to determine the nature of the tumors for all these tumors have similar manifestations on both pre- and post-contrast MRI. For these cases, clinical history and serum tumor markers are important clues for radiologists to get the right diagnosis.

Ovarian germ cell tumors (Figs. 41.7, 41.8, 41.9, and 41.10) are also seen in young girls, especially for girls less than 10 years old [4]. Elevation of serum AFP is an important tumor marker for this kind of disease. They commonly appear as homogeneously solid mass with avid enhancement on contrast-enhanced MRI.

For suspected gynecological diseases in children, MRI provides more information about the extent of disease than the origin, because the children's pelvis and abdomen are small, making the normal adnexal structure shown unclear [2, 3]. For these patients, however, the lesions always have huge size at her first medical consultation. Overall, comprehensive review of both clinical history and imaging data will narrow the possible differential diagnoses. The final diagnosis is determined by histopathological results.

H. Zhang (✉)
Department of Radiology, Obstetrics and Gynecology Hospital, Fudan University, Shanghai, People's Republic of China
e-mail: zhanghe1790@fckyy.org.cn

X. Tao
Department of Pathology, Obstetrics and Gynecology Hospital, Fudan University, Shanghai, People's Republic of China

G. Zhang (ed.), *MRI of Gynaecological Diseases*, https://doi.org/10.1007/978-981-99-3644-1_41

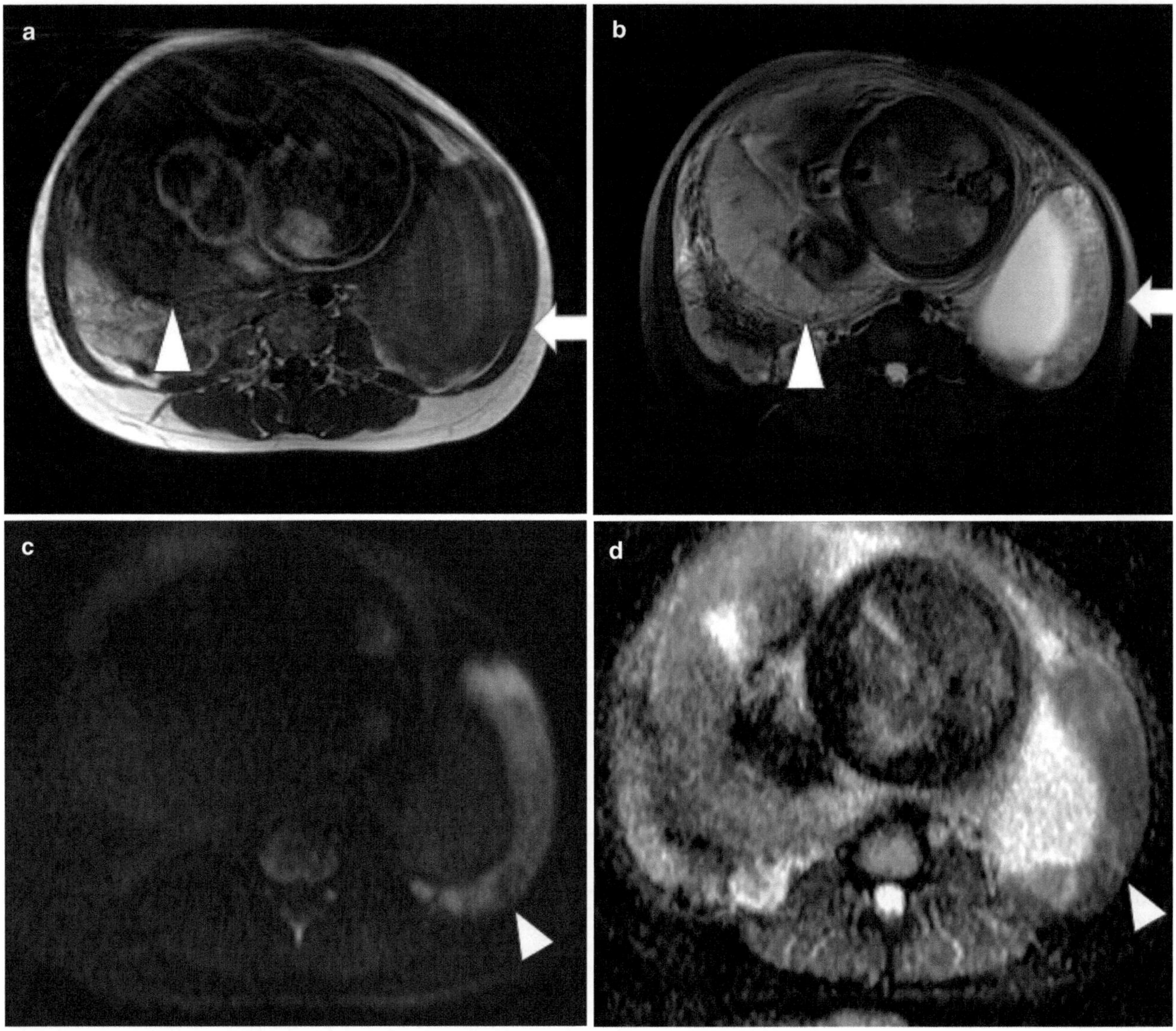

Fig. 41.1 A 25-year-old woman. A woman with a 38 gestational week fetus was accidentally reported a pelvic mass during her routine ultrasonography screening. The surgery was performed after delivery, and pregnancy luteoma was reported. In the left lower abdomen, there was cystic mass (arrow) besides the pregnant uterus (arrowhead), which presumably originating from the left ovary. The mass displayed as iso-hypo intensity signal on T1WI (**a**) and iso-hyper intensity signal on T2WI (**b**). The mass showed slightly high signal on DWI (**c**) and low signal on the corresponding ADC map (**d**)

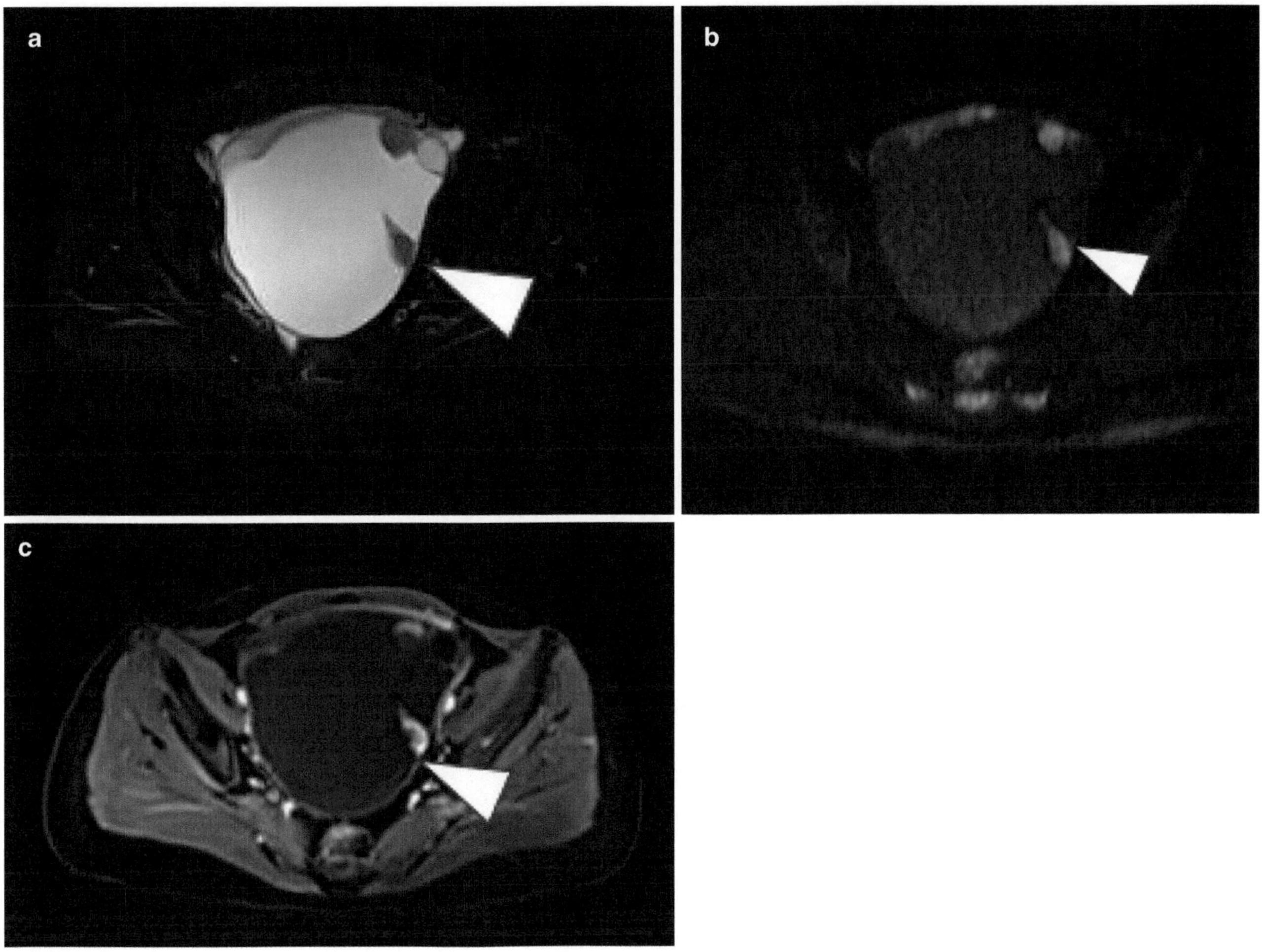

Fig. 41.2 A 23-year-old woman. The patient said she was suggested MRI examination during the routine ultrasonography screening. No abnormal complaints were recorded. The final pathological diagnosis included both ovarian borderline tumors and tiny cancer lesion. The cystic components of the pelvic mass mainly displayed as high signal on T2WI (**a**), and the vegetations (arrowhead) abutting the cystic wall showed medium signal on T2WI and high signal on DWI (**b**) and enhanced significantly after contrast enhancement (**c**)

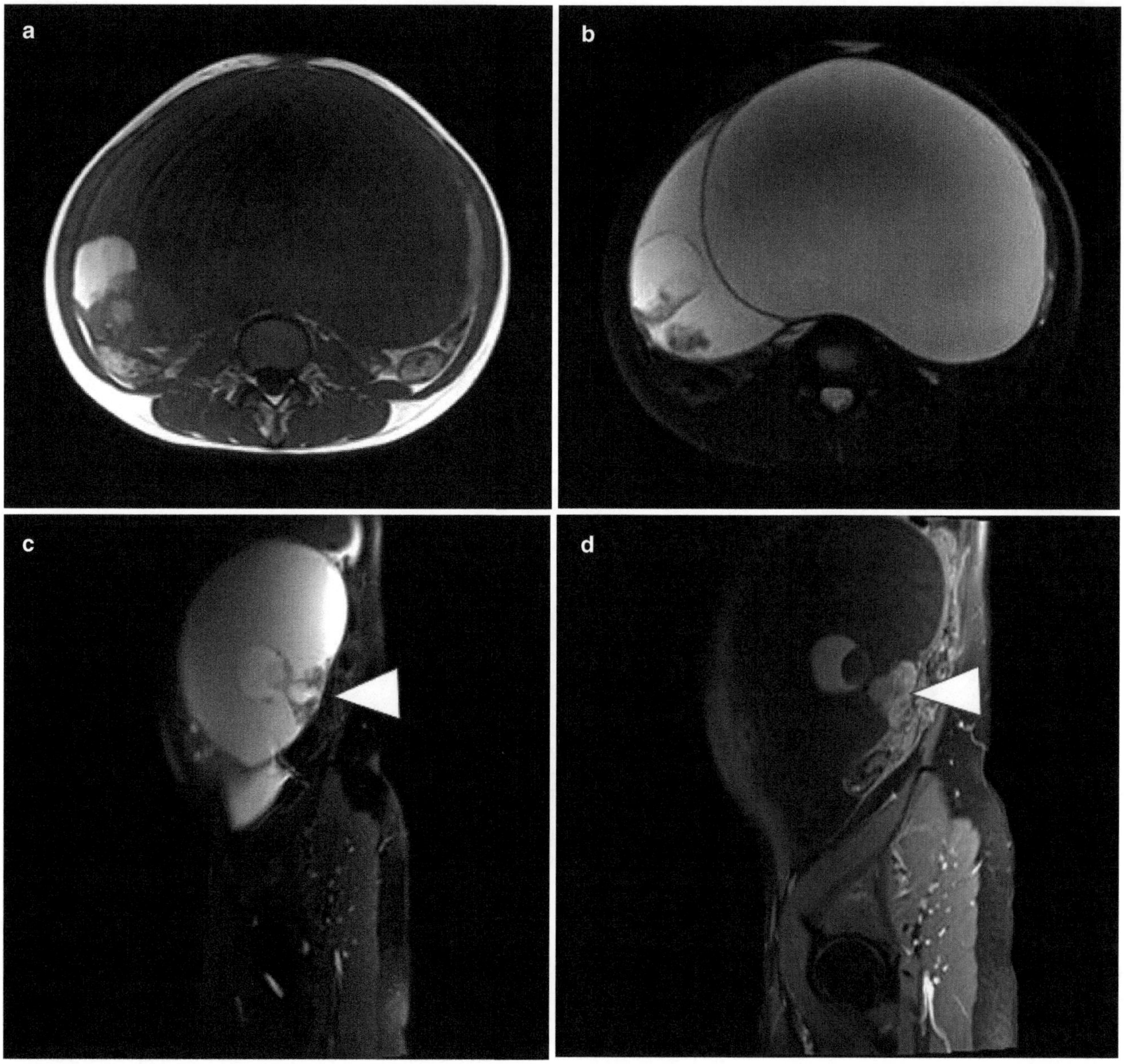

Fig. 41.3 A 18-year-old girl with pathologically proven ovarian borderline tumor mixed with epithelial cancer. She felt abdominal distension almost one month ago, and this condition was obvious in a couple of weeks. A giant cystic mass located in the abdominal and pelvic cavity. The mass mostly manifested as low signal on T1WI (**a**) and high signal on T2WI (**b**). On contrast-enhanced images, the vegetations (arrowhead) abutting right wall of the mass displayed obvious enhancement (**c**, **d**)

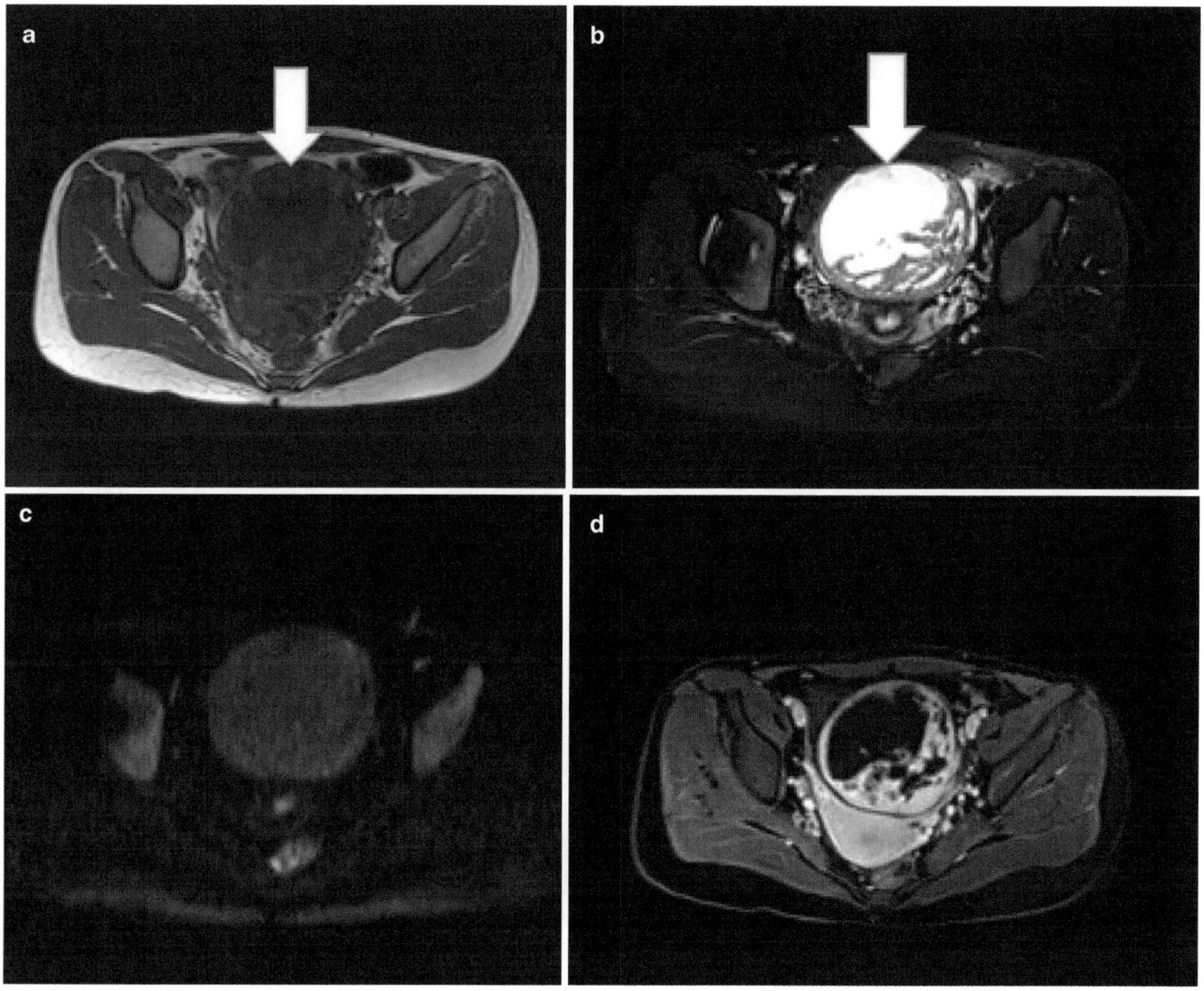

Fig. 41.4 A 21-year-old woman. She complained of feeling a pelvic mass, with regular menstrual period. The final pathological diagnosis was ovarian sclerosing stromal tumor. The round, multilocular mass (arrow) with intact capsule manifested as low signal on T1WI (**a**), high signal on T2WI (**b**), and medium signal on DWI (**c**). The mass enhanced avidly after contrast enhancement (**d**)

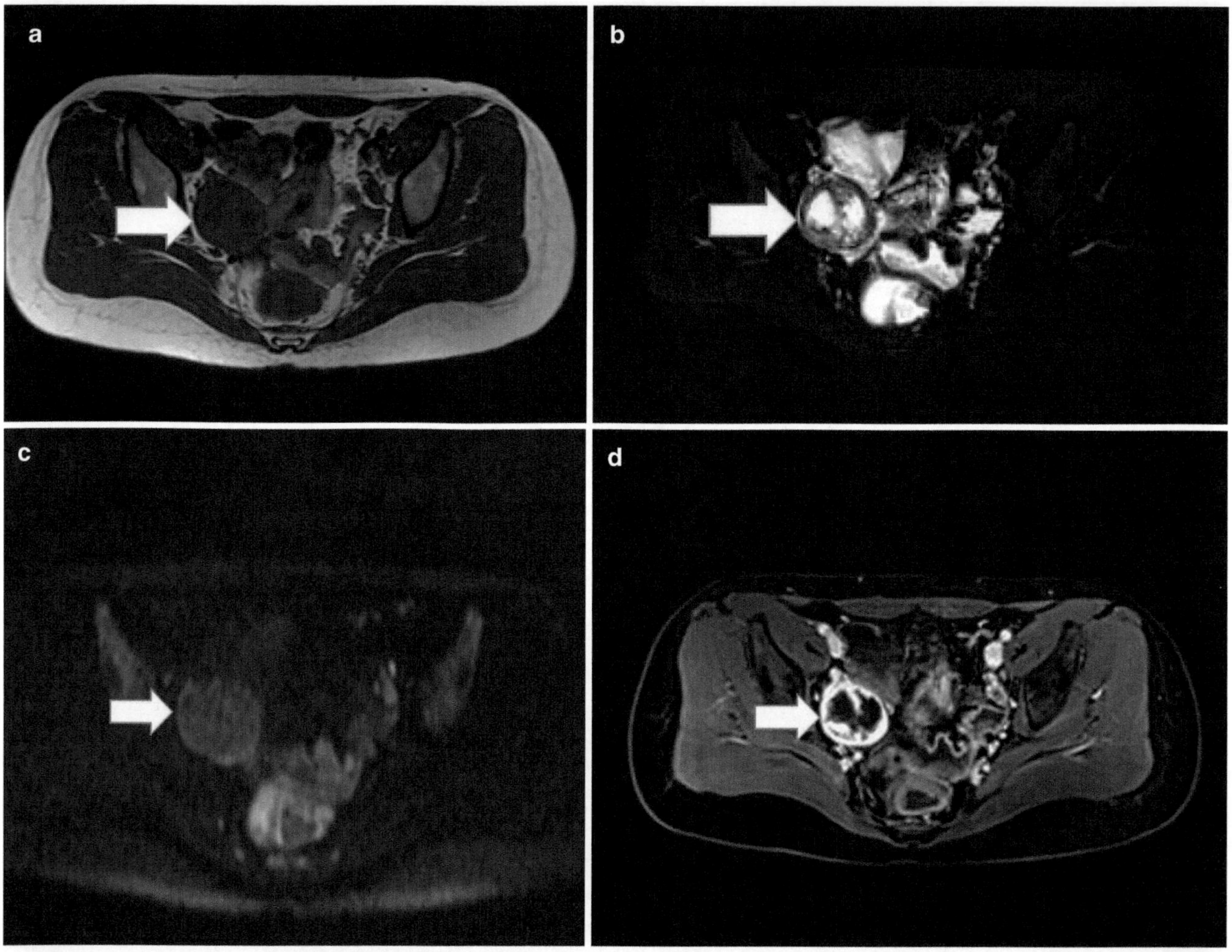

Fig. 41.5 A 24-year-old woman. She complained of having a pelvic mass one month ago without tenderness. Serum tumor markers were all in normal range. MRI: The oval mass (arrow) located in the right adnexa area, showing mainly intermediate signal on T1WI (**a**) and intermediate-high signal on T2WI (**b**). The mass showed relatively low signal on DWI (**c**) and enhanced obviously on contrast-enhanced image (**d**). The final pathological diagnosis was ovarian sclerosing stromal tumor

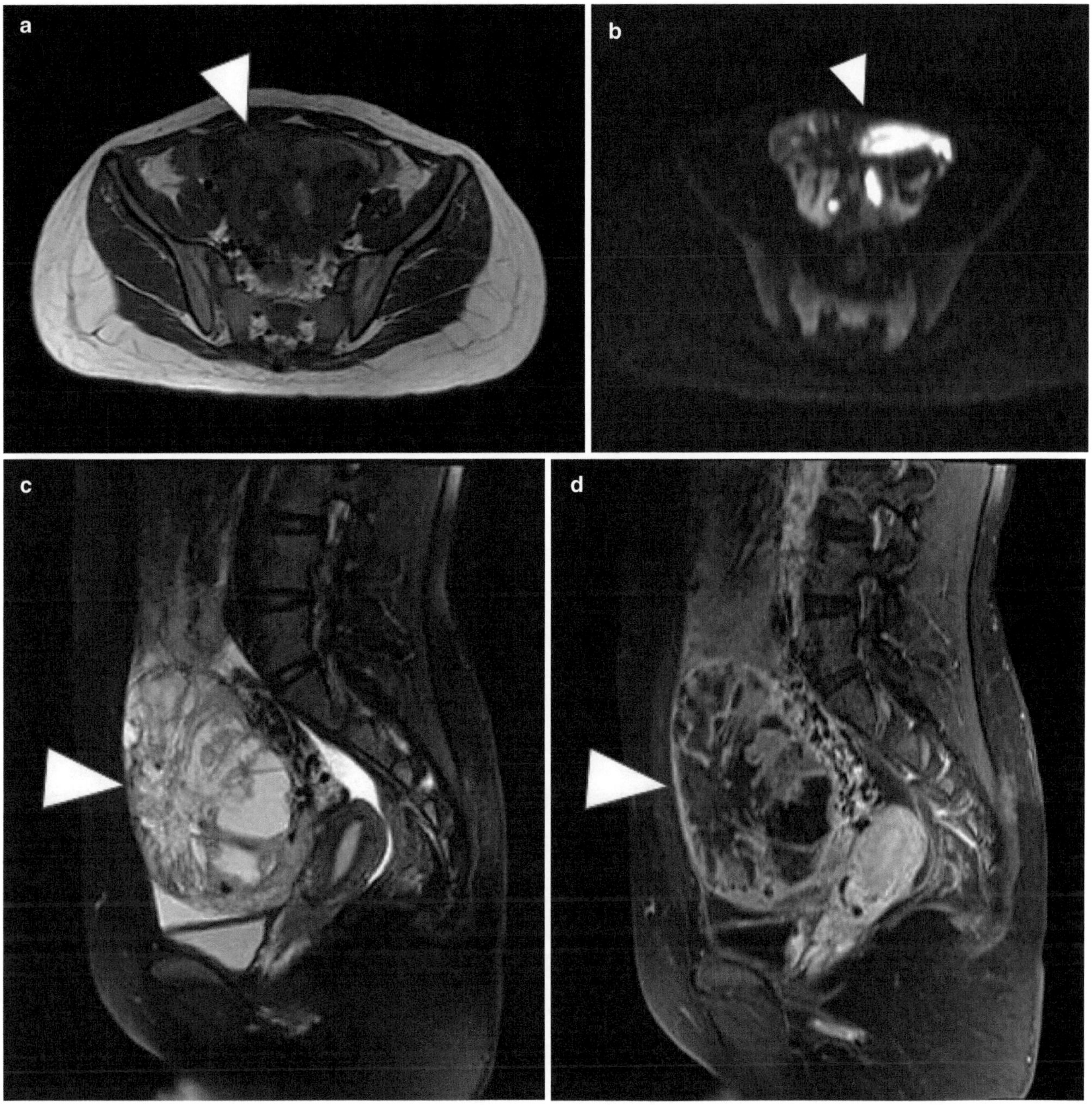

Fig. 41.6 A 13-year-old girl with ovarian juvenile granulosa cell tumor. She complained of an irregular menstrual period for lasting almost 2 months, and ultrasound examination report in the outer hospital revealed a pelvic mass 10 days ago. A giant, cystic mass (arrowhead) displayed as mixed signal on both T1WI (**a**) and DWI (**b**). The multilocular components within the mass were evident on T2WI (**c**); the solid components enhanced avidly like the myometrium (**d**). Microscopic examination revealed tumor cells arrange in nests of various size and irregularity. In the nests, numerous papillae are formed with stroma and vessels in the center (**e**, HE ×5). Tumor cells are small, round, and with a bland nucleus in the center; 1 or 2 small nucleoli are obvious. The nuclear membrane is smooth, without grooves which are typically observed in adult granulosa cell tumor. The tumor cells are arranged in multilayers, with loose intercellular connection (**f**, HE ×20)

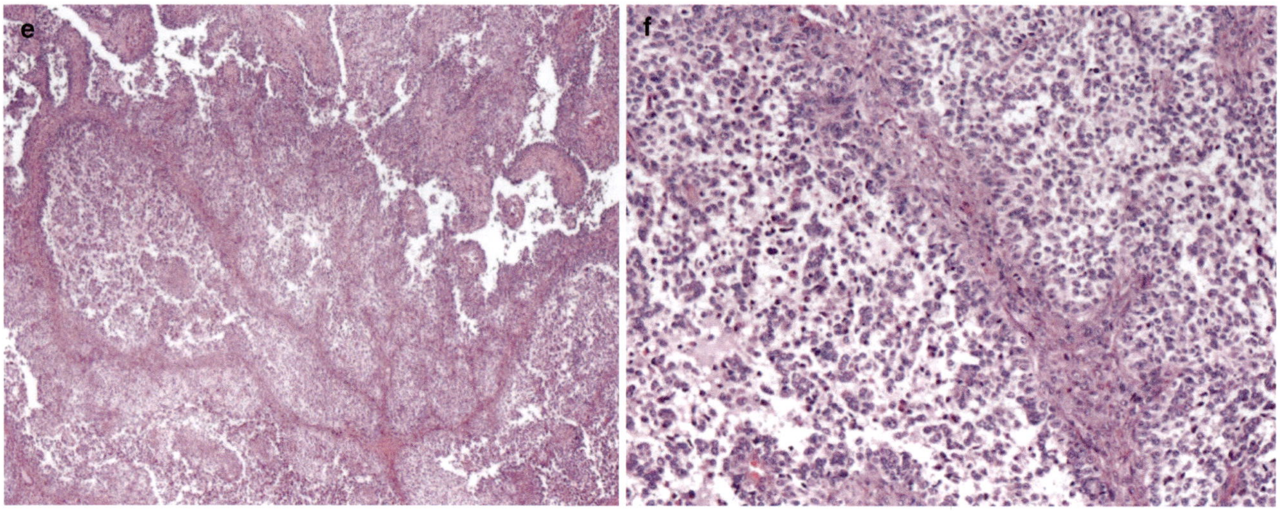

Fig. 41.6 (continued)

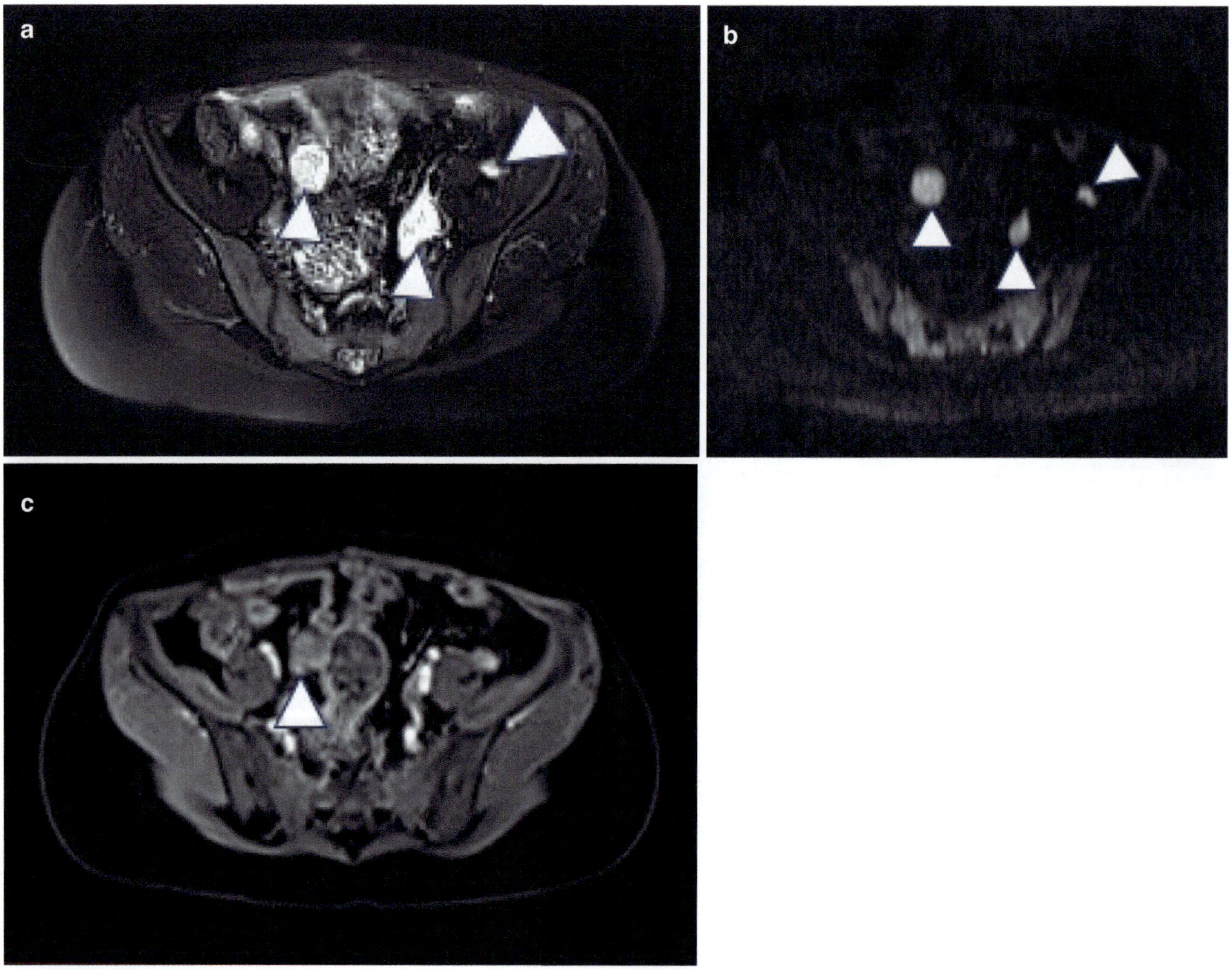

Fig. 41.7 A 26-year-old woman. The patient was diagnosed as ovarian Sertoli-Leydig tumor and underwent two cycles of chemotherapy previously. At the MRI examination, she complained of abdominal pain for several days. The multiple lesions (arrowhead) in pelvis showed relatively high signal on fat suppressed T2WI (**a**) and restricted diffusion signal on DWI (**b**). The mass showed moderate enhancement on contrast-enhanced image (**c**)

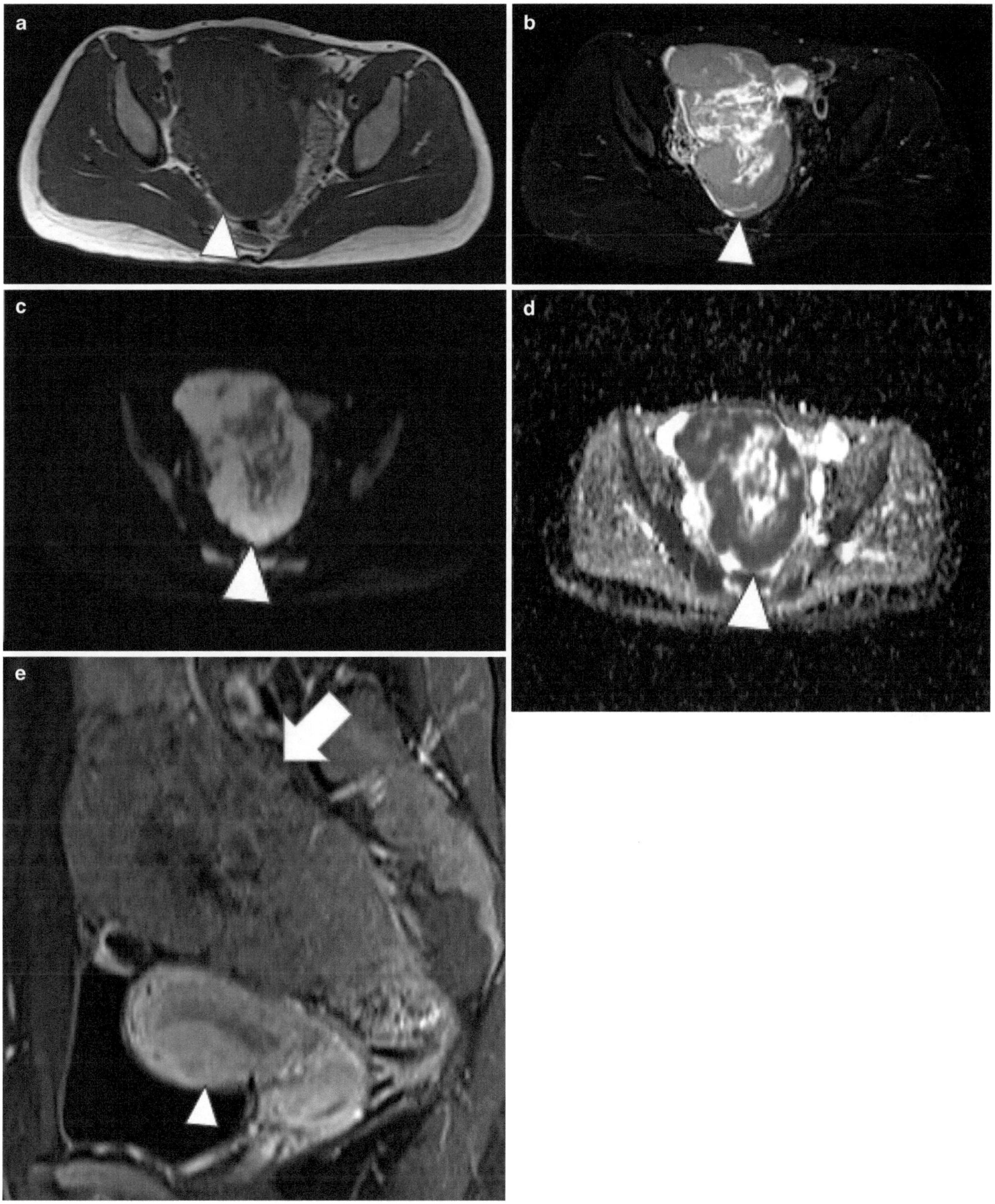

Fig. 41.8 A 21-year-old woman. The patient complained she felt a pelvic mass a decade days ago. Ultrasound examination suggested a solid mass arising from the ovary. CA125: 49.02 U/mL; HE4: 39.6 pmol/L; CA153: 6.40 U/mL; and CA199: <2.00 U/mL, AFP: 1.81 ng/mL. No abdominal pain and distension, fever, abnormal vaginal bleeding, and discharge were reported. The final pathological diagnosis was ovarian dysgerminoma. A giant mass occupied the most part of pelvis with isointense signal on both T1WI (**a**) and T2WI (**b**). The solid components (arrow), showing restricted diffusion signal on DWI (**c**) and the corresponding ADC map (**d**), enhanced less significantly than normal myometrium (arrow, **e**)

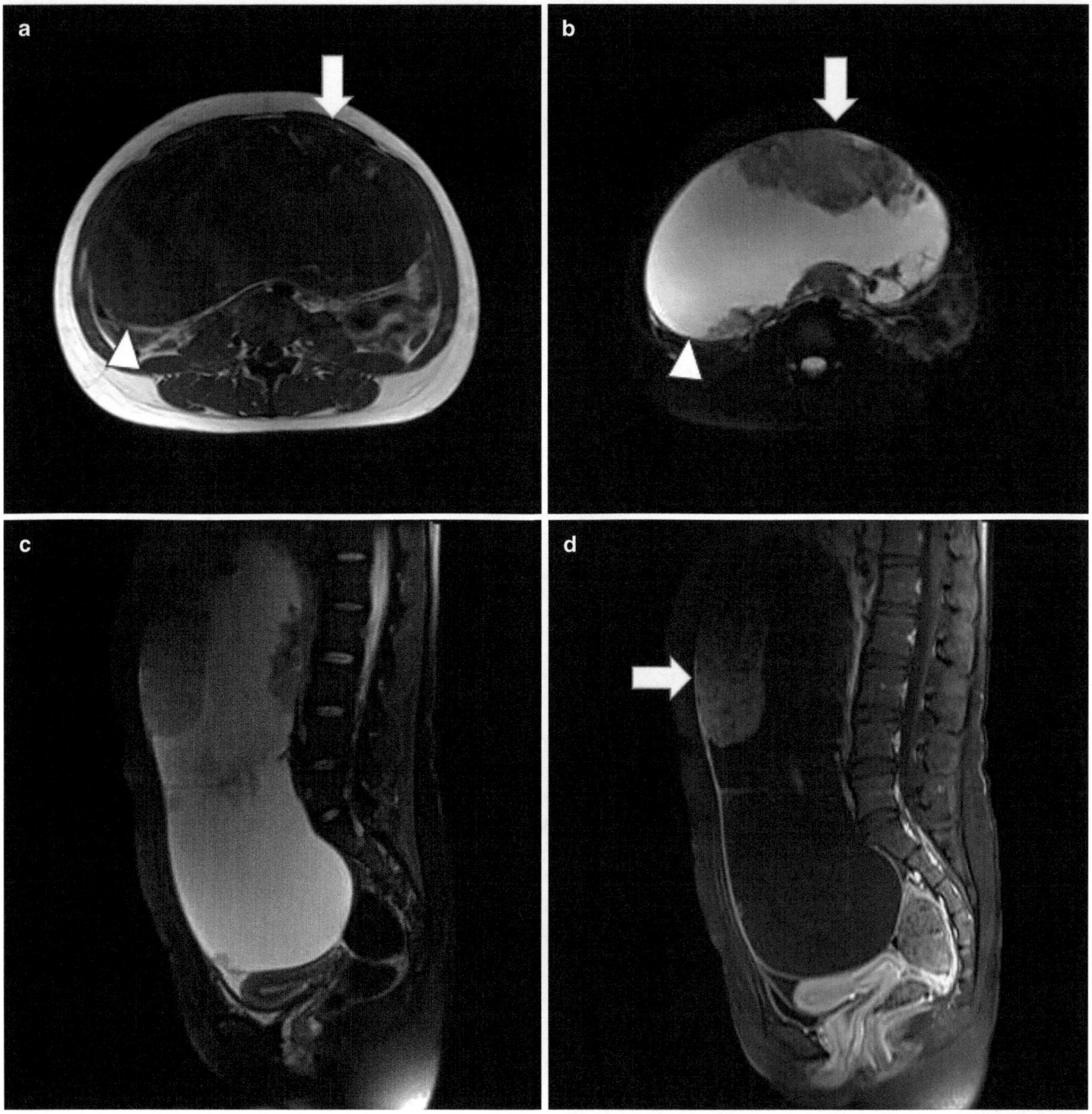

Fig. 41.9 A 20-year-old woman. She complained of abdominal distension, vomiting, diarrhea, and an increase in abdominal girth. CT (the outer hospital) displayed a mass with an average density of 15–28 Hu. Within the mass, there was a patchy of calcification and a strand of low-density components. A month after the CT examination, she underwent an MRI examination. The final pathological diagnosis was ovarian malignant mixed teratoma. MRI: The giant mass occupied the whole abdominal cavity with intact capsule. The cystic components (arrowhead) displayed as low signal on T1WI and high signal on T2WI, while the solid components (arrow) showed intermediate signal on both T1WI (**a**) and T2WI (**b**, **c**). The cystic wall showed weak enhancement after contrast enhancement (**d**)

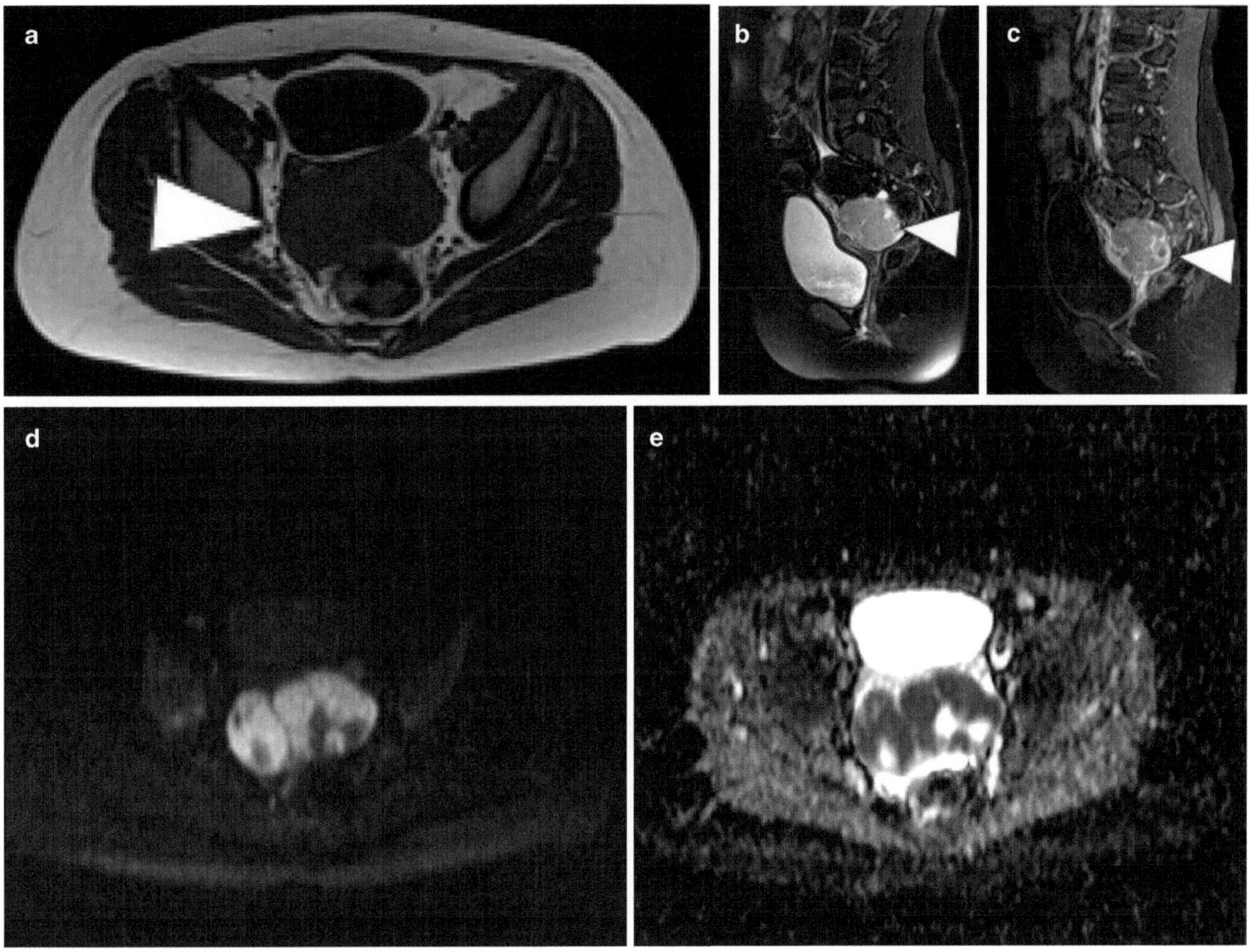

Fig. 41.10 A 9-year-old girl with ovarian dysgerminoma. The patient was admitted to the hospital complaining of abdominal pain and fever for several days. The tumor with homogeneous isointense (**a**, **b**) signal centered in the rectouterine pouch (arrowhead), enhancing obviously on contrast-enhanced image (**c**). The mass showed obvious diffusion restricted signal intensity on DWI (**d**) and displayed as low signal on the corresponding ADC map (**e**)

References

1. Javadi S, Ganeshan DM, Jensen CT, Iyer RB, Bhosale PR. Comprehensive review of imaging features of sex cord-stromal tumors of the ovary. Abdom Radiol (NY). 2021;46:1519.
2. Hanafy AK, Mujtaba B, Yedururi S, Jensen CT, Sanchez R, Austin MT, Morani AC. Imaging in pediatric ovarian tumors. Abdom Radiol (NY). 2020;45(2):520–36.
3. Lala SV, Strubel N. Ovarian neoplasms of childhood. Pediatr Radiol. 2019;49(11):1463–75.
4. Bergeron LM, Bishop KC, Hoefgen HR, Abraham MS, Tutlam NT, Merritt DF, Peipert JF. Surgical management of benign adnexal masses in the pediatric/adolescent population: an 11-year review. J Pediatr Adolesc Gynecol. 2017;30(1):123–7.

Part XI

Pelvic Inflammatory Diseases

42 Pelvic Suppurative Inflammation

Jielin Xie

42.1 Clinical History

Female patient, 69 years old. She was experiencing menopausal 24 years ago; there was no obvious cause of a small amount of vaginal bleeding 10 days ago, accompanied by dull pain and discomfort in the right lower abdomen and no obvious fever. The patient was admitted to our hospital and underwent examination of serum tumor markers: CA125: 37.45 U/mL; CA199: 7.98 U/mL; and CEA: 0.8 ng/mL. Ultrasonography showed ill-defined parenchymal structure in the myometrium of uterus, with abundant blood supply of the lesion. She underwent laparoscopic extensive intestinal adhesiolysis, appendectomy, total hysterectomy, and bilateral salpingo-oophorectomy. During the operation, it was found that there was extensive adhesion and significant pus exudation in pelvic cavity, and diffuse purulent exudation in the myometrium was seen by dissection of uterus.

Postoperative pathological results: acute and chronic inflammation of the myometrium with abscess formation.

42.2 Imaging Analysis

Pelvic suppurative inflammation tends to occur in women of childbearing age, which is mostly developed from acute pelvic inflammation. It can also occur after repeated episodes of chronic pelvic inflammatory disease, and a few can occur in women without symptom [1]. The clinical manifestations are mostly vague pain and dull pain in the lower abdomen, which occur intermittently and may be aggravated during menstrual period or after fatigue, and leukorrhea may increase. The site of the disease is widely distributed. Any part of the pelvic cavity may be affected, mostly in fallopian tube or ovary. MRI may have different findings depending on the stage of suppurative inflammatory abscess formation. In the early stage of abscess formation, MRI shows patchy high-intensity T2WI and low-intensity T1WI foci with fuzzy boundary and unclear boundary with surrounding tissues, and there may be exudate around the lesion. After abscess formation, MRI shows cystic or solid and cystic masses in the pelvic cavity with irregular shape, thick cystic wall, and uneven wall thickness (Figs. 42.1 and 42.2). Cystic fluid mostly shows high signal intensity on T2WI and low signal intensity on T1WI. The lesions adhered to surrounding structures with ill-defined boundary and with septations, and mural nodules can be seen in some lesions (Figs. 42.3 and 42.4), which are significantly enhanced after contrast enhancement (Fig. 42.5). Pneumatosis or gas-liquid stratification may occur in typical abscess formation, but the occurrence is less frequent [2–4].

J. Xie (✉)
Department of Radiology, Obstetrics and Gynecology Hospital, Fudan University, Shanghai, People's Republic of China

G. Zhang (ed.), *MRI of Gynaecological Diseases*, https://doi.org/10.1007/978-981-99-3644-1_42

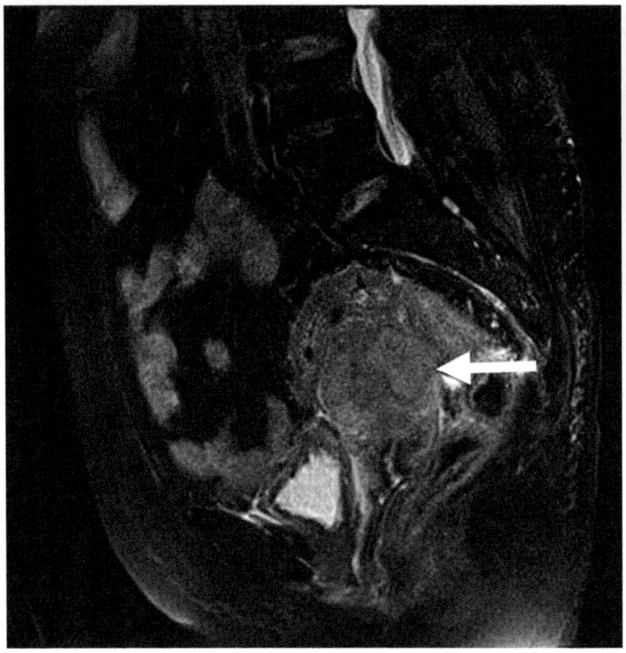

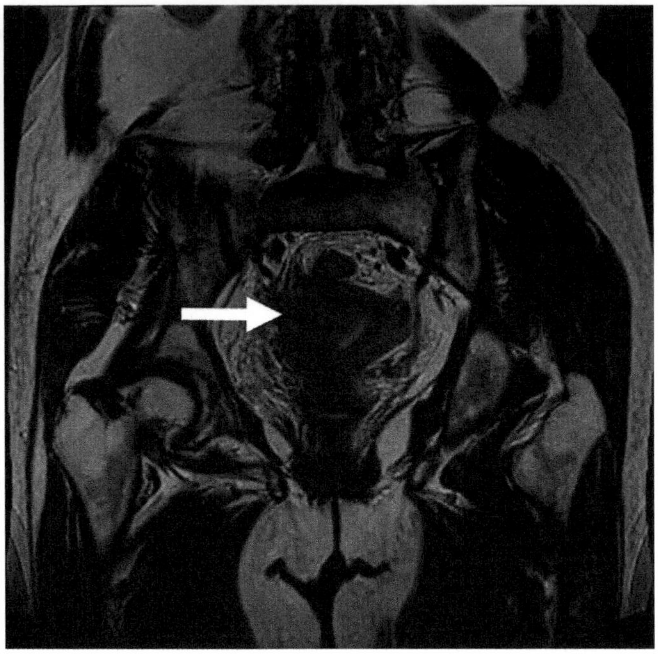

Figs. 42.1 and 42.2 Sagittal pre-contrast fat-suppressed T2WI image: the uterus was inconsistent with menopausal years. The uterus was enlarged, and the myometrium was thickened. The lesion showed slightly high signal intensity on T2WI with ill-defined boundary, and the uterus adhered to surrounding intestinal canal. Coronal pre-contrast T2WI: the muscular layer of right uterine wall was thickened, uterine cavity was compressed, and uterine junctional zone was intact

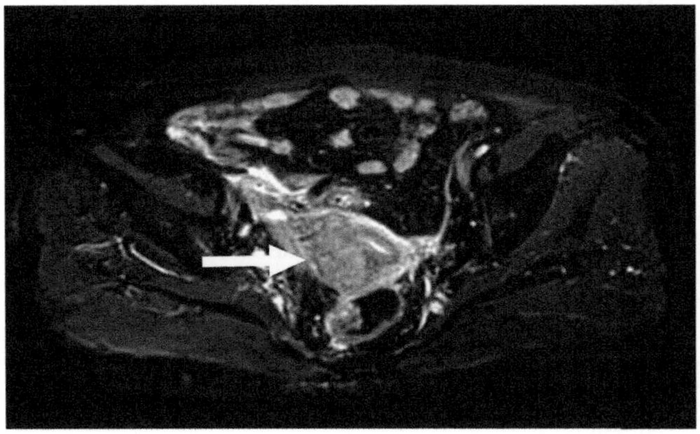

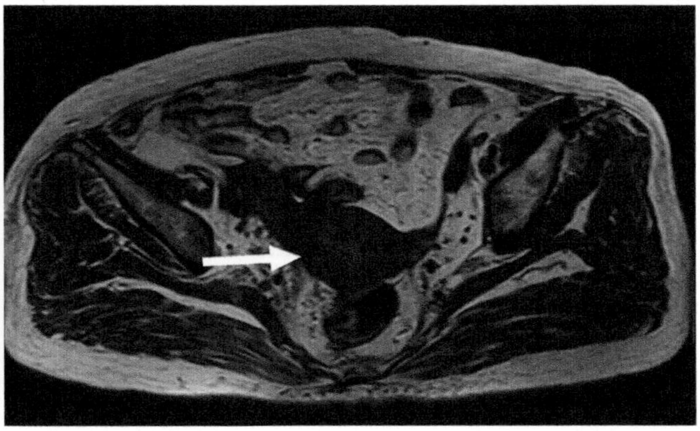

Figs. 42.3 and 42.4 Axial pre-contrast fat-suppressed T2WI image: the lesion was located in the muscular layer of anterior and posterior wall of uterus, with slightly high signal intensity on T2WI and ill-defined boundary. Axial pre-contrast T1WI: the lesion showed iso-signal and slightly high signal intensity

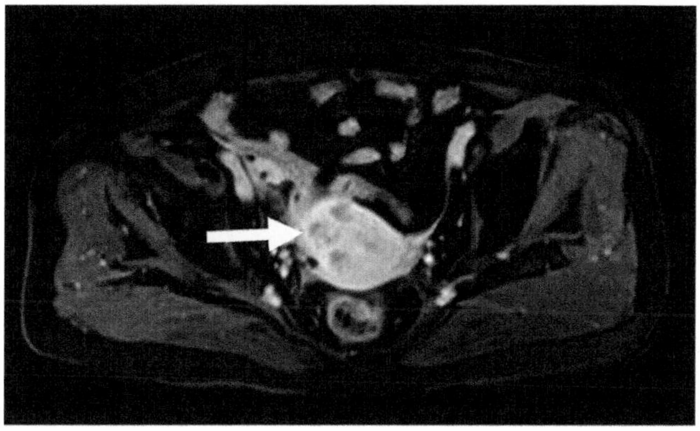

Fig. 42.5 Axial contrast-enhanced T1WI: the lesion showed heterogeneous and significant enhancement, with multiple small patchy foci of mild enhancement

42.3 Differential Diagnosis

Pelvic suppurative inflammation is mainly differentiated from endometriosis, ovarian teratoma, and ovarian cystadenoma. Endometriosis can have abdominal pain, MRI signal intensity is mixed, cystic wall is thick, multiple cysts can be connected, and endometriosis lesions are adhered to surrounding structures. It is difficult to distinguish endometriosis from pelvic abscess. However, endometriosis has hemorrhage signals, and the enhancement degree is less significant, which can be distinguished. Ovarian teratoma mostly has no obvious clinical symptoms such as abdominal pain and mostly contains fat components, and MRI shows reduced signal intensity on fat-suppressed sequences. Ovarian cystadenoma has no clinical manifestations of pelvic inflammatory disease. MRI findings are mostly cystic or solid and cystic masses, with thin cystic wall and clear boundary with surrounding structures, which can be distinguished from pelvic suppurative inflammation [3, 5, 6].

References

1. Curry A, Williams T, Penny ML. Pelvic inflammatory disease: diagnosis, management, and prevention. Am Fam Physician. 2019;100(6):357–64.
2. Chappell CA, Wiesenfeld HC. Pathogenesis, diagnosis, and management of severe pelvic inflammatory disease and tuboovarian abscess. Clin Obstet Gynecol. 2012;55(4):893–903.
3. Kim HY, Yang JI, Moon C. Comparison of severe pelvic inflammatory disease, pyosalpinx and tubo-ovarian abscess. J Obstet Gynaecol Res. 2015;41(5):742–6.
4. Li W, Zhang Y, Cui Y, et al. Pelvic inflammatory disease: evaluation of diagnostic accuracy with conventional MR with added diffusion-weighted imaging. Abdom Imaging. 2013;38(1):193–200.
5. Ueda H, Togashi K, Kataoka ML, et al. Adnexal masses caused by pelvic inflammatory disease: MR appearance. Magn Reson Med Sci. 2002;1(4):207–15.
6. Szklaruk J, Tamm EP, Choi H, et al. MR imaging of common and uncommon large pelvic masses. Radiographics. 2003;23(2):403–24.

43 Pelvic Tuberculosis

Jielin Xie

43.1 Clinical History

Female patient, 20 years old. In December 2020, the patient presented with vague pain in the right lower abdomen for 3 days without obvious inducement and no fever, she underwent no treatment, and self-relieved. In February 2021, she went to a local clinic because of fever and chills. Physical examination showed right lower abdominal tenderness, and anti-inflammatory treatment was given for 3 days. The temperature improved, but there was still lower abdominal tenderness, and she underwent no further treatment. In March 2021, without obvious cause, she developed fever again (38.9 °C) accompanied by persistent lower abdominal and lumbar pain. She was hospitalized in another hospital (details unknown). Hematological examination: CA125: 761.7 U/mL; CA199: 18.47 U/mL; and HCG was normal. Ultrasonography showed bilateral adnexal masses, which adhered to each other and had unclear boundaries with uterus. For further treatment, she was hospitalized in our hospital in May and underwent laparoscopic examination, extensive intestinal adhesion decomposition, pelvic abscess incision and drainage, and peritoneal lesion biopsy. Intraoperative findings: the abdominal and pelvic cavity showed tuberculosis inflammatory miliary changes, normal anatomical structure disappeared, and ovaries and fallopian tubes showed tuberculous inflammatory destructive changes, containing a large amount of caseous tissue.

Postoperative pathological results: connective tissue granulomatous inflammation, considered tuberculous. The patient was recommended to be treated in a specialized hospital.

43.2 Imaging Analysis

Pelvic tuberculosis is the female genital inflammation caused by Mycobacterium tuberculosis, which is common in women of childbearing age and also in postmenopausal elderly women. Pelvic tuberculosis is often a manifestation of systemic tuberculosis, often secondary to tuberculosis elsewhere in the body. The main route of transmission is blood-borne transmission [1].

Clinical manifestations of pelvic tuberculosis are diverse, and some patients may be asymptomatic. Infertility and menstrual disorders are often the main symptoms due to destruction and adhesion of fallopian tube mucosa and endometrium and may be accompanied by lower abdominal pain. If in the active period, there may be general symptoms of tuberculosis, such as fever, night sweating, fatigue, weight loss, etc. [2] MRI manifestations of pelvic tuberculosis mainly include the following: (1) irregular solid and cystic lesions in the pelvic cavity, thick cystic wall, and unclear boundary with surrounding structures (Figs. 43.1 and 43.2). (2) In typical cases, calcification with low signal intensity on both T2WI and T1WI is seen in the solid part of the lesion or in the cystic wall. (3) When tuberculosis affects uterus, endometrial cavity fluid and intrauterine adhesions can be seen. (4) Free fluid can be seen in the pelvic cavity, and greater omentum shows significant cake-like thickening (Fig. 43.3). (5) The cystic wall and solid part of lesions are significantly heterogeneously enhanced after contrast enhancement of solid and cystic lesions in the pelvic cavity (Fig. 43.4). (6) Multiple enlarged lymph nodes can be seen, with ring enhancement after contrast enhancement [3, 4].

J. Xie (✉)
Department of Radiology, Obstetrics and Gynecology Hospital, Fudan University, Shanghai, People's Republic of China

G. Zhang (ed.), *MRI of Gynaecological Diseases*, https://doi.org/10.1007/978-981-99-3644-1_43

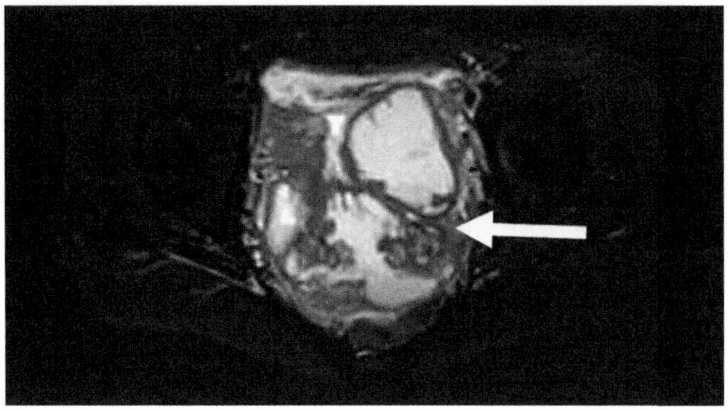

Fig. 43.1 Axial pre-contrast fat-suppressed T2WI image: multiple irregular solid and cystic lesions were found in the pelvic cavity, with thick and uneven cystic walls. The lesions were adhered to each other, and the boundary with surrounding structure was unclear. The cystic fluid showed high signal intensity on T2WI, while the solid part showed slightly high signal intensity on T2WI

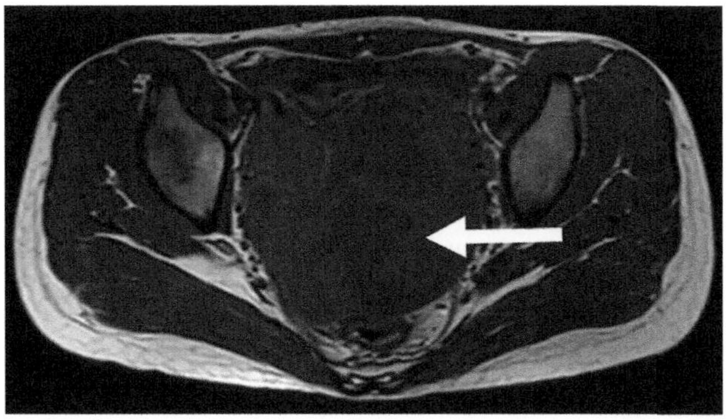

Fig. 43.2 Axial pre-contrast T1WI: the solid part of pelvic lesions showed iso-signal intensity on T1WI, and the cystic fluid showed low signal intensity

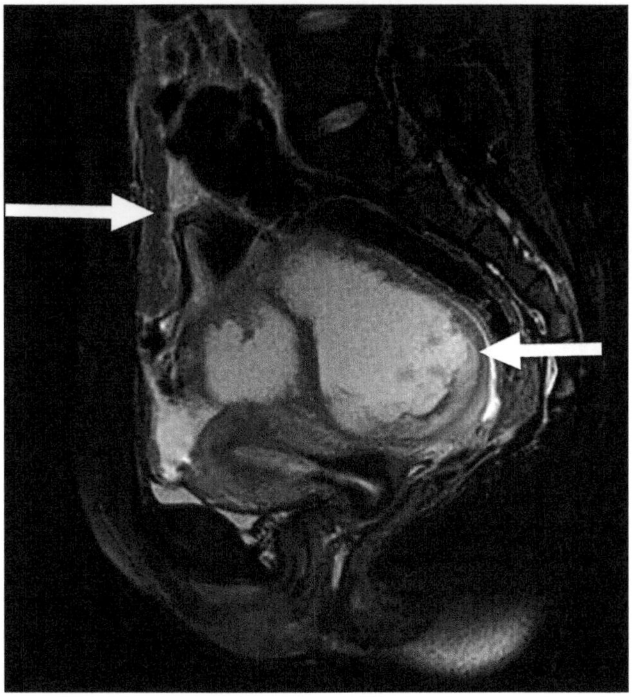

Fig. 43.3 Sagittal pre-contrast fat-suppressed T2WI image: the greater omentum showed significant cake-like thickening, and the boundary between the lesion and uterus was unclear

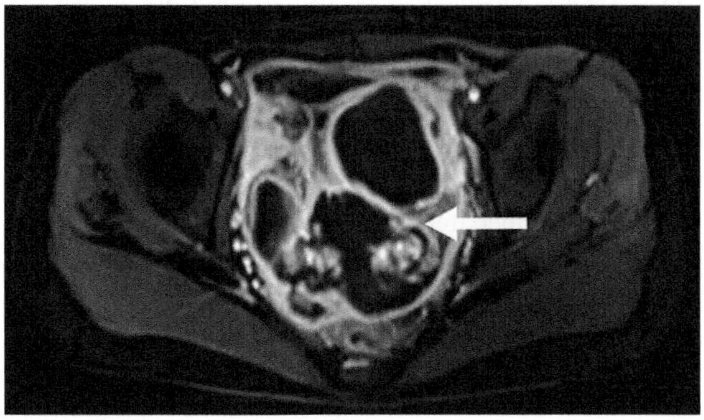

Fig. 43.4 Axial contrast-enhanced T1WI image: the cystic wall and solid part of the lesion were significantly enhanced, and cystic fluid was not enhanced

43.3 Differential Diagnosis

Pelvic tuberculosis is mainly differentiated from ovarian cancer and nonspecific chronic pelvic inflammatory disease. MRI manifestations of pelvic tuberculosis are similar to ovarian cancer, both of which can be characterized by irregular solid and cystic masses with massive ascites. The diagnosis can be differentiated according to the pathogenesis and history of tuberculosis. When the diagnosis is difficult, laparoscopic exploration can be used to confirm the diagnosis. Chronic pelvic inflammatory disease often has a history of abortion or acute pelvic inflammatory disease and generally has large menstrual volume. However, pelvic tuberculosis has menstrual volume reduction, infertility, and other manifestations and can be used to identify when the imaging finding is similar [4, 5].

References

1. Aliyu MH, Aliyu SH, Salihu HM. Female genital tuberculosis: a global review. Int J Fertil Womens Med. 2004;49(3):123–36.
2. Gao LF, Luo X. Reunderstanding of the characteristics of female pelvic and genital tuberculosis. Chinese J Pract Gynecol Obstet. 2008;24(4):261–3.
3. Martingano D, Cagle-Colon K, Chiaffarano J, et al. Pelvic tuberculosis diagnosed during operative laparoscopy for suspected ovarian cancer. Case Rep Obstet Gynecol. 2018;2018:6452721.
4. Abreu N, Serrado MA, Matos R, et al. Pelvic tuberculosis: a forgotten diagnosis—case report. Radiol Case Rep. 2018;13(5):993–8.
5. Sala E, Kataoka MY, Priest AN, et al. Advanced ovarian cancer: multiparametric MR imaging demonstrates response- and metastasis-specific effects. Radiology. 2012;263(1):149–59.

Hydrosalpinx

44

Jielin Xie

44.1 Clinical History

Female patient, 48 years old. The patient complained of an increase in vaginal discharge 1 year ago, which was watery, and she did not seek medical attention. She had menstrual disorders in the past half year and visited a local hospital due to delayed menstruation and underwent ultrasonography, which suggested ovarian cysts. She visited our hospital 1 month later, and ultrasonography showed cystic masses in bilateral adnexa areas. After anti-inflammatory treatment, ultrasound examination showed no significant change. She underwent laparoscopic pelvic adhesiolysis and bilateral salpingectomy. During the operation, bilateral tubal sausage-like thickening and distortion were observed, with dense adhesions to surrounding tissues.

Postoperative pathological results: bilateral hydrosalpinx.

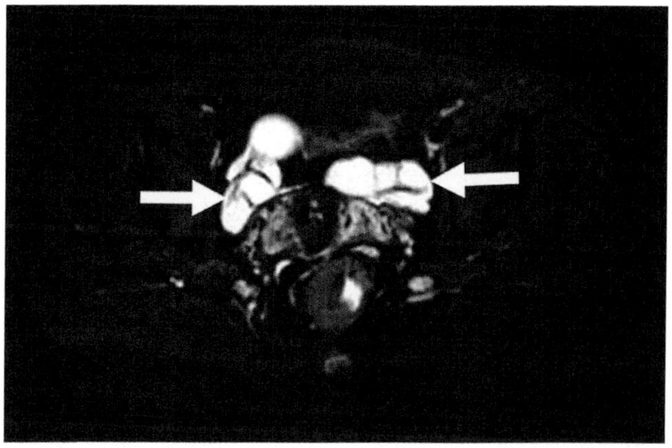

Fig. 44.1 Axial pre-contrast fat-suppressed T2WI image: Tortuous tubular dilated structures were seen in bilateral adnexa areas, with thin wall, and the cystic fluid showed high signal intensity on T2WI

44.2 Imaging Analysis

Hydrosalpinx often occurs in women of childbearing age, mostly bilateral, and is mostly caused by retrograde infection of reproductive tract involving fallopian tubes. Fallopian tubes are slightly or moderately enlarged, fimbria is adherent and atresia, and the effusion accumulates to form hydrosalpinx. The main pathogenic bacteria were *Chlamydia trachomatis* and *Neisseria gonorrhoeae*. Clinically, the systemic symptoms are not obvious, which can be manifested as lower abdominal bulging, leukorrhea increases with watery appearance, and increased menstrual volume, often aggravated after tiredness or sexual intercourse, and are prone to acute or subacute attacks, or accompanied by fatigue, weakness, and low-grade fever, and difficult to be cured completely. It is often discovered accidentally or due to infertility [1]. MRI manifestations of hydrosalpinx mainly include the following: (1) Sausage-like thickening and dilated tubular structure can be seen in bilateral or unilateral adnexa area, with the tip pointing to uterine horn (Fig. 44.1). When the lesion is curled obviously, incomplete septation can be seen, showing multilocular-like changes. (2) The intraluminal fluid mainly shows high signal intensity on T2WI and low signal intensity on T1WI. If protein content of the fluid is high, it shows high signal intensity on both T2WI and T1WI (Fig. 44.2). (3) The wall is thin and uniform, without mural nodules. If accompanied by acute attack, the wall is thickened and edematous,

J. Xie (✉)
Department of Radiology, Obstetrics and Gynecology Hospital, Fudan University, Shanghai, People's Republic of China

G. Zhang (ed.), *MRI of Gynaecological Diseases*, https://doi.org/10.1007/978-981-99-3644-1_44

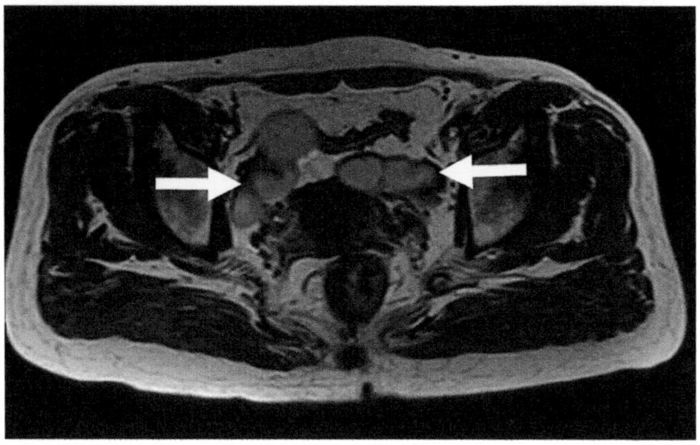

Fig. 44.2 Axial pre-contrast T1WI: The cystic fluid in bilateral adnexal lesions showed high signal intensity on T1WI, which was cystic fluid with high protein content

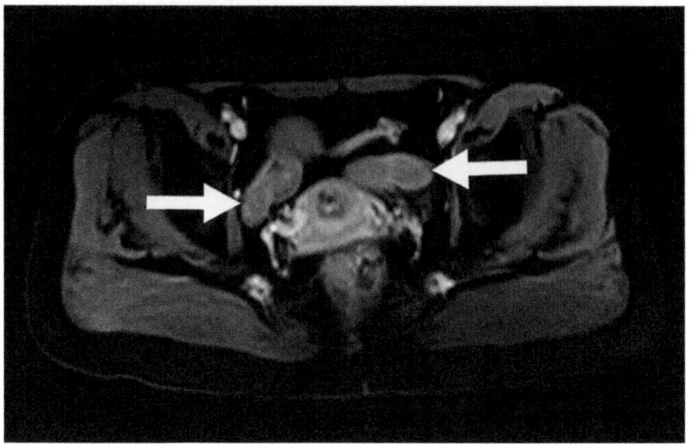

Fig. 44.4 Axial contrast-enhanced T1WI image: The wall of lesions in bilateral adnexa areas was slightly enhanced after contrast enhancement, and no obvious enhancement was observed in the cystic fluid

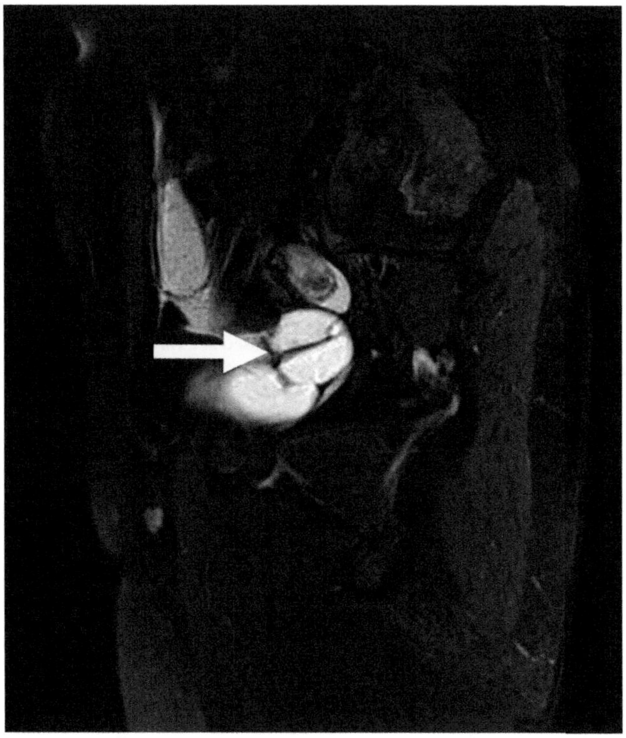

Fig. 44.3 Sagittal pre-contrast fat-suppressed T2WI image: Tortuous tubular dilated structure was seen in the adnexa area, showing high signal intensity on T2WI, with local folding or kinking, and resembling incomplete septation

and the boundary with surrounding structure is unclear (Fig. 44.3). (4) After contrast enhancement, the wall may show mild to moderate enhancement, and there is no enhancement of intraluminal fluid (Fig. 44.4). If there is an acute attack, the degree of enhancement of the wall may increase [2–4].

44.3 Differential Diagnosis

Hydrosalpinx should be differentiated from fallopian tube carcinoma, ovarian cystadenoma, and pelvic encapsulated effusion. Fallopian tube carcinoma can also present as bilateral or unilateral tubal effusion, but the wall thickness is often uneven on MRI, multiple small mural nodules can be seen, and cystic fluid is inhomogeneous. After contrast enhancement, the wall and mural nodules can be significantly enhanced. Severe hydrosalpinx, with significant dilatation of fallopian tube, with local folding or kinking, is easily confused with ovarian multilocular cystadenoma, but the septation of ovarian cystadenoma is generally complete, and the hydrosalpinx septation is incomplete, which is incompletely expanded mucosal folds. Pelvic encapsulated effusion caused by pelvic inflammatory disease is sometimes similar to hydrosalpinx, but the former has no obvious tubular structure, and ovaries can be wrapped around them, accompanied by fluid around [1, 4, 5].

References

1. Mi YK, Sung ER, Soon NO, et al. MR imaging findings of hydrosalpinx: a comprehensive review. Radiographics. 2009;29(2):495–507.
2. Czeyda-Pommersheim F, Kalb B, Costello J, et al. MRI in pelvic inflammatory disease: a pictorial review. Abdom Radiol (NY). 2017;42(3):935–50.
3. Foti PV, Ognibene N, Spadola S, et al. Non-neoplastic diseases of the fallopian tube: MR imaging with emphasis on diffusion-weighted imaging. Insights Imaging. 2016;7(3):311–27.
4. Lin HR, Li YZ, Han JX, et al. MRI diagnosis of fallopian tube hydrosalpinx/pyosalpinx. J Pract Radiol. 2014;30(11):1858–60.
5. Katz SI, Ramchandani P, Torigian DA, et al. Hydrosalpinx in patients with hysterectomy without salpingo-oophorectomy referred for pelvic magnetic resonance imaging. Clin Imaging. 2019;55:95–9.

Part XII

Miscellaneous

45 Cervical Tubular Lobular Hyperplasia

Xuan Yin and Yan Ning

45.1 Clinical History

A 49-year-old female patient complained of vaginal discharge with irregular vaginal bleeding. A test for high-risk strains of human papillomavirus (HPV) was negative. The Pap smear showed a low-grade squamous intraepithelial lesion (ISIL).

MRI: MRI revealed groups of cysts and multilocular cystic lesions in the enlarged uterine cervix, extending from the isthmus to the outside of the cervix, surrounding the cervical canal, and growing in the stroma of the cervix, approximately 40 mm × 50 mm × 45 mm. The larger cysts encircled the smaller cysts in a pattern similar to the "cosmos patterns." Cysts showed low signal intensity on T1WI and hyperintense signal on T2WI (Figs. 45.1 and 45.2). No obvious solid components were clearly identified in the cysts. No restricted diffusion areas were observed on DWI. After contrast enhancement, some cyst walls or septation was moderately enhanced, but no obvious thickening of cyst walls was observed (Figs. 45.3 and 45.4).

Radiologic diagnosis: cervical tubular lobular hyperplasia may be possible; minimal deviation adenocarcinoma or other benign conditions, such as cystic cervicitis or multiple grouped nabothian cysts, could not be excluded.

The patient underwent laparoscopic hysterectomy and bilateral salpingectomy. The ovaries were preserved.

Postoperative pathology: benign cervical glands around the larger glands of the lobules hyperplasia. It appeared to be the multilobular pattern (Figs. 45.5 and 45.6). The glands were lined by mucinous epithelium and were immunopositive for HIK1083 and MUC6. There was no obvious cellular atypia. No interstitial connective tissue hyperplasia was observed. The lesion was confined to the internal wall of the cervix. The final pathological diagnosis was lobular endocervical glandular hyperplasia (LEGH). Ten months postoperatively, the patient remained asymptomatic and showed no signs of disease recurrence.

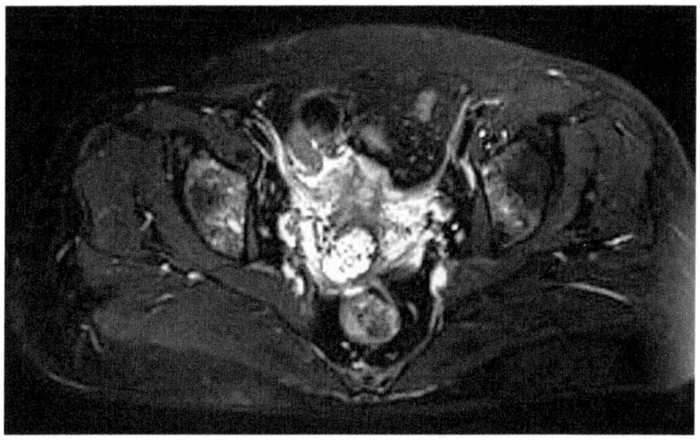

Fig. 45.1 Axial T2-weighted image. This image demonstrated enlarged, well-defined, high-signal intensity multilocular cystic lesions within the stroma of the cervix. A large number of small cysts were partially surrounded by many larger cysts that resemble the "cosmos pattern" described in LEGH

X. Yin (✉)
Department of Radiology, Obstetrics and Gynecology Hospital, Fudan University, Shanghai, People's Republic of China

Y. Ning
Department of Pathology, Obstetrics and Gynecology Hospital, Fudan University, Shanghai, People's Republic of China

G. Zhang (ed.), *MRI of Gynaecological Diseases*, https://doi.org/10.1007/978-981-99-3644-1_45

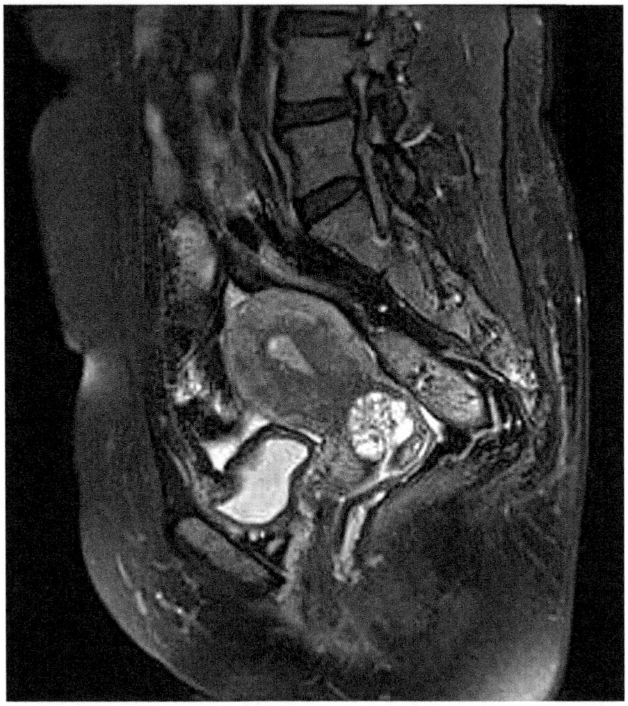

Fig. 45.2 Sagittal T2-weighted image. This image demonstrated enlarged, well-defined, high-signal intensity multilocular cystic lesions within the stroma of the cervix. A large number of small cysts were partially surrounded by many larger cysts that resemble the "cosmos pattern" described in LEGH

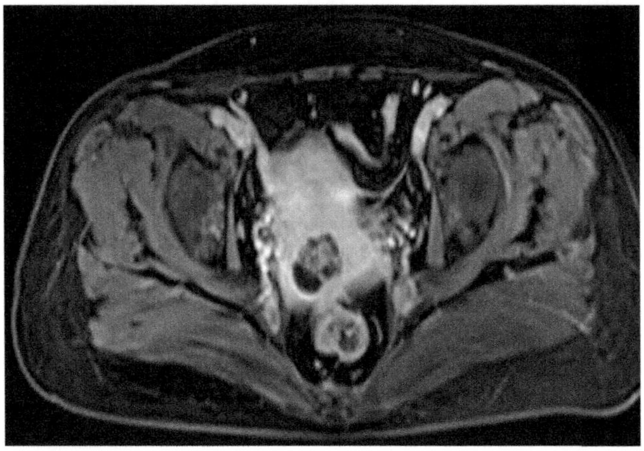

Fig. 45.3 Axial contrast-enhanced fat-suppressed T1-weighted image. In this image, part of the cyst wall or septation was slightly thickened and irregularly enhanced, with no obvious solid component enhancement

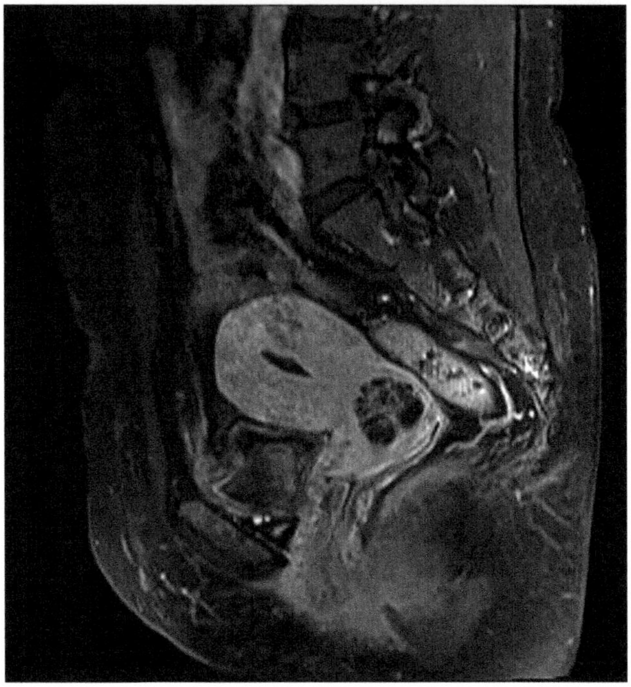

Fig. 45.4 Sagittal contrast-enhanced fat-suppressed T1-weighted image. In this image, part of the cyst wall or septation was slightly thickened and irregularly enhanced, with no obvious solid component enhancement

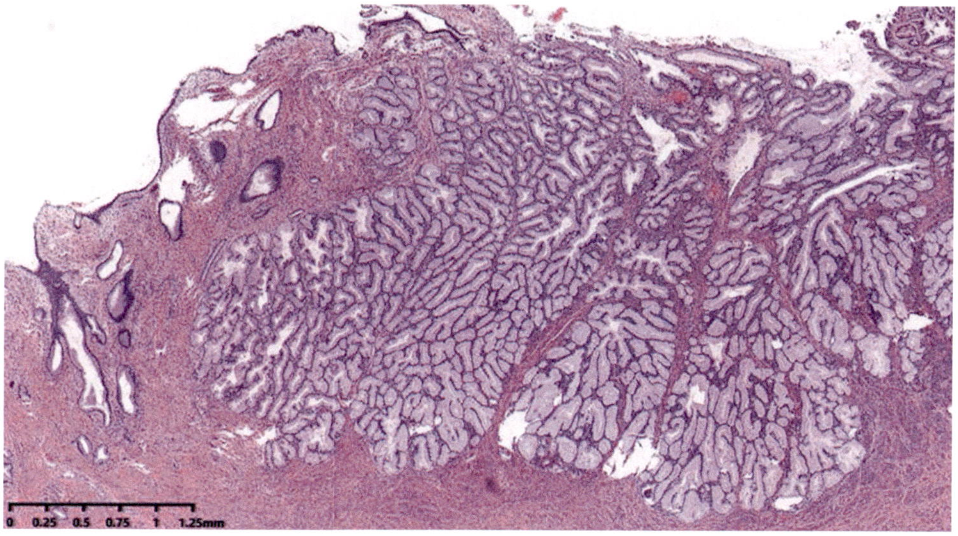

Fig. 45.5 Low-power view of LEGH, showing clusters of small glands surrounding dilated ducts (HE ×25)

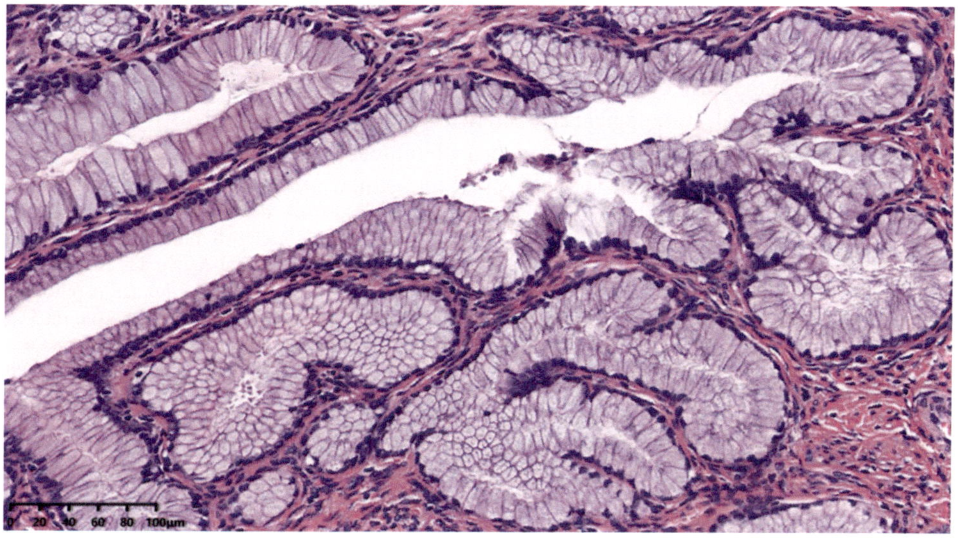

Fig. 45.6 High-power view of LEGH showing bland nuclear morphology of small glands arranged in a lobular manner. Endocervical glands are lined by columnar cells with abundant pale eosinophilic cytoplasm (HE ×200)

45.2 Imaging Analysis

Lobular endocervical glandular hyperplasia (LEGH), also known as cervical hendometrial glandular hyperplasia, is a rare benign lesion characterized by differentiation of cervical glands to gastric mucus glands, whose pathogenesis remains unclear. At present, it is believed that the cervical gland cells are differentiated into gastrointestinal types, which may be related to chronic inflammation. Nucci et al. [1] first proposed the concept of cervical endometrial glandular hyperplasia as a benign lesion. Later researchers classified LEGH into endometrial neoplasia and atypical endometrial neoplasia (ALEGH) and believed that ALEGH was a precursor to minimal deviation/gastric type cervical adenocarcinoma (MDA). In 2014, WHO officially classified it as a benign glandular tumor of the cervix and tumor-like lesions. Such lesions lack specific clinical manifestations and gynecological examination signs, and the positive rate of routine cervical cytology screening is low. The pathological changes are similar to those of cervical and gastric adenocarcinoma, so clinical misdiagnosis and missed diagnosis are often common.

LEGH is a relatively rare benign lobular proliferation of endocervical glands. At present, most studies are small samples or case reports. Matsubara et al. [2] found that the onset of LEGH was related to mutations of GNAS, KRAS, STK11, and other genes, suggesting that LEGH may have the potential to transform into tumors. Hashi et al. [3] tested the expression of HPV-DNA and p16INK4a in LEGH, and the results showed that HPV was negative, suggesting that the onset of LEGH was not related to HPV infection. The positive rate of p16INK4a was 87.5%, suggesting that LEGH was related to cervical malignant tumors. LEGH's glands contain pyloric mucin, which is yellow on a conventional Pap smear and is identified by the HIK1083 labeled latex agglutination test (HIK1083 latex test) on cervical secretions.

LEGH usually occurs in premenopausal women; the age of onset ranges from 37 to 71 years [1]. Its clinical manifestations lack specificity; it may be associated with watery or mucoid vaginal discharge. A few patients presented with cervical mass and irregular vaginal bleeding. Some patients had no obvious clinical symptoms and were found accidentally after total hysterectomy or conization of the cervix. LEGH may be associated with Peutz-Jeghers syndrome (PJS) or ovarian mucinous cystadenoma. These results suggest that LEGH may be a component of mucinous metaplasia and neoplasm occurring simultaneously in the female reproductive tract.

LEGH is usually found incidentally on pathological examination or in the form of a mass or cyst, mostly located in the cervical intraoral. Pathological characteristics are usually centered on a large gastric or pyloric gland differentiated glandular tube, clustered into clusters, and small to medium size glands to form a clear lobulated shape (similar to the nut with fibrous roots hanging fruit, and the central duct as the stem). The lesion is cystic and confined to the superficial 1/2 of the cervix [4].

On MRI, the lesion of LEGH is usually located at the upper part of the cervical canal, presenting multiple cystic lesions. T1WI images show low signal, and T2WI images show multiple small cysts with high signal. Dynamic contrast-enhanced MRI images show reticular enhancement, reflecting the extensive glandular structure of the tumor. It can be divided into two types. "Floral" lesions consist of numerous small cysts surrounded by many large cysts. Takatsu [5] refers to this type as a "cosmos pattern." "Raspberry" lesions are dense clusters of tiny cysts with occasional small cysts [6].

45.3 Differential Diagnosis

Although LEGH is classified as a benign lesion of the cervix, it is often associated with adenocarcinoma in situ or invasive adenocarcinoma of the cervix. The primary differential diagnosis of LEGH is minimal deviation adenocarcinoma (MDA). Adenocarcinoma should be considered when the cyst wall has irregular thickening enhancement. Once LEGH is detected, continuous follow-up is needed to detect early adenocarcinoma.

In summary, LEGH may resemble some cervical malignancies and in some cases may be considered a premalignant lesion. Surgical treatment is the best option to avoid misdiagnosis and malignancy as the disease progresses, but in some cases close follow-up is possible.

References

1. Nucci MR, Clement PB, Young RH. Lobular endocervical glandular hyperplasia, not otherwise specified: a clinicopathologic analysis of thirteen cases of a distinctive pseudo neoplastic lesion and comparison with fourteen cases of adenoma malignum. Am J Surg Pathol. 1999;23(8):886–91.
2. Matsubara A, Sekine S, Ogawa R, et al. Lobular endocervical glandular hyperplasia is a neoplastic entity with frequent activating GNAS mutations. Am J Surg Pathol. 2014;38(3):370–6.
3. Hashi A, Xu JY, Kondo T, et al. p16INK4a overexpression independent of human papillomavirus infection in lobular endocervical glandular hyperplasia. Int J Gynecol Pathol. 2006;25(2):187–94.
4. Nara M, Hashi A, Murata S, Kondo T, Yuminamochi T, Nakazawa K, et al. Lobular endocervical glandular hyperplasia as a presumed precursor of cervical adenocarcinoma independent of human papilloma virus infection. Gynecol Oncol. 2007;106:289–98.
5. Takatsu A, Shiozawa T, Miyamoto T, Kurosawa K, Kashima H, Yamada T, et al. Preoperative differential diagnosis of minimal deviation adenocarcinoma and lobular endocervical glandular hyperplasia of the uterine cervix: a multicenter study of clinicopathology and magnetic resonance imaging findings. Int J Gynecol Cancer. 2011;21:1287–96.
6. Omori M, et al. Utility of imaging modalities for predicting carcinogenesis in lobular endocervical glandular hyperplasia, vol. 14; 2019. p. e0221088.

Rectosigmoid Endometriosis

46

Shouxin Gu and Yan Ning

46.1 Clinical History

In a 28-year-old female patient who had dysmenorrhea for 5 years, a pelvic mass was found 2 years ago, and hematochezia during menstruation was found one year ago. The patient underwent colonoscopy; during the examination, the colonoscopy was blocked and failed when the sigmoid colon was reached. The patient underwent left ovarian endometrioid cyst dissection and decomposition of intestinal adhesion.

Intraoperative findings: The tight adhesion between sigmoid colon and the posterior wall of the uterus was confirmed during laparoscopy (Fig. 46.1). It was confirmed that the sigmoid colon was rigid and adhered to the posterior wall of the uterus.

MRI examination: The sigmoid colon is in close proximity to the posterior wall of the uterus and an intraluminal submucosal mass in the sigmoid colon with low signal intensity on T2WI causing folding of the sigmoid colon (Figs. 46.2 and 46.3). Three-dimensional multiplanar reconstruction sequence can show the lesion from multiple angles, and the details of the lesion can be displayed more clearly (Fig. 46.4).

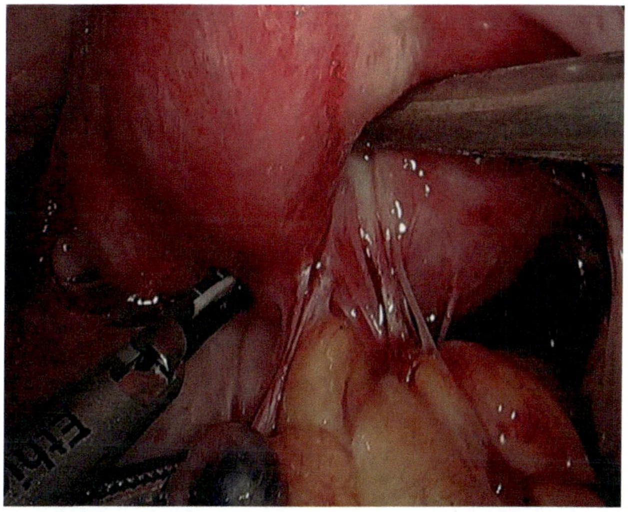

Fig. 46.1 The tight adhesion between sigmoid colon and the posterior wall of the uterus was confirmed during laparoscopy

Deep infiltrating lesion swelling into the lumen led to the narrowing of sigmoid colon involved, which was also the cause of the failure of colonoscopy.

S. Gu (✉)
Department of Radiology, Obstetrics and Gynecology Hospital, Fudan University, Shanghai, People's Republic of China

Y. Ning
Department of Pathology, Obstetrics and Gynecology Hospital, Fudan University, Shanghai, People's Republic of China

G. Zhang (ed.), *MRI of Gynaecological Diseases*, https://doi.org/10.1007/978-981-99-3644-1_46

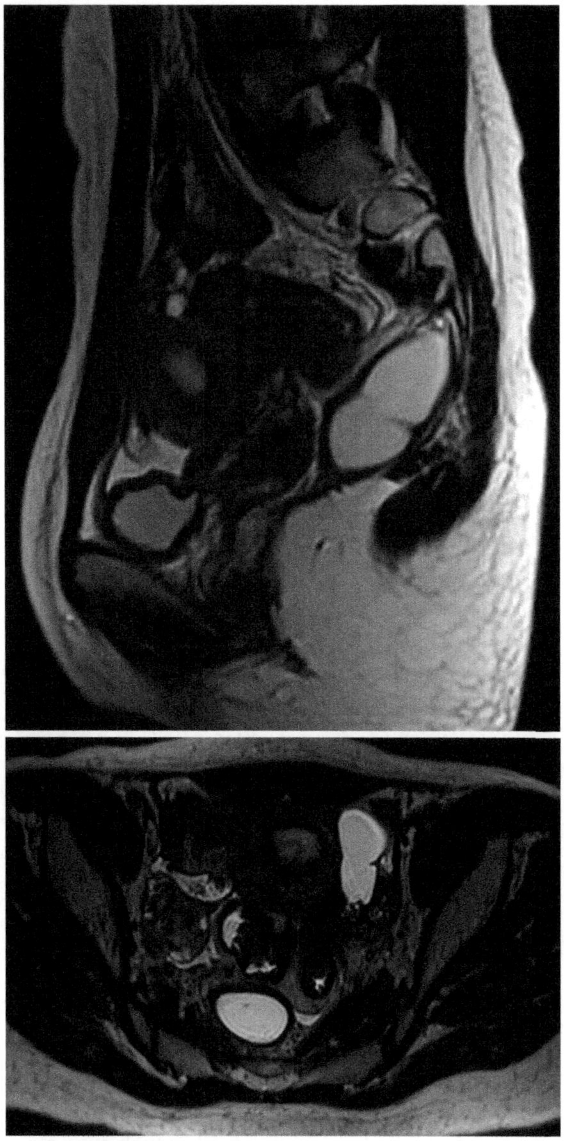

Figs. 46.2 and 46.3 Sagittal T2WI shows a close relationship between sigmoid colon and the posterior wall of the uterus with an intraluminal sigmoid mass with low signal intensity on T2WI. The 3D-space sequence, which can be reconstructed in multiple planes, shows the pelvic cavity in clearer detail

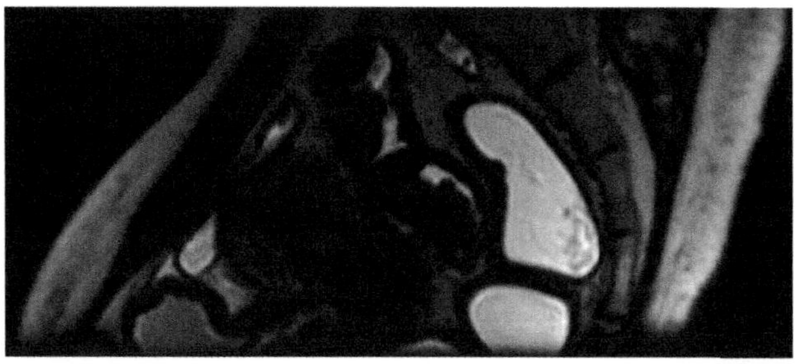

Fig. 46.4 Sagittal T2WI based on high resolution images (the 3D-space sequence) better showed the lesion details

46.2 Imaging Analysis

Intestinal tract is a common site of pelvic extragenital endometriosis, which is found in up to 37% of patients with deep endometriosis, among which rectum and sigmoid colon are the most vulnerable sites, due to proximity to the uterus [1, 2]. Rectum and rectosigmoid junction are the preferential localizations of bowel endometriotic sites, the latter being the most common site of extragenital endometriosis and one of the most severe forms of deep infiltrating endometriosis (DIE). Hypointense signal of the anterior wall of rectosigmoid involved by endometriosis on T2-weighted images disappeared, and a soft mass forming an obtuse angle with the wall of the rectosigmoid, extending to the anterior wall of rectum and the inferior wall of sigmoid colon, was manifested [3].

Imaging has been shown to be accurate in diagnosing this subtype of endometriosis, among which MRI has been well studied for the assessment of rectosigmoid endometriosis and shown consistent accuracy in detection of lesions in the rectum and rectosigmoid [2]. Typical imaging features of MRI showed homogeneous low signal nodules on T2WI images, and cystic lesions were rare [1]. A recent Cochrane systematic evaluation showed that MRI had a sensitivity of 0.92 (95% CI: 0.86–0.99) and a specificity of 0.96 (95% CI: 0.93–0.98) for detecting rectosigmoid endometriosis [4].

46.3 Differential Diagnosis

Bowel endometriosis should be differentiated with colonic malignancy or malignant implant metastasis. As with "mushroom cap" sign, which is an important and specific imaging feature on T2WI image representing deep rectosigmoid endometriosis with submucosal infiltration, the dark submucosal nodule on T2WI is characteristic of fibromuscular proliferation from deep endometriosis. However, primary colon malignancy or peritoneal carcinomatosis demonstrates intermediate signal on T2WI. In patients with endometriosis, or history of previous surgery for endometriosis, the shape of the colonic lesion causing folding of the sigmoid colon with a T2WI hypointense core on MRI helps in diagnosing deep colonic endometriosis and avoiding the misdiagnosis between them [5, 6] (Figs. 46.5 and 46.6).

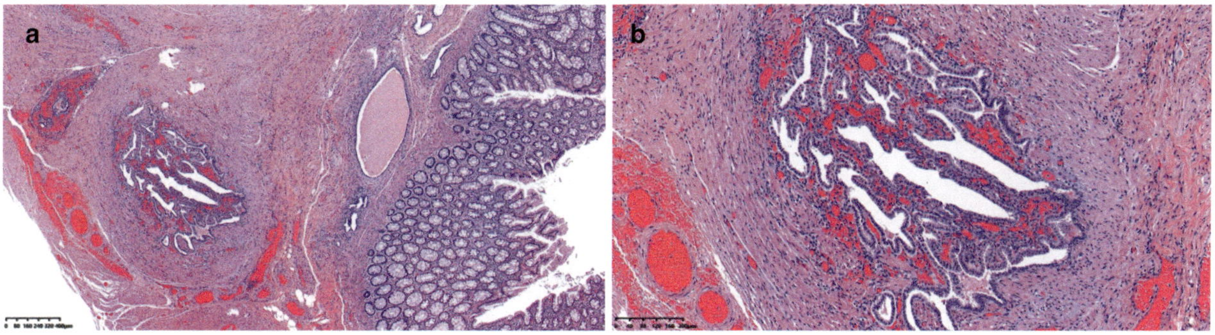

Figs. 46.5 and 46.6 (**a**) Endometriosis involving the sigmoid colon. endometrial glandular and stromal elements within the muscular layer and an intact colonic mucosa (HE × 40). (**b**) A higher magnification of endometriosis revealing endometrial glands surrounded by a hemorrhagic stroma within fibromuscular tissue. (HE ×100)

References

1. Jha P, Sakala M, Chamie LP, et al. Endometriosis MRI lexicon: consensus statement from the society of abdominal radiology endometriosis disease-focused panel. Abdom Radiol (NY). 2020;45(4):1552.
2. Jaramillo-Cardoso A, Shenoy-Bhangle AS, VanBuren WM, Schiappacasse G, Menias CO, Mortele KJ. Imaging of gastrointestinal endometriosis: what the radiologist should know. Abdom Radiol (NY). 2020;45(6):1694–710. https://doi.org/10.1007/s00261-020-02459-w. PMID: 32236651.
3. Netter A, D'Avout-Fourdinier P, Agostini A, et al. Progression of deep infiltrating rectosigmoid endometriotic nodules. Hum Reprod. 2019;34(11):2144–52.
4. Bazot M, Kermarrec E, Bendifallah S, et al. MRI of intestinal endometriosis. Best Pract Res Clin Obstet Gynaecol. 2021;71:51–63.
5. Varela C, Zulfiqar M, Schiappacasse G, et al. 'Fortune cookie sign': a variant of mushroom cap sign on T2 weighted MRI for deep sigmoid endometriosis. Abdom Radiol (NY). 2020;46:1272.
6. Robinson KA, Menias CO, Chen L, Schiappacasse G, Shaaban AM, Caserta MP, Elsayes KM, VanBuren WM, Bolan CW. Understanding malignant transformation of endometriosis: imaging features with pathologic correlation. Abdom Radiol (NY). 2020;45(6):1762–75. https://doi.org/10.1007/s00261-019-01914-7. PMID: 30941451.

47 Cesarean Scar Pregnancy

Jia Liu

47.1 Clinical History

A 35-year-old female patient presented to the outpatient department with a small amount of vaginal bleeding after more than one month of menopause. She had a history of cesarean section. The patient had regular menstruation with moderate amount and no dysmenorrhea and the presence of mild vaginal bleeding with positive result of a pregnancy test. Ultrasonography had shown cystic structure at the cesarean section incision, with a size of 6 mm × 5 mm × 3 mm, and abundant color blood flow around.

Histopathological results: Decidua tissue and villi could be seen in uterine cavity.

47.2 Imaging Analysis

In recent years, owing to the increased cesarean delivery rate, the incidence of cesarean scar pregnancy (CSP) has risen significantly. The clinical manifestations of CSP are nonspecific. Asymptomatic abdominal discomfort and vaginal bleeding are the most common manifestations. With the prolongation of pregnancy, it may lead to life-threatening complications, such as uterine rupture, massive bleeding, etc. Therefore, early diagnosis and prompt treatment are crucial for patients with CSP. Ultrasonography is the most common diagnostic modality for CSP. MRI, with its excellent soft tissue resolution, non-ionizing radiation, and multiplane imaging, can be an effective complementary method for ultrasound examination of suspected CSP. MRI images of incisional pregnancy can show the signal characteristics of cesarean incision diverticulum, gestational sac, and decidua, respectively [1].

The main clinical manifestations of CSP are menopause and elevated serum β-hCG concentration in women of childbearing age. The imaging diagnosis was based on the presence of a gestational sac in the lower anterior uterine wall (Figs. 47.1 and 47.2) and the loss of normal myometrium between the gestational sac and bladder. As pregnancy progresses, there are three types of gestational sac (GS): (1) cystic gestational sac: There was no visible contents in the sac. MRI showed low signal on T1WI and high signal on T2WI; (2) embryo sac: The gestational sac had a small and regular content, such as a yolk sac or embryo, with homogeneously significant enhancement after contrast enhancement on MRI; (3) hybrid sac: GS contained a large, irregular hybrid mass with a heterogeneously intense signal with inhomogeneous enhancement. This may be due to bleeding or medical treatment in early pregnancy. The diverticulum of the cesarean scar was seen between the gestational sac and bladder. The diverticulum wall showed relatively low signal on T2WI. The cesarean scar diverticulum may be cystic or fissure shaped, with similar signal intensity compared to the myometrium of uterus. Besides, decidua tissue can be seen between the diverticulum and the gestational sac (Fig. 47.3). The intensity of T2WI signal was between the gestational sac and the diverticulum with homogeneous enhancement on MRI. K.-W. Peng et al. [2] suggested that the detection of decidua signals may be the basis for the diagnosis of placental implantation.

J. Liu (✉)
Department of Radiology, Obstetrics and Gynecology Hospital, Fudan University, Shanghai, People's Republic of China

G. Zhang (ed.), *MRI of Gynaecological Diseases*, https://doi.org/10.1007/978-981-99-3644-1_47

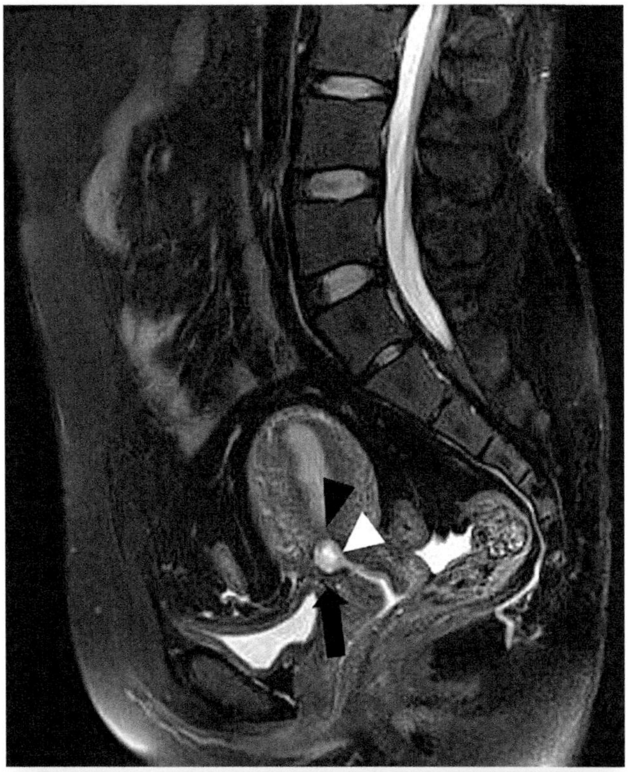

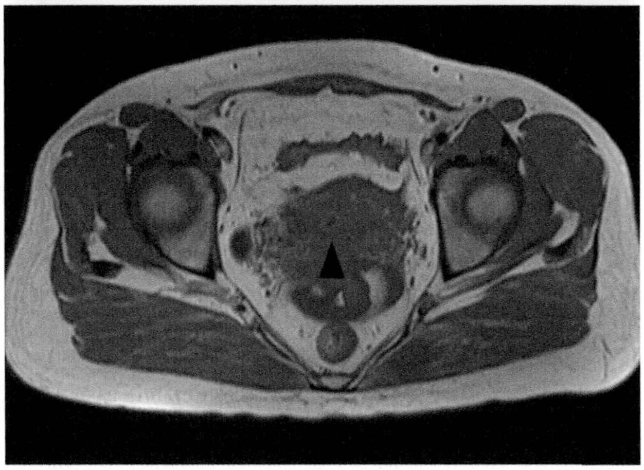

Figs. 47.1 and 47.2 The gestational sac in the lower part of the uterus displays iso- and high signal intensity on T1-weighted and T2-weighted sagittal imaging (black arrowhead), respectively, surrounded by moderate high signal intensity. The cesarean incision diverticulum wall between the gestational sac and the bladder was seen, presenting with hypo-signal intensity on T2WI (black arrow). The decidua of moderate high signal intensity was seen between the diverticulum and the gestational sac (white arrowhead)

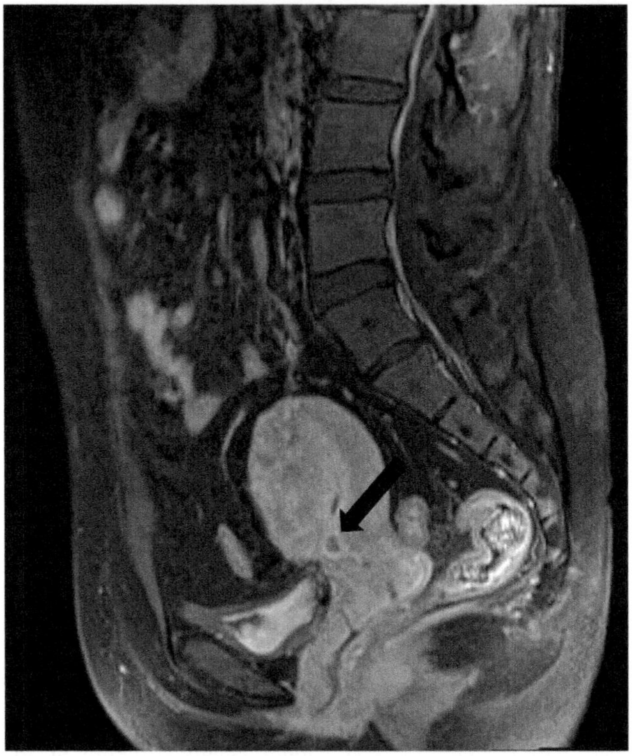

Fig. 47.3 After contrast enhancement, the cesarean incision diverticulum wall and decidua showed hyperintense signal on sagittal T1WI, while gestational sac showed a relatively low signal intensity (long black arrow)

47.3 Differential Diagnosis

CSP needs to be differentiated from leiomyoma of uterine isthmus and gestational trophoblastic disease. Leiomyoma of uterine isthmus showed uniform low signal on T2WI with clear boundary; homogeneous enhancement with the signal after contrast enhancement was similar to that of the myometrium. Gestational trophoblastic disease is an ill-defined mass that invades uterine structures. The lesion showed "insect erosion" changes, and the blood supply was abundant after contrast enhancement. The diagnosis of CSP can be made based on menopause, elevated blood β-hCG, and a history of cesarean section, combined with ultrasonography and/or MRI findings.

References

1. Huang Q, Zhang M, Zhai R-Y. The use of contrast-enhanced magnetic resonance imaging to diagnose cesarean scar pregnancies. Int J Gynecol Obstet. 2014;127:144–6.
2. Peng K-W, Lei Z, Xiao T-H, et al. First trimester caesarean scar ectopic pregnancy evaluation using MRI. Clin Radiol. 2014;69:123–9.

48 Angular Pregnancy

Jia Liu and Yan Ning

48.1 Clinical History

A 31-year-old female patient who had 50 days of menopause with vaginal bleeding for more than half a month. The patient has regular menstruation accompanied by mild dysmenorrhea. The last menstruation was on April 2. The presence of mild vaginal bleeding with positive result of a pregnancy test on April 23 was found. An elevated β-hCG level of 6731 mIU/mL was shown after two times curettage. Ultrasonography had shown a medium low echo at left horn of the uterus with a size of 19 mm × 15 mm × 13 mm.

Histopathological results: left angular pregnancy (Figs. 48.1 and 48.2).

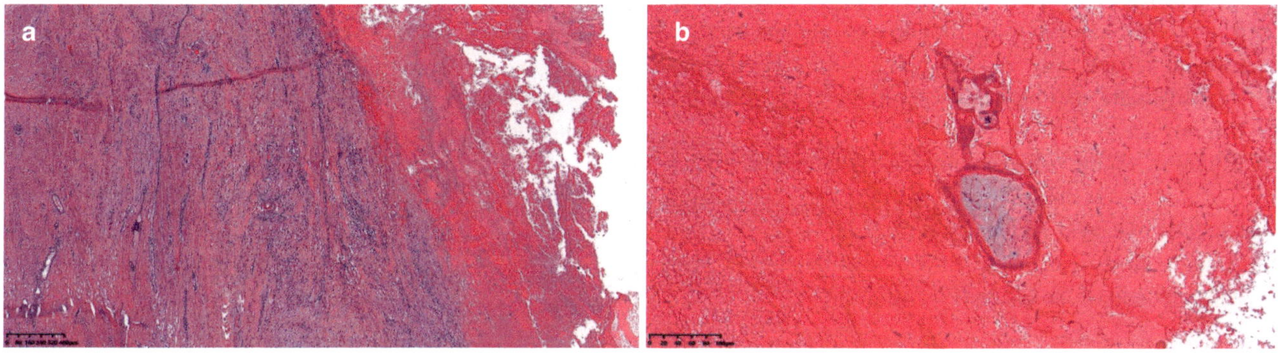

Figs. 48.1 and 48.2 Uterine cornual pregnancy. (**a**) Low-power view of cornual pregnancy showing large hemorrhage region (HE ×40). (**b**) High-power view of cornual pregnancy showing chorionic villi ghost in hemorrhage region (right, HE ×200)

J. Liu (✉)
Department of Radiology, Obstetrics and Gynecology Hospital, Fudan University, Shanghai, People's Republic of China

Y. Ning
Department of Pathology, Obstetrics and Gynecology Hospital, Fudan University, Shanghai, People's Republic of China

G. Zhang (ed.), *MRI of Gynaecological Diseases*, https://doi.org/10.1007/978-981-99-3644-1_48

48.2 Imaging Analysis

The incidence of angular pregnancy is about 2–4.7% of ectopic pregnancies [1]. This type of pregnancy is associated with high rates of spontaneous abortion, uterine rupture, and placenta accrete. An accurate diagnosis and timely treatment are very important to these patients. In women of reproductive age, menopause, elevated blood β-hCG, and absence of gestational sac in the uterus are important diagnostic criteria for ectopic pregnancy.

MR imaging can provide images with high soft tissue contrast in multiple plane without ionizing radiation or the use of intravenous contrast agents. In the setting of suspected ectopic pregnancy, MRI is an effective supplementary examination method for ultrasonography. T2WI sequences can clearly show the high-signal endometrium and the relatively low-signal muscular layer of the uterus, while T1WI sequences are helpful for the detection of hemorrhage. The main MRI findings of angular pregnancy are as follows [2]:

1. The circular gestational sac is located in the angular region with a heterogeneously intense signal. The size of it varies with pregnancy.
2. The gestational sac is surrounded by endometrium of high signal intensity on T2WI (Fig. 48.3). High signal intensity in the uterine wall itself can represent intramural hemorrhage.
3. Thinning of the adjacent myometrium and/or unclear boundary between the lesion and the local myometrium suggests placental implantation (Fig. 48.4).
4. Axial contrast-enhanced T1W imaging showed ring enhancement of the lesion (Fig. 48.5).

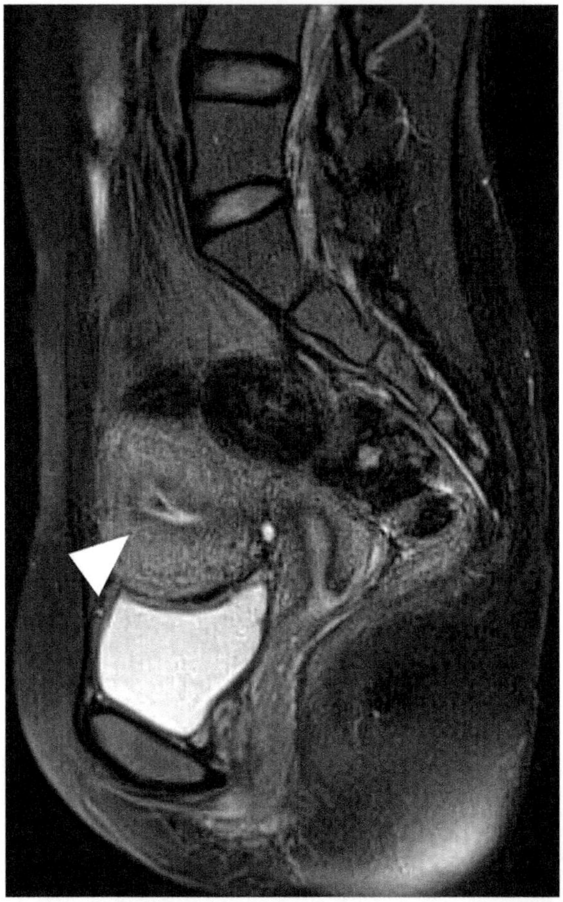

Fig. 48.3 Axial and sagittal fat suppressed T2WI showed a gestational sac with isointensity surrounded by uterine myometrium of hyperintensity (white arrowhead). Thinning of the adjacent myometrium was observed, and the boundary between local myometrium and lesion was unclear

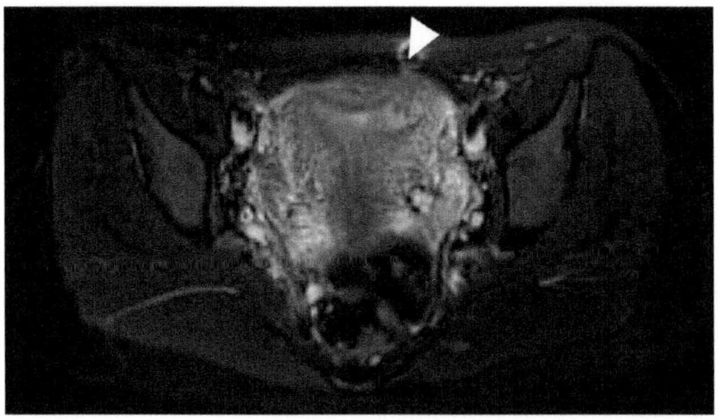

Fig. 48.4 Axial fat suppressed T2WI showed a gestational sac at the left corna

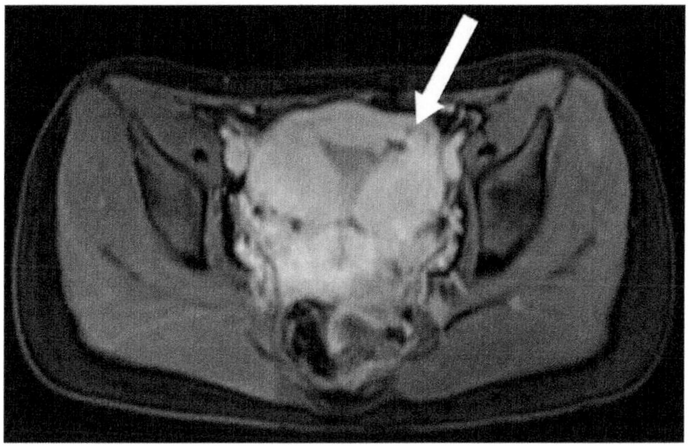

Fig. 48.5 Axial contrast-enhanced T1W imaging showed ring enhancement of the lesion (white arrow)

48.3 Differential Diagnosis

Angular pregnancy mainly needs to be differentiated from interstitial pregnancy, uterine horn gestational trophoblastic disease, and uterine fibroids [3]. Interstitial pregnancy is frequently confused with angular pregnancy. Interstitial pregnancy refers to implantation in the most proximal segment of the fallopian tube, while angular pregnancy is defined as implantation in one of the lateral angles of the uterus. The gestational sac will not develop toward uterine cavity. The differential diagnosis is important for angular pregnancy can sometimes be carried to term. On MRI, interstitial pregnancy shows heterogeneous mass with high T2 signal intensity located lateral to the uterine horn. On T2WI, the lesion is mainly surrounded by the myometrium with relatively low signal, and/or there is an intact zone of low signal between the lesion and the endometrium. When the gestational sac is larger, the junctional zone may move towards the uterine cavity. Distinction between them can sometimes be difficult, when an angular pregnancy is fully implanted into the myometrium. Gestational trophoblastic disease is characterized by multiple, ill-defined mass of invasive growth that destroys uterine structures. The presence of flow-void often can be seen in the lesion, showing "insect erosion" change, with abundant blood supply after contrast enhancement. Most uterine fibroids have clear boundaries and relatively low signal on T2WI. The signal intensity of myometrium is similar to that of myometrium after contrast enhancement. The diagnosis can be made based on whether the patient has menopause and elevated blood β-hCG.

References

1. Elizabeth KA, Ersilia MD. Cornual, interstitial, and angular pregnancies: clarifying the terms and a review of the literature. Clin Imaging. 2014;38(6):763–70.
2. Parker RA III, Yano M, Tai AW, et al. MR imaging findings of ectopic pregnancy: a pictorial review. Radiographics. 2012;32:1445–60.
3. Finlinson AR, Bollig KJ, Schust DJ, et al. Differentiating pregnancies near the uterotubal junction (angular, cornual, and interstitial): a review and recommendations. Fertil Res Pract. 2020;6(8):1–8.

Pelvic Floor Dysfunction

49

Jia Liu

Pelvic floor dysfunction (PFD) is a general term for a variety of clinical disorders, including urinary incontinence (UI), pelvic organ prolapsed (POP) (Fig. 49.1), fecal dysfunction, lower urinary tract sensory and emptying abnormalities, sexual dysfunction, and some chronic pelvic pain syndromes. More than 15% of multiparous women are affected by the disease. The risk factors for PFD include vaginal delivery, multiparity, hysterectomy, advanced age, and chronic obstructive pulmonary disease, among which vaginal delivery and advanced age are the most correlated risk factors [1]. With increasing life expectancy, the negative effect of PFD on the health care system in terms of cost, productivity, and quality of life is critical. The clinical evaluation of PFD is mainly performed by using the POP quantification system, which demonstrated low sensitivity and specificity for the diagnosis of complex alterations [2]. The accuracy of clinical diagnosis directly affects the formulation of surgical plan, which is also one of the important reasons for associated surgical failure and high recurrence rates. Traditional techniques for PFD include assessment of the bladder and levator ani muscle (Fig. 49.2) by transvaginal ultrasonography (US), urodynamic test, and vesicovaginal defecography. During the past decade, three-dimensional (3D) and four-dimensional (4D) translabial ultrasonography and magnetic resonance imaging (MRI) have been used to accurately assess pelvic floor anatomy and function, enabling evaluation of all three pelvic compartments simultaneously. MRI has excellent soft tissue and time resolution and can evaluate the organs, muscles, and ligaments in the pelvic cavity in multiplanar without ionizing radiation.

J. Liu (✉)
Department of Radiology, Obstetrics and Gynecology Hospital, Fudan University, Shanghai, People's Republic of China

G. Zhang (ed.), *MRI of Gynaecological Diseases*, https://doi.org/10.1007/978-981-99-3644-1_49

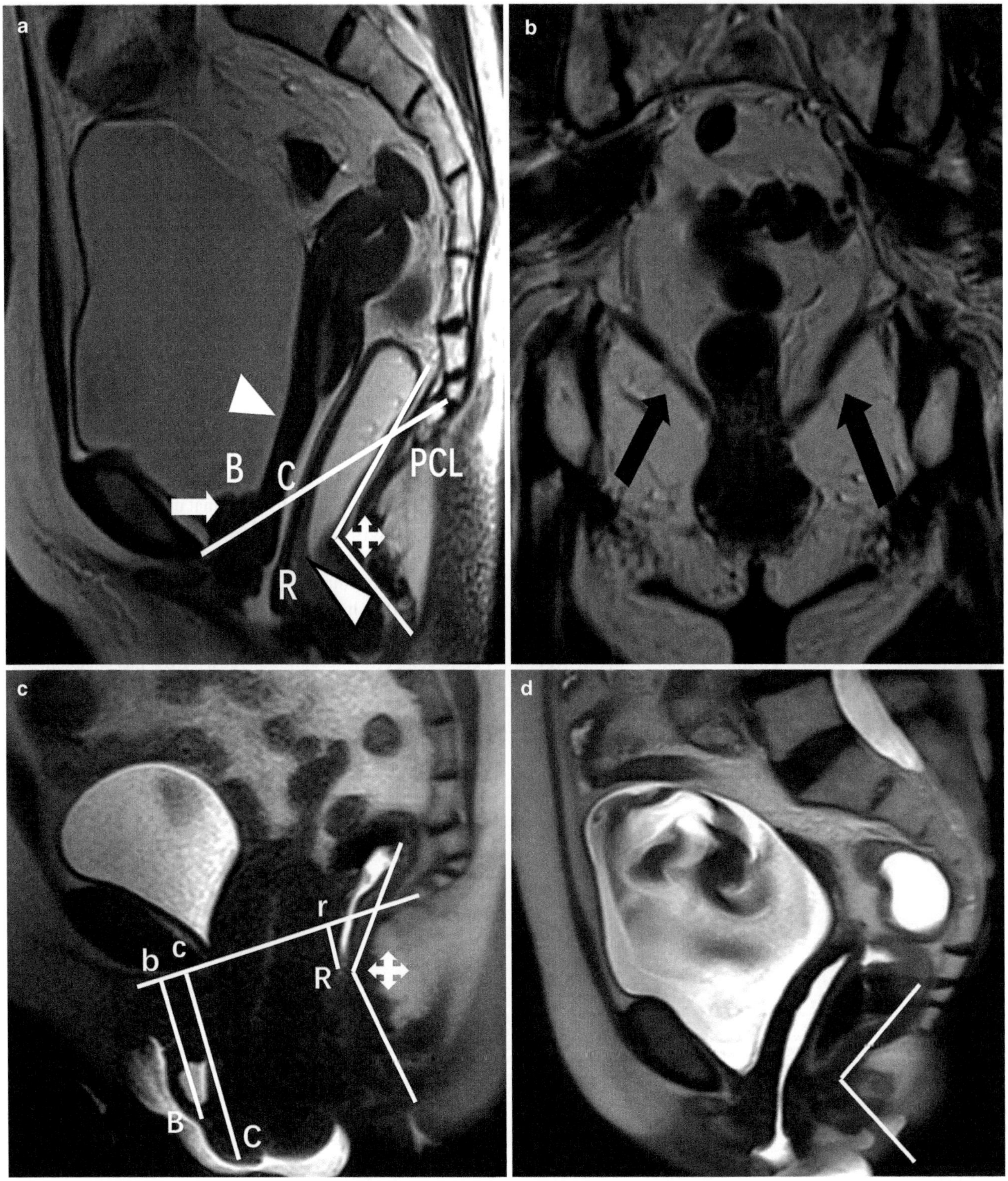

Fig. 49.1 Multiplanar MRI images of a female patient with pelvic organ prolapse (POP). (**a**) Midline sagittal section of a female patient at rest, this section should encompass the pubic symphysis, bladder neck, vagina, rectum, and coccyx. "PCL" line is the line from the lower border of the pubic symphysis to the last coccygeal joint, representing the level of the entire pelvic floor. Letter "B" in figures represents the lowest point of bladder neck (white arrow); letter "C" in figures represents the most inferior and anterior point of the cervix (white arrowhead); letter "R" in figures stands for anorectal junction (black framed arrowhead). The anorectal angle is within the normal range (asterisk). (**b**) Coronal T2WI obtained at rest of a 60-year-old female patient with POP. The iliococcygeus muscle and pubococcygeus muscle (black arrow) can be seen lost its horizontal configuration. (**c**) Sagittal T2WI HASTE obtained during straining. The vortices of urine in the bladder are caused by maximal straining of patient. The lowest point "B" of the bladder and the lowest point "C" of the anterior lip of the cervix changed obviously relative to the PCL. The anorectal angle becomes more obtuse during squeezing (asterisk). (**d**) Sagittal T2WI HASTE obtained during squeezing. The anorectal joint is higher and the angle becomes more acute than that in **a**. (**e**) Deformation of the vaginal fornix (asterisk)

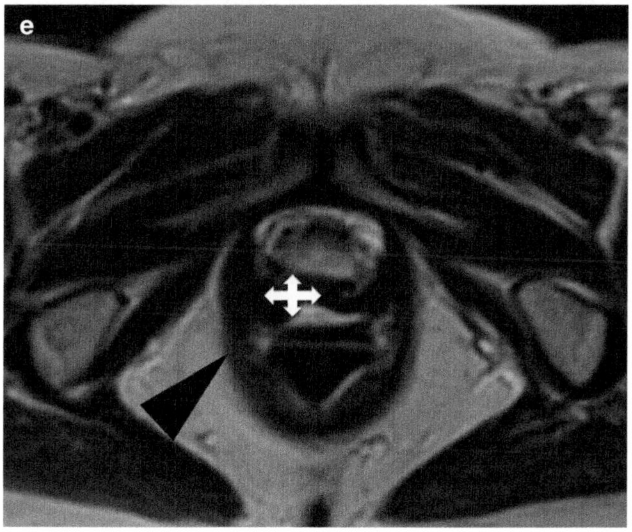

Fig. 49.1 (continued)

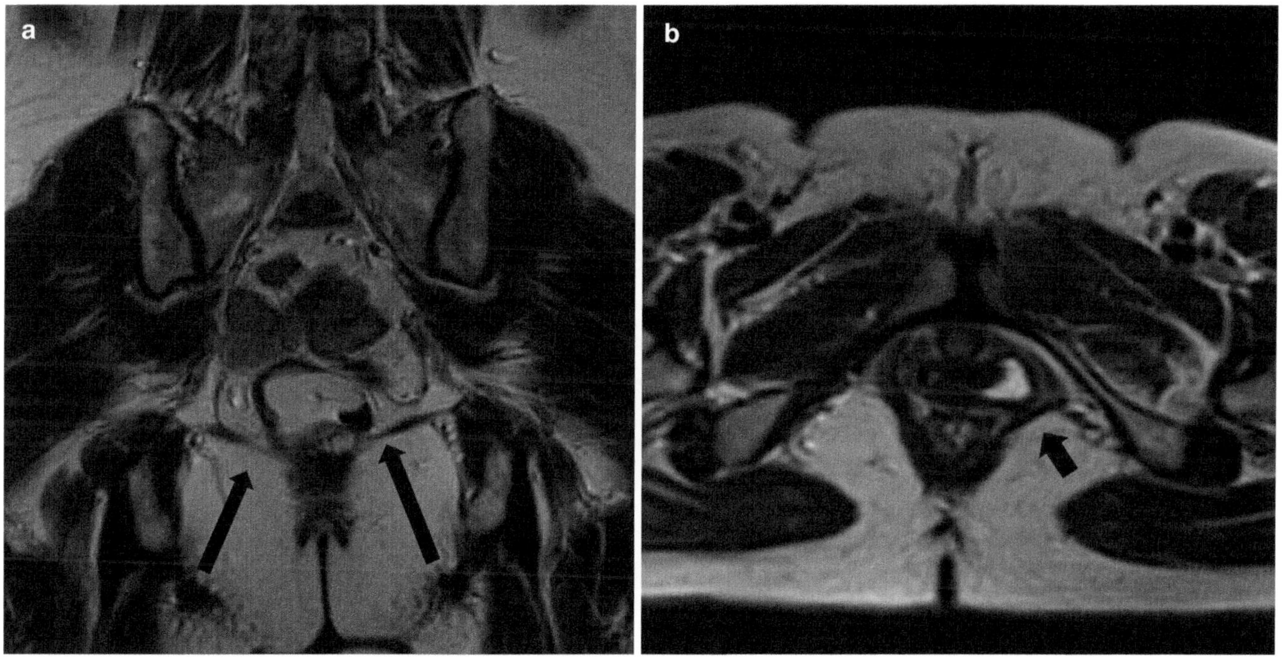

Fig. 49.2 Imaging anatomy of levator ani muscle. (**a**) Coronal T2WI obtained at rest of a 52-year-old healthy woman. The bilateral iliococcygeus muscle and pubococcygeus muscle can be seen clearly (black long arrow), which having a horizontal orientation. The "U" shape of the puborectalis muscle with detachment of the right aspect of it can be seen in an axial T2WI (**b**). (**c**) Midsagittal T2WI. The levator plane is seen posterior to the rectum and anterior to the coccyx (white arrowhead)

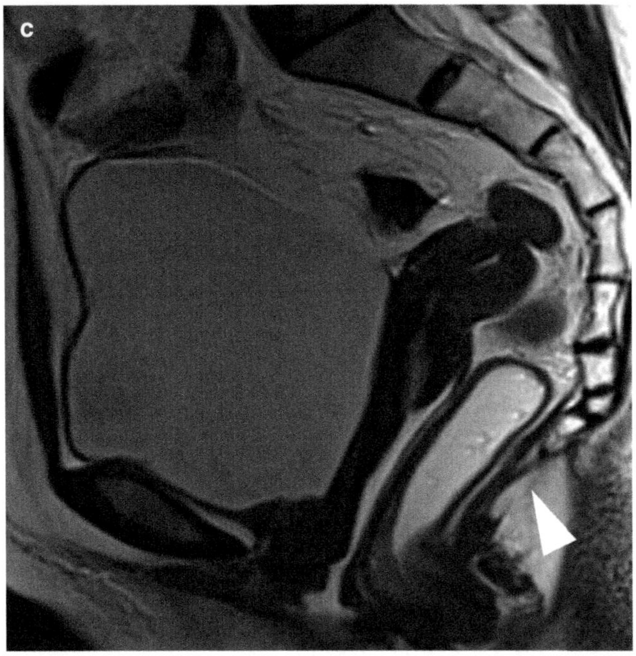

Fig. 49.2 (continued)

49.1 Imaging Analysis

The pelvic floor is a dynamically balanced three-dimensional structure. The pelvic floor is divided into three major compartments: (1) anterior: urinary bladder, urethra, and urethral support system; (2) middle: vagina (anterior and posterior wall) and uterocervical support; and (3) posterior: rectum and support structure. The main support structures are the endopelvic fascia and ligaments, the pelvic diaphragm, and the urogenital diaphragm from cranial to caudal. The support structures of the pelvic floor consist of a complex interaction among the bones, muscles, ligaments, and organs. The pathological features of PFD generally affect the interrelated network of them and result in structural damage and dysfunction in three pelvic compartments [3].

MRI protocols of PFD consist of static sequences and dynamic sequences. Dynamic MRI examination is performed while the patient is squeezing, straining, and defecation. The findings seen on high-resolution T2-weighted images obtained at rest are helpful for anatomic evaluation. This mainly include puborectalis muscle, pubococcygeus muscle, iliac coccygeus muscle, levator plate, etc. The assessment should be focused on: (1) the structural and signal intensity, symmetry, and thickness of bilateral puborectalis muscle, pubococcygeus muscle, and iliac coccygeus muscle; (2) the levator plate tends to be vertical and is no longer roughly parallel to the upper half of the vagina; and (3) vagina loses its "H" shape on axial images [4].

Steady state (e.g., FISP, GRASS, FFE, PSIF, SSFP, T2-FFE) or balanced state free precession sequences (e.g., True-FISP, FIESTA, B-FFE) in sagittal plane is recommended for dynamic sequences (squeezing and straining) and evacuation sequence [5]. Interpretation of pelvic floor MRI requires a standardized approach. At present, pubococcygeal line (PCL) is the most widely accepted reference line. It extends from the inferior border of the pubic symphysis to the last coccygeal joint in the midsagittal plane, represents the level of the pelvic floor. Before MRI examination, approximately 180 mL of warm ultrasound gel is injected into the vagina and rectum in our institution to better display the organ reference point. In the anterior compartment of the pelvis, the reference point is the most inferior aspect of bladder base. In the middle compartment of the pelvis, the reference point is the most anterior and inferior aspect of the cervix or the vaginal posterior apex in patients who have undergone a hysterectomy. In the posterior compartment of the pelvis, the reference point is the anterior aspect of anorectal junction. The vertical distance from each reference point to PCL should be measured. In women with a normal pelvic floor anatomy, these organ reference points are located at or above the PCL level. Even in the case of maximum abdominal pressure, the range of variation not more than 1 cm below the PCL is considered normal. The severity of pelvic floor organ prolapse can be graded according to "Rule of three": prolapse of an organ below the PCL by 3 cm or less is mild, between 3 cm and 6 cm is moderate, and more than 6 cm is severe [6, 7]. The change of the anorectal angle was observed, while the patient is resting and squeezing. This angle is drawn between the longitudinal axis of the anal canal and the posterior rectal wall. It normally measures 108°–127° at rest and varies between 15° and 20° during contraction or defecation. Failure of the anorectal angle to open (become more obtuse) during defecation and prolonged and incomplete evacuation of the rectal gel (less than two-third gel evacuated in more than 30 s) are suggestive of spastic pelvic floor syndrome.

The anterior compartment organ prolapse mainly includes cystocele (Fig. 49.3) and urethral hypermobility (Fig. 49.4). Cystocele is defined as greater than 1 cm descent of the posterior bladder wall or bladder neck below the PCL. The grading standard follows "Rule of three." Clinically, eversion of the vaginal mucosa can be seen, and severe cystocele may cover up urethral hypermobility and impair bladder voiding. In healthy women, the urethral axis maintains vertical orientation. In patients with urethral hypermobility, there is a more drastic horizontal clockwise rotation greater than 30° during strain/evacuation, which can lead to stress urinary incontinence [8]. Moderate to severe bladder prolapse is usually associated. It is secondary to loss of periurethral and paraurethral support. Urethral hypermobility and funneling

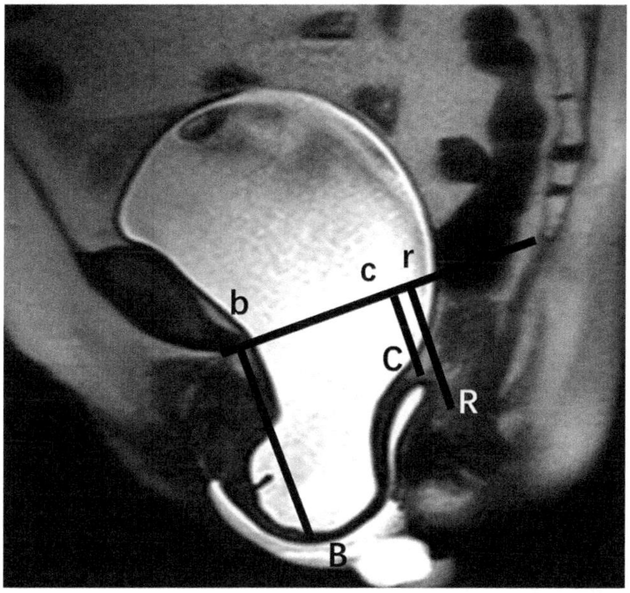

Fig. 49.3 Cystocele. Sagittal HASTE image obtained during straining of a 55-year-old woman with cystocele. The "PCL" line is drawn from the inferior border of the pubic symphysis to the last coccygeal joint. Sagittal T2WI image showed the lowest point of the bladder (B), the vaginal vault (C), and the anorectal junction (R) all located below the PCL. The distance of Bb was 4.5 cm

are associated with stress-induced urinary incontinence and can lead to urinary tract infections.

The middle compartment organ prolapse mainly includes uterine prolapse (Fig. 49.5) or vaginal vault prolapse and peritoneocele. Uterine or vaginal vault prolapse is measured perpendicularly from the most anterior and inferior aspect of the cervix or the vaginal posterior apex to the PCL. Grading of the prolapse is severity according to "Rule of three." In healthy women, the pouch of Douglas is normally located at the level of the posterior vagina fornix. Peritoneocele can be diagnosed when peritoneal fat and small bowel loop appeared between rectum and vagina, and the position of small bowel loop was lower than PCL. These hernias are named according to their content (peritoneal fat, small bowel loop, or sigmoid colon). On dynamic MRI, peritoneocele manifests at the end of the evacuation phase after emptying of the bladder and rectum [3].

The middle compartment organ prolapse mainly includes rectocele (Fig. 49.6) and intussusception (Fig. 49.7). The most common measurement of rectocele on MRI is the depth of wall protrusion beyond the expected margin of the normal anorectal wall. It usually occurs in the anterior wall of the rectum and occasionally involves the posterior and lateral

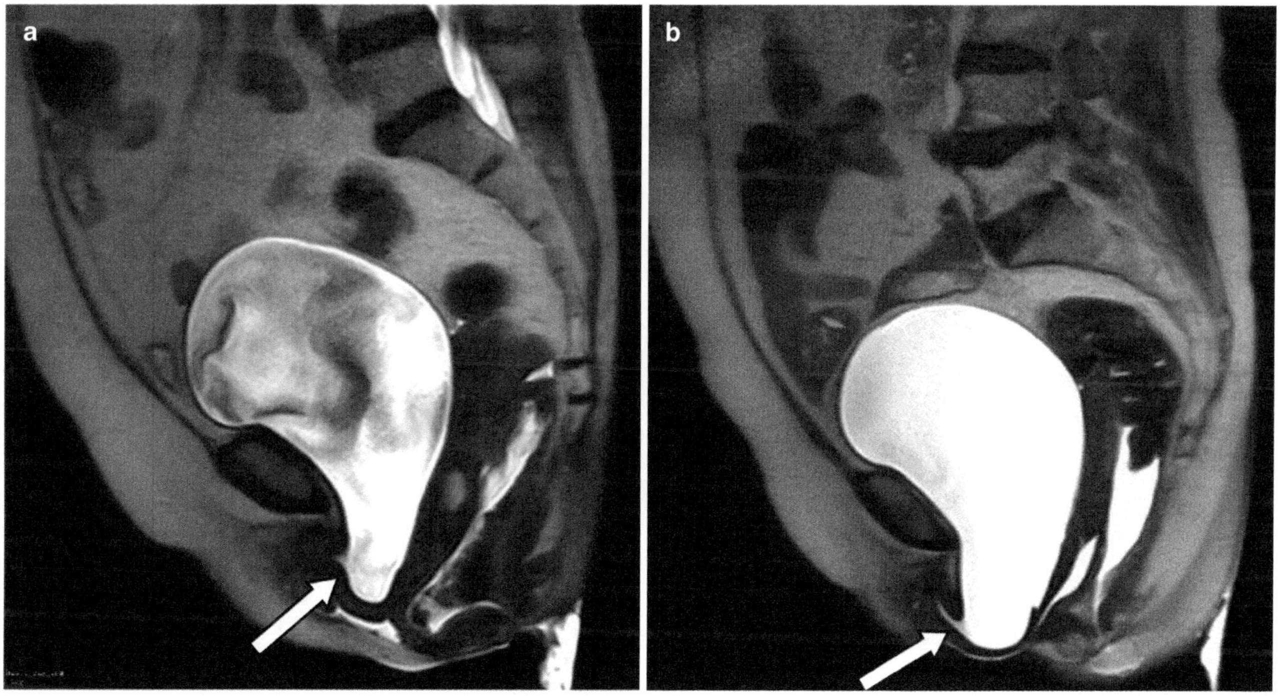

Fig. 49.4 Urethral hypermobility and urethral funneling. (**a, b**) Sagittal HASTE images obtained during straining of a 70-year-old woman and 65-year-old woman with cystocele, respectively. (**a**) Rotation of the urethral axis, even beyond the horizontal position. (**b**) Dilation of the proximal urethral lumen and apparent shortening of the urethra

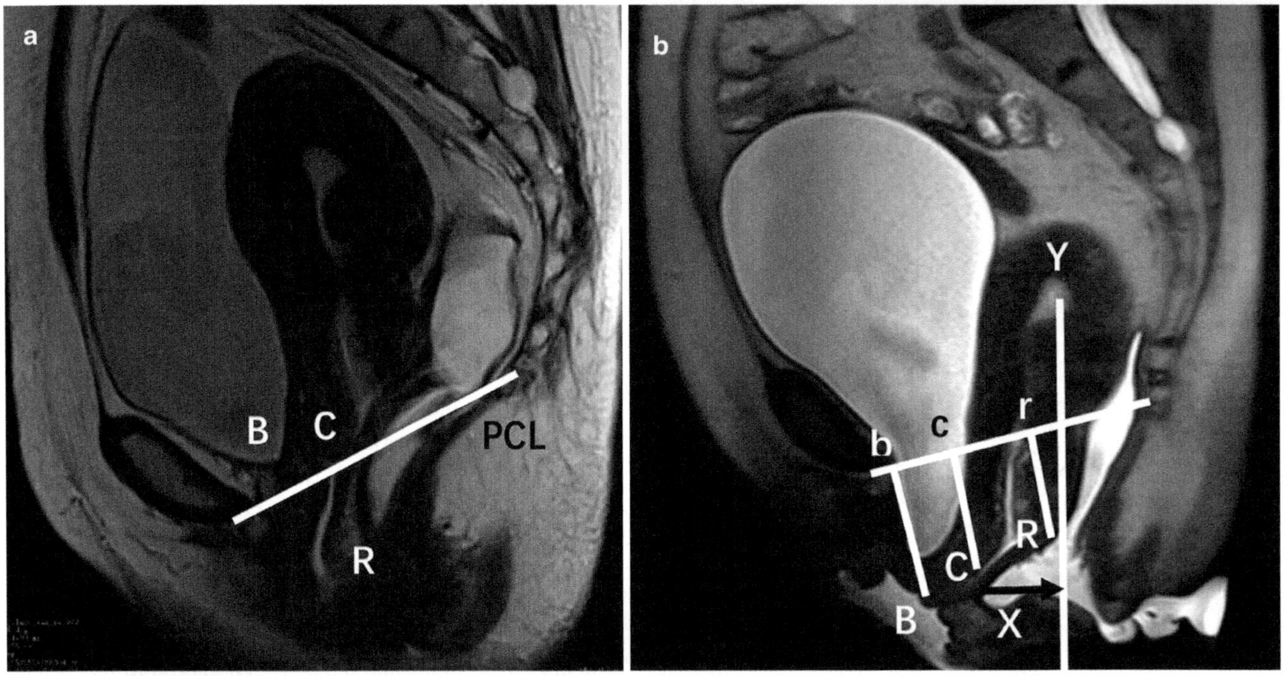

Fig. 49.5 Uterine prolapse. A 46-year-old woman with uterine prolapse. The sagittal T2WI image (**a**) obtained at rest showed the lowest point of bladder base (letter "B") and cervix (letter "C") located above the PCL, while the anorectal junction (letter "R") located below it. The T2WI HASTE image obtained during straining (**b**) showed all the point B, C, R located below PCL obviously. Bb, Cc, Rr represent their vertical distances to PCL, respectively. Rectocele also could be seen in (**b**). The Y line represents the expected margin of the normal anorectal wall. The X line represents the depth of wall protrusion beyond the expected margin of the normal anorectal wall

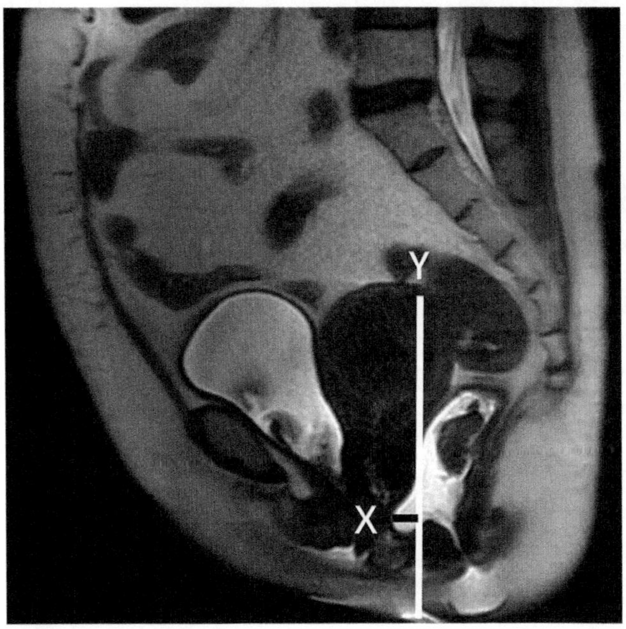

Fig. 49.6 Rectocele. A HASTE T2WI image of a 52-year-old woman with rectocele. The Y line represents the expected margin of the normal anorectal wall. The X line represents the depth of wall protrusion beyond the expected margin of the normal anorectal wall

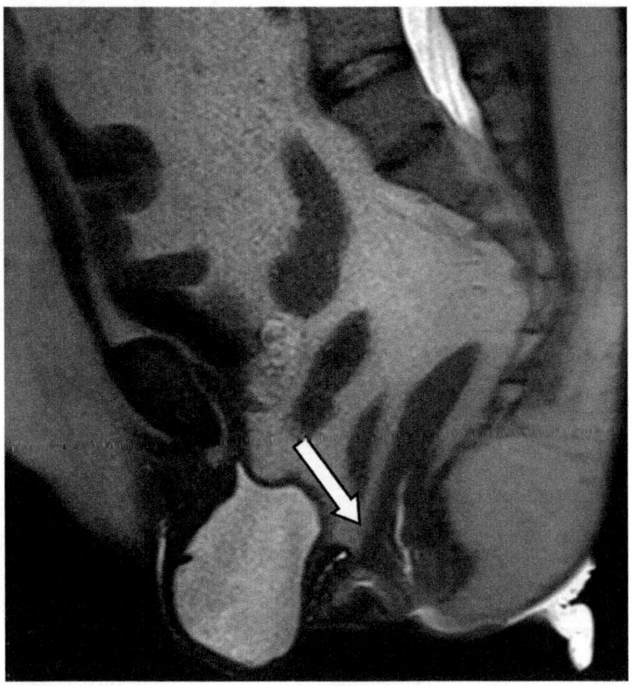

Fig. 49.7 Intussusception. A 65-year-old woman with intussusception. A sagittal True-FISP image during defecation showed a full-thickness rectal wall prolapse intra-anal involving both the mucosa and muscular layer. Cystocele also could be seen

walls. When the outpouching of the rectal wall is less than 2 cm, the rectocele is termed mild, while 2–4 cm is termed moderate, and greater than 4 cm is severe. Mild rectocele is more common, with a range of ≤3 cm, and these are considered clinically significant only when symptoms develop [9]. Intussusception and rectal prolapse are an invagination of the rectal wall and can be internal or external. The distance of parietal inversion from the anal verge can be classified as intrarectal, intra-anal, or extra-anal. MR defecography has the potential advantage of clearly distinguishing between rectal mucosal intussusception and rectal full-thickness intussusception [10]. An intussusception is commonly only visible at the end of defecation phase, when the gel is evacuated [11].

Dynamic MRI is a helpful diagnostic tool for patients with multicompartmental pelvic floor abnormalities, or for those with prior surgical repairs. It has unique advantage over traditional examinations. Dynamic MR imaging of the pelvic floor is valuable for selecting candidates for surgical treatment and for indicating the most appropriate surgical approach. A standardized MR imaging and reporting of PFD is crucial to enhance effective communication between the radiologist and the clinician for the sake of patients' benefit.

References

1. Mant J, Painter R, Vessey M. Epidemiology of genital prolapse: observations from the Oxford Family Planning Association Study. Br J Obstet Gynaecol. 1997;104(5):579–85.
2. Woodfield CA, Hampton BS, Sung V, Brody JM. Magnetic resonance imaging of pelvic organ prolapse: comparing pubococcygeal and midpubic lines with clinical staging. Int Urogynecol J Pelvic Floor Dysfunct. 2009;20(6):695–701.
3. Chamié LP, Ribeiro DMFR, Caiado AHM, Warmbrand G, Serafini PC. Translabial US and dynamic MR imaging of the pelvic floor: normal anatomy and dysfunction. Radiographics. 2018;38(1):287–308.
4. El Sayed RF. Magnetic resonance imaging of the female pelvic floor: anatomy overview, indications, and imaging protocols. Radiol Clin North Am. 2020;58(2):291–303.
5. El Sayed RF, Alt CD, Maccioni F, et al. Magnetic resonance imaging of pelvic floor dysfunction – joint recommendations of the ESUR and ESGAR pelvic floor working group. Eur Radiol. 2017;27:2067–85.
6. Garcia del Salto L, de Miguel CJ, Aguilera del Hoyo LF, et al. MR imaging-based assessment of the female pelvic floor. Radiographics. 2014;34(5):1417–39.
7. Colaiacomo MC, Masselli G, Polettini E, et al. Dynamic MR imaging of the pelvic floor: a pictorial review. Radiographics. 2009;29(3):e35.
8. Gupta AP, Pandya PR, Nguyen M-L, et al. Use of dynamic MRI of the pelvic floor in the assessment of anterior compartment disorders. Curr Urol Rep. 2018;19:112.
9. Alapati S, Jambhekar K. Dynamic magnetic resonance imaging of the pelvic floor. Semin Ultrasound CT MRI. 2017;38:188–99.
10. Mortele KJ, Fairhurst J. Dynamic MR defecography of the posterior compartment: indications, techniques and MRI features. Eur J Radiol. 2007;61(3):462–72.
11. MRI of the pelvic floor and MR defecography. Hodler J, et al. editors. Diseases of the abdomen and pelvis 2018–2021, IDKD Springer Series.

GPSR Compliance

The European Union's (EU) General Product Safety Regulation (GPSR) is a set of rules that requires consumer products to be safe and our obligations to ensure this.

If you have any concerns about our products, you can contact us on ProductSafety@springernature.com

In case Publisher is established outside the EU, the EU authorized representative is:

Springer Nature Customer Service Center GmbH
Europaplatz 3
69115 Heidelberg, Germany

Batch number: 09231230

Printed by Printforce, the Netherlands